The Addison-Wesley Manual of

PEDIATRIC
NURSING
PROCEDURES

Kathleen M. Speer, PhD, MSN, RN

A DIVISION O... ..., INC.

SPONSORING EDITOR: Mark McCormick
PRODUCTION COORDINATOR: Alyssa Wolf
BOOK DESIGNER: Paula Schlosser
COVER DESIGNER: John Martucci
PHOTOGRAPHER: Chris Reynolds
ILLUSTRATORS: Mary Ann Zapalac and Katie Schatzlein
COPYEDITOR: Barbara Fuller
PROOFREADER: Elizabeth Wiltsee
INDEXER: William J. Richardson Associates
MANUFACTURING SUPERVISOR: Merry Free Osborn
COMPOSITION: The Clarinda Company

Care has been taken to confirm the accuracy of information represented in this book. The authors, editors, and publisher, however, cannot accept responsibility for errors or omissions or for consequences from application of the information in this book and make no warranty, express or implied, with respect to its contents.

The authors and publisher have exerted every effort to ensure that drug selections and dosages set forth in this text are in accord with current recommendations and practice at the time of publication. However, in view of ongoing research, changes in government regulations, and the constant flow of information relating to drug therapy and drug reactions, the reader is urged to check the package inserts of all drugs for any change in indications of dosage and for added warnings and precautions. This is particularly important when the recommended agent is a new and/or infrequently employed drug. Mention of a particular generic or brand name drug is not an endorsement, nor an implication that it is preferable to other named or unnamed agents.

Library of Congress Cataloging-in-Publication Data

Speer, Kathleen Morgan.
    The Addison-Wesley manual of pediatric nursing procedures /
Kathleen M. Speer, Carolyn L. Swann.
       p.   cm.
    Includes index.
    ISBN 0-8053-7645-3
    1. Pediatric nursing—Handbooks, manuals, etc.   I. Swann, Carolyn
L. II. Title. III. Title: Pediatric nursing procedures.
    [DNLM: 1. Pediatric Nursing—methods.   WY 159 S742a]
RJ245.S62   1993
610.73'62—dc20
DNLM/DLC
for Library of Congress   92-49339
                                             CIP

ISBN 0-8053-7645-3
1 2 3 4 5 6 7 8 9 10 AL 95949392

Addison-Wesley Nursing
A Division of The Benjamin/Cummings Publishing Company, Inc.
390 Bridge Parkway
Redwood City, California 94065

Preface

PHILOSOPHY

There are many procedure textbooks on the market, however, very few are exclusively for use in pediatric nursing. The procedure textbooks that do address pediatric procedures are either limited in scope or have placed the procedure in a care plan format, which makes the essential steps more difficult to access. The authors developed a procedure textbook specifically for nurses and students that is both comprehensive and easy to use. This textbook can serve as a source to staff nurses and students to assist in providing safe, specialized care to children.

ORGANIZATION

Procedures are organized alphabetically and the procedural format is consistent throughout the book.

Each procedure includes the following components:

- Psychosocial considerations—explained in the Features section below.

- Length of time to perform the procedure if applicable—the time for performance of a procedure will vary depending on the expertise of the practitioner. The times given are for nurses who have had experience performing that particular procedure. Set-up times will also vary and add to the total time of the procedure.

- The purpose and objectives—give an overview of the procedure and the expected outcomes.

- An equipment list—this list may vary depending on the individual hospital's policies.

- Safety issues—an important part of this textbook. Potential safety issues related to each individual procedure are discussed. Highlighted and placed before the steps, nurses and students will see these first and be aware of any potential problems.

- Essential steps—a clear, concise and organized guide through the actual performance of each procedure.

- Lab values if applicable—reviews the normal lab values for children.

- Documentation—nurses may have questions as to what should be documented following a procedure. This section is provided to facilitate complete, efficient documentation.

- Potential related medical and nursing diagnoses—to increase the book's reference value and to help clarify which diagnoses may be associated with a particular procedure.

- References—to provide a base for further reading if desired.

- Checklists—explained in the Features section below.

FEATURES
Special features include:

- Psychosocial considerations—We added this unique feature to highlight the special considerations nurses must be aware of when performing procedures with children. For example, nurses need to avoid certain language that might have mixed meanings for a child. Also, it is important to provide appropriate explanations to the child and his or her family.

- Skills Checklist—In each procedure there is a checklist that the nurse may use to quickly review the steps in each procedure. The checklist may also be used by the faculty or preceptor to evaluate the performance of students or other nurses.

ACKNOWLEDGEMENTS

We would like to express our appreciation to all the individuals who have worked on the policies and procedures at Children's Medical Center of Dallas which formed the base for our work. We would like to offer our special thanks to Michele Faxel and Elizabeth Simone who were key contributors on this project. In addition, reviews were solicited from all areas of the country including Illinois, Iowa, Louisiana, Michigan, New Hampshire, North Carolina, North Dakota, South Carolina, and Wisconsin. We wish to recognize and thank these individuals for their time and expertise: Ann Batchelder; Kathy Bradley; Mary Ellen Brown; Sandy Chacko; Dan Chausse; Florencetta Gibson; Lilly Lee; Marie Simmons; Susan Sorenson.

CONTRIBUTORS

Michele Faxel
Children's Hospital Oakland
747 52nd Street
Oakland, CA 94609
(510)428-3000

Elizabeth L'Estrange Simone
11855 Laurel Road (home)
Chesterland, OH 44026
(216)729-8209

REVIEWERS

Anne Batchelder
New Hampshire Technical College/
  Manchester
1066 Front Street
Manchester, NH 03102
(603)668-6706

Mary Ellen Howell (née Brown)
Women's Center of Carolina Hospital
  System
Box 5906 (home)
Florence, SC 29502
(803)393-5350

Kathy Bradley
Mercy College of Detroit
820 W. Outer Drive
Famington Hills, MI 48018
(313)993-6055

Lilly Lee
Illinois Central College
1 College Drive
East Peoria, IL 61635
(309)694-5011

Sandy Chacko
Des Moines Area Community College
1125 Hancock Drive
Boone, IA 50036
(515)432-7203

Marie Simmons
Surry Community College
Box 304
Dobson, NC 27017
(919)386-8121

Daniel Chaussee
University of Mary
7500 University Drive
Bismark, ND 58504
(701)255-7500

Susan Sorenson
Bellin College
929 Cass Street
Green Bay, WI 54301
(414)433-3560

Florencetta Gibson
Northeast Louisiana University
700 University Avenue
Monroe, LA 71209
(318)342-1640

Contents

1 Admission Procedures

Scale

Thermometer

Blood-pressure equipment

Stethoscope

Tape measure

Otoscope/ophthalmoscope (optional)

Admission packet

    Visiting/rooming-in information

    Information about the hospital

        Parking

        Cafeteria

        Ronald McDonald House, if available

        Hotels

Forms

    Nursing assessment

    Growth and development chart

    Height and weight graph

PSYCHOSOCIAL CONSIDERATIONS: The child may be fearful of the actual hospitalization and of physical harm. Provide information in developmentally appropriate terms. Do not appear rushed, as doing so may frighten or overwhelm the child. Do not immediately obtain vital signs or perform a physical assessment unless the child is unstable. Allow the child to play with equipment to decrease fear. Do not separate the child from parents during admission procedures unless absolutely necessary. Parents are often overwhelmed and may need additional support.

TIME: 30 minutes to 1 hour

PURPOSE

To give effective physical and emotional care to the child and psychological support to the family.

To exchange information about the child and the hospital procedures in a professional manner.

To begin intervention for acute and/or chronic dysfunction.

OBJECTIVES

- To prepare the child for hospitalization.
- To decrease anxiety and fear.
- To provide information about the hospital to the child and family.
- To assess the child's physical and psychosocial status.

ESSENTIAL STEPS

1. Prepare the child and family for admission.
2. Assemble the equipment.
3. Wash hands.
4. Obtain vital signs.
5. Obtain initial admission history:

    History of present illness.

    Current health status, including immunizations and exposure to communicable diseases.

    Significant past history.

    Growth and development milestones.

    Current medications.

    Birth history.

Family members' history.

Psychosocial status, including information about support systems.

Health concerns.

Nutritional information.

6. Perform physical assessment, including evaluations of the following:

Eyes, ears, nose, mouth, and throat.

Neurological system.

Respiratory system.

Cardiovascular system.

Gastrointestinal system.

Genitourinary system.

Musculoskeletal system.

Integumentary system.

7. Explain

Plans of medical and nursing care.

Visiting hours.

Meal times.

Routine procedures.

Equipment in the room.

Procedure for calling for help.

8. Tour the unit and any area in which the child may be located, such as the intensive care unit, the surgery room, and/or the recovery room. Point out the following areas:

Playroom.

Parent lounge.

Bathrooms.

Telephone.

Kitchen.

Skills Checklist

☐ Prepare the child and family.
☐ Assemble the equipment.
☐ Wash hands.
☐ Obtain vital signs.
☐ Obtain history and perform physical assessment.
☐ Orient the child and family to the room and hospital.
☐ Conduct a tour, if applicable.
☐ Document.

DOCUMENTATION

- Time and mode of arrival.
- Reason for admission.
- History.
- Physical assessment.
- Child and family coping techniques.
- Child's routine.
- Child's preferred name.
- Hospital routines explained and orientation of child/family to room.
- Tour, if applicable.
- Responsible adults accompanying the child and their response.
- Initiation of plan of care.

POTENTIAL RELATED NURSING DIAGNOSES

Coping, ineffective individual

Family processes, altered

Fear

Anxiety

Social isolation

POTENTIAL RELATED MEDICAL DIAGNOSES

Universal application

REFERENCES

Mott, S., James, S., and Sperhac, A. 1990. *Nursing care of children and families.* Redwood City, Calif.: Addison-Wesley.

Bathing the Child: Tub or Basin

PSYCHOSOCIAL CONSIDERATIONS: Explain the procedure to the child in developmentally appropriate terms. Older children may be fearful of a stranger seeing or touching genitalia. Allow the child as much independence in taking the bath as possible. Also allow flexibility of times; many children bathe in the evening, not in the morning. Do not drain the bathtub when a young child is in it. Young children may not be able to conceptually differentiate themselves from the water and may feel they too will go down the drain.

TIME: 15 to 20 minutes

PURPOSE

To facilitate personal hygiene and allow thorough assessment of skin integrity.

OBJECTIVES

- To maintain hygiene.
- To assess the child.
- To prevent injury.

EQUIPMENT

Basin or tub
Washcloths
Shampoo, as appropriate
Soap
Towels
Lotion or bath oil, such as Alpha Keri, as appropriate

SAFETY ISSUES

- **Place a towel on the bottom of the tub or basin to prevent the child from slipping.**
- **Ensure that room temperature is warm to prevent chilling.**
- **Do not bathe infants in the sink. A very young infant may be sponge-bathed. Immersion in a tub is rarely appropriate before the cord has dropped off. For safety purposes, tub baths often may not start until the infant is between 3 and 6 months of age.**

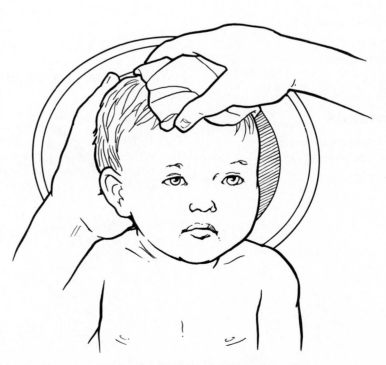

FIGURE 2.1 *Supporting the head and keeping the scalp clean.*

- Do not leave a young child under 7 years of age alone in a tub. Children over 7 years may require supervision, depending on developmental level or medical condition.
- To prevent burns, run cold water through the tap to cool the faucet before placing a child in a tub.

ESSENTIAL STEPS

1. Prepare the child and family.
2. Assemble the equipment.
3. Wash hands.
4. Run water. Check the water temperature by submerging a wrist in the water.
5. Shampoo hair. Wash the scalp of an infant less than 1 year of age as necessary. Pour water over the head. Apply soap or shampoo and rinse. Avoid water or soap or shampoo in the eyes. (See Figs. 2.1 and 2.2)
6. Bathe, starting with the eyes and ending with the perineal area. Do not allow the child to become chilled. Wrap immediately in a towel when finished.
7. Dry with a towel.
8. Apply lotion, as needed.
9. Teach hygiene practices to the child and parents as needed: cleaning genitalia, shampooing hair, bathing frequently enough, and so on.

DOCUMENTATION

- Personal hygiene care completed.
- Significant observations made.
- Teaching done.

POTENTIAL RELATED NURSING DIAGNOSES

Body temperature, altered: *high risk*

Skin integrity, impaired: *high risk*

Self-care deficit, bathing and/or hygiene

POTENTIAL RELATED MEDICAL DIAGNOSES

Universal application

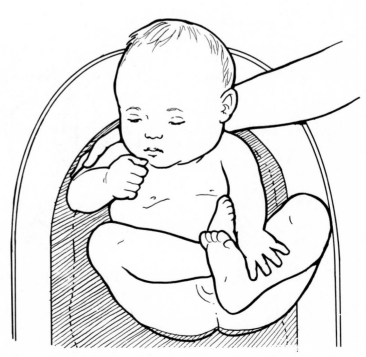

FIGURE 2.2 *Supporting the body of the infant.*

3) Blood Administration: Cryoprecipitate

- Check for informed consent.
- Cryoprecipitate is issued non–type specific. The blood bank may require an ABO group and an Rh factor for each patient receiving blood products.
- Cryoprecipitate administration must be completed within 1 hour after blood is obtained from the blood bank.
- Cryoprecipitate is not to be placed in the blood refrigerator.
- Cryoprecipitate expires 6 hours after thawing and 4 hours after pooling.

PSYCHOSOCIAL CONSIDERATIONS: Explain the procedure in developmentally appropriate terms. Avoid using terms with mixed meanings, such as *stick* and *shot*. A child who has had a transfusion reaction may fear another such occurrence. Explain the screening process to detect the HIV virus, if appropriate; some parents may be fearful of AIDS.

TIME: Up to 1 hour

PURPOSE

To provide a source of Factor VIII and fibrinogen for Factor VIII deficiencies, von Willebrand's disease, and afibrinogenemia. (Note: Alternate blood products or other treatment measures are usually preferred; cryoprecipitate should rarely be used in current practices.)

OBJECTIVES

- To administer cryoprecipitate safely.
- To prevent injury.

EQUIPMENT

Cryoprecipitate

Blood administration set

Gloves, nonsterile

Needle to cap intravenous tubing, sterile

Stopcock and extension tubing, if appropriate

Normal saline (0.9% sodium chloride), 5 ml syringe, and needle, sterile

ESSENTIAL STEPS

1. Prepare the child and family. Refer to "Blood Administration: General Procedure."
2. Assemble the equipment.
3. Wash hands.
4. Obtain the cryoprecipitate. If several pooled units are to be given, sequence the pickup times so each bag is administered within the 1-hour hang time.
5. Check the cryoprecipitate label and blood request form. Refer to "Blood Administration: General Procedure."
6. Put on gloves and prime the administration set.
7. Identify the child by checking the identification band.
8. Obtain baseline vital signs.
9. Refer to "Blood Administration: General Procedure" for steps to initiate the administration of blood/blood products.
10. Turn off the infusing IV solution and disconnect the tubing. Cap the IV tubing with a sterile needle.

11. Add extension tubing and a stopcock to the hub of the IV device, if appropriate. Use the second port on the stopcock for the normal saline line or normal saline syringe.

12. Flush the IV cannula with 3 to 5 ml of normal saline.

13. Connect the administration set to the stopcock or the hub of the IV device.

14. Infuse the cryoprecipitate.

15. When the cryoprecipitate bag is empty, wash the bag and flush the blood administration set using 10 to 15 ml of normal saline to completely remove all of the product from the system.

16. If giving several units in sequence, use the same blood administration set without normal saline flushing between units. The filter and/or administration set should hang no longer than 4 hours.

17. Carefully observe for transfusion reaction. Refer to "Blood Administration: Transfusion Reaction."

18. Discard the bag and administration set in an appropriate manner.

DOCUMENTATION

- Name of blood product.
- Start time.
- Baseline and serial vital signs.
- Amount infused.
- Child's response.
- Amount of any normal saline flushes.
- Completion time.

Skills Checklist

☐ Prepare the child and family; check for informed consent.
☐ Assemble the equipment.
☐ Wash hands.
☐ Obtain cryoprecipitate.
☐ Check the label and verify that the blood product is correct.
☐ Put on gloves and prime the tubing.
☐ Identify the child by checking the identification band.
☐ Obtain baseline vital signs.
☐ Turn off the infusing IV solution.
☐ Disconnect the tubing.
☐ Add extension tubing, if appropriate.
☐ Flush the IV line with normal saline.
☐ Administer cryoprecipitate.
☐ Monitor vital signs.
☐ Put on gloves and flush the IV line with normal saline.
☐ Disconnect the administration set and reconnect the IV.
☐ Discard the bag and administration set.
☐ Document.

POTENTIAL RELATED NURSING DIAGNOSES

Fear

Anxiety

Tissue perfusion, altered, peripheral

Infection: *high risk*

Hyperthermia

POTENTIAL RELATED MEDICAL DIAGNOSES

Hemophilia

REFERENCES

American Association of Blood Banks. 1989. *Circular of information for the use of human blood and blood components.* Arlington, Va.: American Association of Blood Banks.

Mott, S., James, S., and Sperhac, A. 1990. *Nursing care of children and families.* Redwood City, Calif.: Addison-Wesley.

National Blood Resource Education. 1991. Choosing blood components and equipment. *AJN* 91, no. 6: 42–52.

4 Blood Administration: Factor VIII

- **Check for informed consent.**
- **The blood bank usually requires only one ABO group and Rh factor on record for each patient to whom Factor VIII is administered. (Cross-matching is not necessary.)**
- **Factor VIII deficiency should be proven prior to administration of Factor VIII.**
- **Although Factor VIII should be used promptly after reconstitution, it can hang for up to 24 hours as a constant infusion.**
- **A parent or child instructed in home hemophilia care can give Factor VIII.**

PSYCHOSOCIAL CONSIDERATIONS: Explain the procedure in developmentally appropriate terms. Avoid using terms with mixed meanings, such as *stick* and *shot*. A child who has had a transfusion reaction may fear another such occurrence. Explain the screening process to detect the HIV virus, if appropriate; some parents may be fearful of AIDS.

TIME: Up to 24 hours

PURPOSE

To safely administer a commercially prepared concentrate of human antihemophiliac Factor VIII (AHF) for the treatment of bleeding episodes in classical Type A hemophilia; not effective in the treatment of von Willebrand's disease.

To prophylactically administer AHF to Type A hemophiliac patients preoperatively.

OBJECTIVES

- To administer Factor VIII safely.
- To prevent injury.

EQUIPMENT

Gloves, nonsterile

Factor VIII

Povidone-iodine swabs *or* alcohol swabs

Plastic syringes and needles, appropriate size

23g or 25g butterfly (if no preexisting IV)

Normal saline (0.9% sodium chloride), 5 ml syringe, and needle, sterile

ESSENTIAL STEPS

1. Prepare the child and family. Refer to "Blood Administration: General Procedure."
2. Assemble the equipment.
3. Wash hands and put on gloves.
4. After the physician has ordered the *approximate* number of units needed, call the blood bank to determine the units per vial available. (Each lot number has varying units per vial.) Once given this information, the physician will amend the order so that entire vials are given (such as Factor VIII, 5 vials of 240 units per vial given via IV).
5. In order to reduce the child's risk and exposure to viral agents, request that the blood bank supply all vials from the same lot number.
6. Obtain Factor VIII.
7. Check the vial label(s) and request form. Refer to "Blood Administration: General Procedure."

8. Remove the tops of vials and clean the stoppers with povidone-iodine swabs. Inject the supplied diluent slowly to avoid foaming. Do not shake. *Gently* swirl or roll the vial between the hands until the Factor VIII is dissolved.

9. Do not refrigerate reconstituted Factor VIII.

10. Attach the supplied filter needle to the sterile syringe and withdraw the solution. *Remove the filter needle.* (Do not administer solution through this needle.)

11. Identify the child by checking the identification band.

12. Refer to "Blood Administration: General Procedure" for steps to initiate the administration of blood/blood products.

13. Establish an IV line with butterfly, if no preexisting IV device. Flush with normal saline.

14. Factor VIII can be given IV push at a maximum rate of 1 to 10 ml per minute, by retrograde (small volume) or, if continuous infusion is needed, via metriset (buretrol).

15. Follow Factor VIII with a normal saline flush.

16. After Factor VIII administration, observe and record signs and symptoms of continued or decreased bleeding and check bleeding times. Check the infusion site for bleeding.

17. Discard the bag and administration set in an appropriate manner.

DOCUMENTATION

- Name of blood product.
- Start time.
- Vital signs.
- Lot number, volume (in milliliters), and units infused.
- Child's response.
- Amount of any normal saline flushes.
- Completion time.

Skills Checklist

- ☐ Prepare the child and family; check for informed consent.
- ☐ Assemble the equipment.
- ☐ Wash hands and put on gloves.
- ☐ Obtain Factor VIII.
- ☐ Verify that the blood product is correct.
- ☐ Reconstitute Factor VIII.
- ☐ Identify the child by checking the identification band.
- ☐ Obtain baseline vital signs.
- ☐ Flush the IV line with normal saline.
- ☐ Administer Factor VIII.
- ☐ Flush the IV line with normal saline.
- ☐ Discard the bag and equipment.
- ☐ Document.

POTENTIAL RELATED NURSING DIAGNOSES

Tissue perfusion, altered, peripheral

Fear

Anxiety

Injury: *high risk*

POTENTIAL RELATED MEDICAL DIAGNOSES

Hemophilia

REFERENCES

Mott, S., James, S., and Sperhac, A. 1990. *Nursing care of children and families.* Redwood City, Calif.: Addison-Wesley.

National Blood Resource Education. 1991. Choosing blood components and equipment. *AJN* 91, no. 6: 42–52.

Pisciotto, P., ed. 1989. *Blood transfusion therapy.* Arlington, Va.: American Association of Blood Banks.

Lab Values

Prolonged Prothrombin Time—Normal: 11–15 seconds.
Prolonged Partial Thromboplastin Time—Normal: 60–85 seconds.
Increased Thromboplastin Generation Test—Normal: 8–16 seconds.

5 Blood Administration: Frozen Plasma

PSYCHOSOCIAL CONSIDERATIONS: Explain the procedure in developmentally appropriate terms. Avoid using terms with mixed meanings, such as *stick* and *shot*. A child who has had a transfusion reaction may fear another such occurrence. Explain the screening process to detect the HIV virus, if appropriate; parents may be fearful of AIDS.

TIME: 30 minutes to 6 hours

PURPOSE

Fresh Frozen Plasma (FFP), frozen by the blood bank *within 6 hours of collection*:

- Primarily to supply clotting factors (including labile Factors V and VIII and fibrinogen). May be used in patients with congenital or acquired bleeding disorders when specific plasma factor concentrates are not available. When available, a specific plasma clotting factor concentrate (such as Factor VIII) is used to replace a specific factor deficit.
- Occasionally to provide other specific plasma proteins for patients with congenital or acquired deficiencies.
- As a volume expander.

Aged Frozen Plasma (AFP), frozen by the blood bank *within 26 days of collection*:

- To provide plasma proteins for volume expansion in patients with severe hypoproteinemia. (Note: The treatment of choice in such situations, however, is plasma protein fraction or albumin, both of which are heat treated and free of the risk of hepatitis.)

OBJECTIVES

- To administer frozen plasma safely.
- To prevent injury.

EQUIPMENT

Frozen plasma

Gloves, nonsterile

Plasma administration set

Infusion pump, if appropriate

Needle to cap intravenous tubing, sterile

SAFETY ISSUES

- **Check for informed consent.**
- **Type and cross-match.**
- **Frozen plasma expires 24 hours after thawing.**

ESSENTIAL STEPS

1. Prepare the child and family. Refer to "Blood Administration: General Procedure."
2. Assemble the equipment.
3. Wash hands.
4. Obtain the plasma.

   Request frozen plasma.

   Indicate the quantity of plasma needed in ml or units.

   Indicate if the physician's plan of care is for FFP or AFP.

   Allow 30 minutes to 1 hour to type the child's blood and to thaw the frozen plasma.

   If the child's blood has been previously typed, allow 30 minutes to thaw the plasma.

5. Check the plasma bag label and blood request form. Refer to "Blood Administration: General Procedure."

6. Put on gloves and prime the plasma administration set.

7. Identify the child by checking the identification band.

8. Refer to "Blood Administration: General Procedure" for steps to initiate the administration of blood/blood products.

9. Administer the plasma.

Hang the plasma within 30 minutes of the time it leaves the blood bank. If this is not possible, return the plasma to the blood bank. Do not freeze, refrigerate, or warm plasma.

Begin transfusion. A normal saline flush is not required before or after plasma.

If giving more than 1 unit of plasma, change the administration set after each *3rd unit* or after the set has hung for *6 hours*.

10. Monitor the child for signs and symptoms of a blood transfusion reaction. Refer to "Blood Administration: Transfusion Reaction." Observe for fluid volume overload.

11. Discard the bag and administration set in an appropriate manner.

DOCUMENTATION

- Name of blood product.
- Start time.
- Baseline and serial vital signs.
- Amount infused.
- Child's response.
- Completion time.

Skills Checklist

☐ Prepare the child and family.
  • Check for informed consent.
  • Premedicate.
☐ Assemble the equipment.
☐ Wash hands.
☐ Obtain the plasma.
☐ Verify that the blood product is correct.
☐ Put on gloves and prime the tubing.
☐ Identify the child by checking the identification band.
☐ Obtain baseline vital signs.
☐ Administer frozen plasma.
☐ Monitor vital signs.
☐ Discard the bag and administration set.
☐ Document.

POTENTIAL RELATED NURSING DIAGNOSES

Hyperthermia

Infection: *high risk*

Skin integrity, impaired: *high risk*

Fluid volume deficit

POTENTIAL RELATED MEDICAL DIAGNOSES

Bleeding disorders

Sepsis

Hypovolemia

REFERENCES

American Association of Blood Banks. 1989. *Circular of information for the use of human blood and blood components.* Arlington, Va.: American Association of Blood Banks.

Landier, W., Barrell, M., and Styffe, E. 1987. How to administer blood components to children. *MCN* (May/June): 178–84.

National Blood Resource Education. 1991. Choosing blood components and equipment. *AJN* 91, no. 6: 42–52.

Pisciotto, P., ed. 1989. *Blood transfusion therapy.* Arlington, Va.: American Association of Blood Banks.

6 Blood Administration: General Procedure

PSYCHOSOCIAL CONSIDERATIONS: Explain the procedure in developmentally appropriate terms. Avoid using terms with mixed meanings, such as *stick, shot,* and *take blood.* Explain to younger children immediately prior to the procedure to prevent prolonged anxiety. Be honest about potential discomfort. The child may have magical thinking and be concerned about receiving someone else's blood. An older child may fear AIDS. If the child inquires, explain the screening techniques used to detect the HIV virus. Discuss this screening process with parents, if appropriate. Preschool and school-aged children may benefit from seeing and handling the equipment.

TIME: See the procedure for the specific blood product

PURPOSE

To obtain, safely administer, and document blood/blood products.

OBJECTIVES

- To administer blood products safely.
- To prevent injury during administration.

EQUIPMENT

Blood/blood product

Gloves, nonsterile

Appropriate administration set and filter. Refer to the procedure for administration of a specific blood product.

Normal saline (0.9% sodium chloride), 5 ml syringe, and needle, sterile

Stopcock and extension tubing, if appropriate

Infusion pump, if appropriate

Medication, if ordered

Needle to cap intravenous tubing, sterile

Appropriate documentation form(s)

 SAFETY ISSUES

- Check for informed consent.
- If a blood bag is leaking or is accidentally punctured, return it immediately to the blood bank.
- Do not add IV additives or medications to blood/blood products. Flush the line with 3 to 5 ml of normal saline to give medication, if necessary. Do not interrupt the transfusion for more than 1 hour.
- Flush the IV line with normal saline before and after administering blood products.
- If a reaction occurs, stop the blood transfusion immediately and notify the physician.
- Use an infusion pump to administer blood/blood products through central lines, except when administering platelets.

1. Prepare the child and family.

   Check for informed consent.

   Determine if the child has received a previous transfusion and has had a transfusion reaction. Consult the physician if the child has had a previous reaction.

   Administer premedication per the physician's plan of care.

2. Assemble the equipment.

3. Wash hands.

4. Obtain the blood/blood product.

5. Verify that the blood/blood product is correct.

   Check the blood product against the physician's plan of care.

   Two RNs should check in blood products; one of these two starts the transfusion.

   Both RNs observe the product for abnormal color, clumping, gas bubbles, or extraneous material.

   Both RNs check the blood bag label and blood request form for

Skills Checklist

☐ Prepare the child and family.
   • Check for informed consent.
   • Premedicate.
☐ Assemble the equipment.
☐ Wash hands.
☐ Obtain blood/blood product.
☐ Verify that the blood product is correct.
☐ Put on gloves and prime tubing.
☐ Identify the child by checking the identification band.
☐ Obtain baseline vital signs.
☐ Flush the IV line with normal saline.
☐ Administer blood product.
☐ Monitor vital signs.
☐ Put on gloves and flush the IV line with normal saline.
☐ Discard the blood bag and administration set.
☐ Document.

   The appropriate product name.

   The *donor's* number, ABO group, and Rh factor.

   The volume in the unit.

   The expiration date.

   The child's name and medical record number.

   The *child's* ABO group and Rh factor.

   If there is any discrepancy, do not hang the blood; call the blood bank.

6. Put on gloves and prime the appropriate blood administration set with the blood/blood product. (See Fig. 6.1)

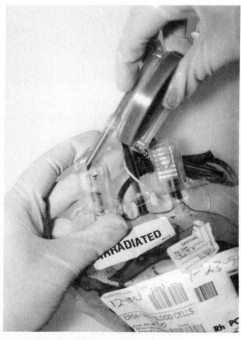

FIGURE 6.1 *Spiking the blood bag with the filter and tubing.*

7. Identify the child. The medical record number on the bag label and blood request form will match the medical record number on the child's identification band.

8. Obtain baseline vital signs. Warm the blood, if necessary.

9. Flush the IV with 3 to 5 ml normal saline to clear any existing IV solution or medication, except when administering plasma.

10. Connect the blood administration set to the hub of the IV device. (Add extension tubing and a stopcock to the hub of the IV device prior to connecting the blood administration set, if necessary.) Use of a stopcock allows connection of a normal saline line for flushing or infusion should a reaction occur.

11. Begin the transfusion. Run at a slow rate for the first 15 minutes, except in an emergency situation when the physician orders push. Observe the child continuously for the first 5 minutes.

12. Take and record vital signs every 15 minutes for the first hour. Then check vital signs hourly or per the physician's plan of care throughout the transfusion. Refer to the procedure for administration of a specific blood product.

13. Flush the IV line with 3 to 5 ml normal saline after transfusion and prior to starting the IV fluid or medication.

14. Discard the blood bag and administration set in an appropriate manner.

DOCUMENTATION

- Name of blood product.
- Start time.
- Baseline and serial vital signs.
- Amount of normal saline flush(es).
- Signs and symptoms relevant to administration of the blood product, such as bleeding if platelets or plasma have been given.
- Time and name of physician notified, signs and symptoms of reaction, and interventions taken if an untoward response occurs. Refer to "Blood Administration: Transfusion Reaction."
- Amount of blood/blood product infused.
- Completion time.

POTENTIAL RELATED NURSING DIAGNOSES

Anxiety

Fear

Fluid volume excess: *high risk*

Hyperthermia

Injury: *high risk*

Fluid volume deficit: *high risk*

Gas exchange, impaired

POTENTIAL RELATED MEDICAL DIAGNOSES

Preoperative preparation

Hemorrhage

Anemia

Leukemia/childhood cancers

REFERENCES

American Association of Blood Banks. 1989. *Circular of information for the use of human blood and blood components.* Arlington, Va.: American Association of Blood Banks.

Hahn, K. 1989. Monitoring a blood transfusion. *Nursing 89* 19, no. 10: 20–21.

Landier, W., Barrell, N., and Styffe, E. 1987. How to administer blood components to children. *MCN* (May/June): 178–84.

Mott, S., James, S., and Sperhac, A. 1990. *Nursing care of children and families.* Redwood City, Calif.: Addison-Wesley.

National Blood Resource Education. 1991. Choosing blood components and equipment. *AJN* 91, no. 6: 42–52.

7 Blood Administration: Granulocyte Transfusion

PSYCHOSOCIAL CONSIDERATIONS: Explain the procedure in developmentally appropriate terms. Avoid using terms with mixed meanings, such as *stick* and *shot*. A child who has had a transfusion reaction may fear another such occurrence. Explain the screening process to detect the HIV virus, if appropriate; some parents may be fearful of AIDS.

TIME: Optimally, up to 6 hours; 24 hours maximum

PURPOSE

To safely administer irradiated granulocytes to a child with clinical sepsis, severe neutropenia, and/or granulocyte storage pool depletion.

OBJECTIVES

- To administer granulocytes safely.
- To prevent complications.
- To prevent or monitor reactions.

EQUIPMENT

Granulocytes

Gloves, nonsterile

Granulocyte administration set, which includes a platelet filter recipient set (175-micron filter)

Syringe pump, if appropriate

Normal saline (0.9% sodium chloride), 5 ml syringe, and needle, sterile

Medication, if ordered

Needle to cap IV tubing, sterile

SAFETY ISSUES

- Check for informed consent.
- Bone marrow aspiration may be performed to determine depletion of neutrophil storage pool in addition to peripheral neutrophil counts.
- Immediately prior to granulocyte transfusion, the physician should order a type and cross-match (T&C) and a complete blood count. Obtain repeat T&C every 48 hours during the days of granulocyte administration.
- For maximum effectiveness, administer granulocytes immediately upon receipt. Effectiveness decreases progressively with the age of the granulocytes, which should be transfused within 6 hours after collection for best therapeutic results. However, the permissible storage time is up to 24 hours. Do not use granulocytes more than 24 hours old.
- The physician orders the granulocyte administration rate. Administer slowly, usually over a 2- to 4-hour period, or as tolerated by the child.
- Do not use infusion pumps; they destroy white blood cells. A syringe pump is acceptable if the child's vein is too small for infusion by gravity alone.

ESSENTIAL STEPS

1. Prepare the child and family. Refer to "Blood Administration: General Procedure." The physician may order premedication for discomfort and/or temperature control.
2. Assemble the equipment.
3. Wash hands.
4. Obtain granulocytes.
5. Check the granulocyte bag or syringe label and blood request form.

Check granulocytes derived from washed whole blood (usually in a syringe) for ABO compatibility. (May give Type O to anybody; no A or B antibodies because no plasma.) Verify with the blood bank that these granulocytes have been filtered and that no filter is required for administration.

Check granulocytes derived from apheresis (usually in a bag) for type specificity (unwashed, unfiltered). (Must give type A blood to type A patient.) Filter before administration.

Verify that granulocytes are irradiated.

6. Put on gloves and prime the administration set.

7. Identify the child by checking the identification band.

8. Refer to "Blood Administration: General Procedure" for steps to initiate the administration of blood/blood products.

9. Measure and record baseline vital signs. Check vitals every 15 minutes for the first hour, every 30 minutes thereafter.

10. Infuse unit at ordered rate or as tolerated, usually 1 pheresis unit over a 2- to 4-hour period.

11. Observe for signs and symptoms of granulocyte reaction:

    Fever, which may be diminished with decreased infusion rate.

    Pulmonary edema, which may occur with rapid infusion.

    Anaphylaxis.

    Other: refer to "Blood Administration: Transfusion Reaction."

12. Discard the bag and administration set in an appropriate manner.

Skills Checklist

☐ Prepare the child and family.
- • Check for informed consent.
- • Premedicate.

☐ Assemble the equipment.

☐ Wash hands.

☐ Obtain granulocytes.

☐ Verify that the blood product is correct.

☐ Put on gloves and prime the administration set.

☐ Identify the child by checking the identification band.

☐ Obtain baseline vital signs.

☐ Flush the IV line with normal saline.

☐ Administer granulocytes.

☐ Monitor vital signs.

☐ Discard the bag and administration set.

☐ Document.

DOCUMENTATION

- Name of blood product.
- Start time.
- Baseline and serial vital signs.
- Amount infused.
- Child's response.
- Completion time.

POTENTIAL RELATED NURSING DIAGNOSES

Hyperthermia

Infection: *high risk*

Skin integrity, impaired: *high risk*

POTENTIAL RELATED MEDICAL DIAGNOSES

Cancer

Aplastic anemia

Sepsis

REFERENCES

American Association of Blood Banks. 1989. *Circular of information for the use of human blood products and blood components.* Arlington, Va.: American Association of Blood Banks.

National Blood Resource Education. 1991. Choosing blood components and equipment. *AJN* 91, no. 6: 42–52.

8 Blood Administration: Immune Globulin

PSYCHOSOCIAL CONSIDERATIONS: Explain the procedure in developmentally appropriate terms. Avoid using terms with mixed meanings such as "little stick" or "bee sting."

TIME: 1 to 6 hours

PURPOSE

To provide for the safe administration of intravenous immune globulin (IVIG).

OBJECTIVES

- To safely administer IVIG.
- To prevent injury.

EQUIPMENT

Gloves, nonsterile

IVIG utilizing tubing with filter, as provided by manufacturer; refer to the drug insert

IV set, as needed

IV pump, as needed

Normal saline (0.9% sodium chloride), if necessary

- Adverse reactions to IVIG are related to the rate of infusion, not the dose. Therefore, orders should be written for a full vial (that is, in multiples of 2.5, 3.0, 5.0 or 6.0 g). Concentration and rate should be specified. Dose range is 200 to 1,000 mg/kg.
- Store IVIG at room temperature, not to exceed 25°C (72°F). Administer within 6 hours after reconstitution.

ESSENTIAL STEPS

1. Prepare the child and family.
2. Assemble the equipment.
3. Wash hands and put on gloves.
4. Obtain IVIG. Check vial(s) and blood request form. Refer to "Blood Administration: General Procedure."
5. Reconstitute IVIG according to the package insert. Do not shake the vial.
6. Prime the administration set.
7. Identify the child by checking the identification band.

8. Refer to "Blood Administration: General Procedure" for steps to initiate the administration of blood/blood products.

9. Infuse IVIG.

10. If adverse reactions occur (refer to drug insert), slow the infusion rate, obtain vital signs, and notify the physician. If an adverse reaction results in a significant change in vital signs:

   Stop the infusion.

   Notify the physician immediately.

   Start a normal saline infusion at a keep-vein-open rate.

11. Discard vial(s) and the administration set in an appropriate manner.

DOCUMENTATION

- Name of blood product.
- Start time.
- Baseline and serial vital signs.
- Rate of infusion and amount infused.
- Child's response.
- Completion time.

POTENTIAL RELATED NURSING DIAGNOSES

Anxiety

Fear

Injury: *high risk*

Fluid volume excess

Skin integrity, impaired: *high risk*

Skills Checklist

☐ Prepare the child and family.
☐ Assemble the equipment.
☐ Wash hands and put on gloves.
☐ Obtain IVIG and verify that the blood product is correct.
☐ Reconstitute IVIG.
☐ Prime the administration set.
☐ Identify the child by checking the identification band.
☐ Obtain baseline vital signs.
☐ Administer IVIG.
☐ Monitor vital signs.
☐ Discard the vial(s) and administration set.
☐ Document.

POTENTIAL RELATED MEDICAL DIAGNOSES

Immunosuppression

Hepatitis

REFERENCES

Pisciotto, P., ed. 1989. *Blood transfusion therapy*. Arlington, Va.: American Association of Blood Banks.

National Blood Resource Education. 1991. Choosing blood components and equipment. *AJN* 91, no. 6: 42–52.

Wasserman, R. L. 1988. Antibody deficiency states. In *Current therapy in pediatric infectious disease*, edited by J. D. Nelson. Philadelphia: B. B. Decker.

9 Blood Administration: Neonatal Transfusion

PSYCHOSOCIAL CONSIDERATIONS: Explain the procedure to the parents. Discuss the reasons for the transfusion. Often transfusions are associated with blood loss, and parents have not witnessed this in their child. Explain the screening process to detect the HIV virus, if appropriate; parents may be fearful of AIDS. Allow parents to see and touch the child prior to the procedure and to hold and comfort the child during the procedure, if possible.

TIME: 10 minutes to 1 hour

PURPOSE

To administer blood products to infants less than 4 months of age. Procedure decreases neonatal blood loss by using maternal rather than neonatal blood sample in screening for maternal red blood cell antibodies.

OBJECTIVES

- To administer a blood transfusion safely.
- To prevent injury.

EQUIPMENT

Tube for infant's 0.5 ml sample

Tube for mother's 7.5 ml sample (or mother's blood sample from transferring hospital)

Gloves, nonsterile

Appropriate administration set

Neonatal bag or syringe of blood

Leukocyte filter, if needed

Normal saline (0.9% sodium chloride), 5 ml syringe, and needle, sterile

Stopcock and extension tubing, if appropriate

Infusion pump, if appropriate

Needle to cap IV tubing, sterile

 SAFETY ISSUES

- **Check for informed consent.**
- **Blood/blood products may be irradiated.**
- **Red blood cells (RBCs) are usually provided as follows:**

    RBCs will be either Group O Rh positive or Group O Rh negative, washed, leukocyte poor, and antigen negative for any clinically significant maternal antibody detected. Check that the syringe or bag containing the RBCs is labeled "LPF" (leukocyte poor filtered).

RBCs can be ordered by the ml and received in a syringe. An extra 15 ml of blood will be added to purge IV tubing. RBCs received in a syringe are prefiltered.

RBCs may also be ordered by the bag (usually for surgery); in this case, they need to be filtered at the time of administration.

Preparation of RBCs takes approximately 60 minutes.

ESSENTIAL STEPS

1. Prepare the child and family. Refer to "Blood Administration: General Procedure." Confirm that the infant is less than 4 months of age.

2. Assemble the equipment. If samples are needed:

    Affix a label to the blood tube for the baby's blood that indicates:

    Infant's name.

    Medical record number (MR#).

    Date, time, and signature of the person drawing the sample.

    Affix a label to the blood tube for the mother's blood that indicates:

    Infant's name and MR#.

    "Mother's blood" clearly labeled.

    Date, time, and signature of the person drawing the sample or of the nurse if the blood has come from a transferring hospital.

Skills Checklist

☐ Prepare the child and family:
  • Check for informed consent.
  • Confirm that the infant is less than 4 months of age.
☐ Assemble the equipment.
☐ Wash hands.
☐ Obtain blood/blood product.
☐ Verify that the blood product is correct.
☐ Put on gloves and prime tubing.
☐ Identify the infant by checking the identification band.
☐ Obtain baseline vital signs.
☐ Flush the IV line with normal saline.
☐ Administer blood/blood product.
☐ Monitor vital signs.
☐ Put on gloves and flush the IV line with normal saline.
☐ Disconnect the blood administration set and reconnect the IV.
☐ Discard the blood bag or syringe and administration set.
☐ Document.

3. Wash hands.

4. Obtain blood/blood product.

5. Check the blood bag or syringe label and the blood request form. Refer to "Blood Administration: General Procedure."

6. Put on gloves and prime the blood administration set. Include a leukocyte filter, if necessary. Use an extension tube to connect a syringe to the IV line.

7. Identify the infant by checking the identification band.

Lab Values

NORMAL

Bleeding Time: 2 minutes
Partial Thromboplastin Time (PTT): <90 seconds
Prothrombin Time (PT): <17 seconds
Hemoglobin (Hgb): 14–23 g/dL (birth–1 month)
Hematocrit (Hct): 43%–75% (birth–1 month)

8. Refer to "Blood Administration: General Procedure" for steps to initiate the administration of blood/blood product.

9. Infuse blood/blood product. Refer to the procedure regarding the specific blood product for infusion steps. (See Figs. 9.1 and 9.2)

10. Carefully observe for a transfusion reaction. Refer to "Blood Administration: Transfusion Reaction."

11. Discard the syringe or bag and administration set in an appropriate manner.

DOCUMENTATION

- Name of blood/blood product.
- Start time.
- Baseline and serial vital signs.
- Amount infused.
- Child's response.
- Amount of any normal saline flushes.
- Completion time.

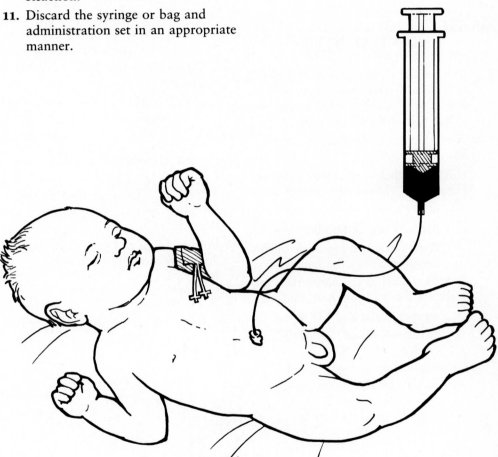

FIGURE 9.1 *Administering blood from a syringe.*

POTENTIAL RELATED NURSING DIAGNOSES

Infection: *high risk*

Hypothermia

Tissue perfusion, altered, cardiopulmonary

Anxiety

Fear

Coping, ineffective family, compromised

POTENTIAL RELATED MEDICAL DIAGNOSES

Anemia

Intraventricular hemorrhage

Hemorrhage

Infection/sepsis

REFERENCES

National Blood Resource Education. 1991. Choosing blood components and equipment. *AJN* 91, no. 6: 42–52.

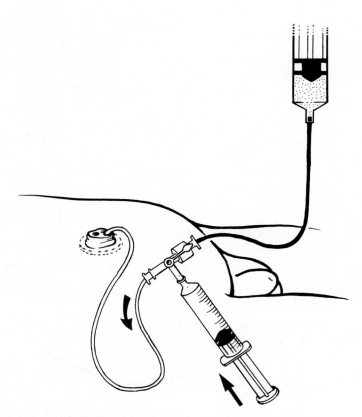

FIGURE 9.2   *Flushing with normal saline.*

10 Blood Administration: Platelets

PSYCHOSOCIAL CONSIDERATIONS: Explain the procedure in developmentally appropriate terms. Avoid using terms with mixed meanings, such as *stick* and *shot*. A child who has had a transfusion reaction may fear another such occurrence. Explain the screening process to detect the HIV virus, if appropriate; some parents may be fearful of AIDS.

TIME: Up to 4 hours

PURPOSE

To safely and adequately provide functioning platelets to patients with thrombocytopenia or dysfunctioning platelets.

OBJECTIVES

- To administer platelets safely.
- To prevent injury.

EQUIPMENT

Platelets

Gloves, nonsterile

Platelet administration set

Needle to cap intravenous tubing, sterile

Stopcock and extension tubing, if appropriate

Normal saline (0.9% sodium chloride), 5 ml syringe, and needle, sterile

Medication, if ordered

- Check for informed consent.
- Blood cross-matching is not necessary prior to platelet administration. ABO type-specific platelets are preferable but not required.
- Blood typing is *recommended* before the administration of platelets. In an emergency situation, ABO/Rh typing of platelets is not necessary. Once the child's ABO/Rh group has been determined, typing for repeated platelet administration is not necessary.
- A physician who determines that excess plasma should be removed from a unit of platelets prior to transfusion may contact the blood bank or write an order indicating such.
- If the physician orders "leukocyte poor" blood product, obtain a leukocyte filter. Change the filter after each pool of 6 to 10 units.
- Hang platelets within 30 minutes of receiving them. Do not store them in the blood refrigerator. If unable to hang platelets immediately, return to the blood bank.
- Do not use infusion pumps to administer platelets. Syringe pumps may be used; roll the syringe every 30 minutes to prevent platelets from settling.
- Hang platelets no longer than 4 hours.
- The physician may order an antipyretic (acetaminophen) and antihistamine (diphenhydramine) before infusion to reduce the possibility of a transfusion reaction.

Essential Steps

1. Prepare the child and family. Refer to "Blood Administration: General Procedure."
2. Assemble the equipment.
3. Wash hands.
4. Obtain the platelets. Indicate if the platelets are to be pooled and/or concentrated.
5. Check the platelet bag label and blood request form. Refer to "Blood Administration: General Procedure."
6. Put on gloves and connect the platelet administration set to the bag of platelets.
7. Prime the platelet administration set, making sure that platelets completely cover the filter in the drip chamber in order to prevent platelet destruction. (See Fig. 10.1)

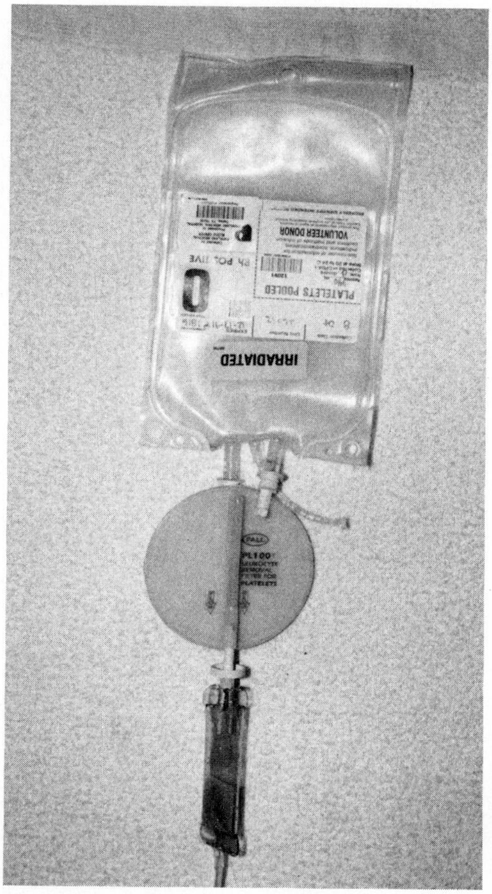

FIGURE 10.1 *Platelet filter.*

Skills Checklist

- ☐ Prepare the child and family.
  - Check for informed consent.
  - Premedicate.
- ☐ Assemble the equipment.
- ☐ Wash hands.
- ☐ Obtain platelets.
- ☐ Verify that the blood product is correct.
- ☐ Put on gloves and prime the tubing.
- ☐ Identify the child by checking the identification band.
- ☐ Obtain baseline vital signs.
- ☐ Disconnect and cap tubing of the infusing IV.
- ☐ Flush the IV line with normal saline.
- ☐ Administer platelets.
- ☐ Monitor vital signs.
- ☐ Put on gloves and flush the IV line with normal saline.
- ☐ Disconnect the platelet administration set and reconnect the IV.
- ☐ Discard the bag and administration set.
- ☐ Document.

Lab Values

PLATELET COUNTS—NORMAL

Birth–1 month: 84–478 × 10^9/L
Other ages: 150–400 × 10^9/L

8. Identify the child by checking the identification band.

9. Refer to "Blood Administration: General Procedure" for steps to initiate the administration of blood/blood products.

10. Turn off the infusing IV solution and disconnect the tubing. Cap the IV tubing with a sterile needle.

11. Add extension tubing and a stopcock to the hub of the IV device, if appropriate. Use the second port on the stopcock for a normal saline line or a normal saline syringe.

12. Flush the IV with 3 to 5 ml of normal saline to clear any existing IV solution or medication.

13. Connect the platelet administration set to the stopcock or the hub of the IV device.

14. Infuse the platelets as rapidly as possible or according to the physician's plan of care for a specific flow rate. Platelets should hang no more than 4 hours because their function decreases with time.

15. After the *ordered* amount has been administered, put on gloves and flush the IV cannula or extension tubing with normal saline.

16. Disconnect the platelet administration set and connect the IV fluid administration set.

17. Discard the empty bag and administration set in an appropriate manner.

18. Observe the child closely for 2 hours posttransfusion. Platelet reactions can occur up to 2 hours posttransfusion and are febrile and nonhemolytic in nature. Refer to "Blood Administration: Transfusion Reaction."

DOCUMENTATION

- Name of blood product.
- Start time.
- Baseline and serial vital signs.
- Amount infused.
- Child's response.
- Amount of any normal saline flushes.
- Completion time.

POTENTIAL RELATED NURSING DIAGNOSES

Hyperthermia

Infection: *high risk*

Skin integrity, impaired: *high risk*

POTENTIAL RELATED MEDICAL DIAGNOSES

Thrombocytopenia

Bleeding disorders

REFERENCES

American Association of Blood Banks. 1989. *Circular of information for the use of human blood and blood components.* Arlington, Va.: American Association of Blood Banks.

Mott, S., James, S., and Sperhac, A. 1990. *Nursing care of children and families.* Redwood City, Calif.: Addison-Wesley.

National Blood Resource Education. 1991. Choosing blood components and equipment. *AJN* 91, no. 6: 42–52.

11 Blood Administration: Prothrombin Complex Concentrate

- Check for informed consent.
- Blood typing and cross-matching are not necessary prior to administration of PCC. The blood bank may require an initial ABO group and Rh factor on each child to whom blood products are administered.
- Factor II, VII, IX, and/or X deficiency and/or the presence of inhibitor should be proven prior to the administration of PCC.
- Although stable at room temperature for 12 hours after reconstitution, PCC should be administered promptly. Do not refrigerate after reconstitution.
- Give entire vials of PCC. Never discard part of a vial.
- Fresh Frozen Plasma (FFP) is the treatment of choice when diagnosis is unproven for infants, and for milder Factor IX patients. (Use FFP to decrease the risk of exposure to viral agents.)
- A child, parent, or guardian instructed in home hemophilia care can give PCC.

PSYCHOSOCIAL CONSIDERATIONS: Explain the procedure in developmentally appropriate terms. Avoid using terms with mixed meanings, such as *stick* and *shot*. A child who has had a transfusion reaction may fear another such occurrence. Explain the screening process to detect the HIV virus, if appropriate; some parents may be fearful of AIDS.

TIME: Up to 12 hours

PURPOSE

To safely administer a commercially prepared concentrate of human prothrombin complex concentrate (PCC) for the treatment of bleeding episodes in congenital or acquired deficiencies of Factor II, VII, IX, and/or X, and/or for treatment of Factor VIII deficiency with an inhibitor.

To prophylactically administer PCC to patients preoperatively who are deficient in Factor II, VII, IX and/or X, and/or have a Factor VIII deficiency with an inhibitor.

OBJECTIVES

- To administer PCC safely.
- To prevent injury.

EQUIPMENT

Gloves, nonsterile

PCC with filter needle and diluent

Povidone-iodine swabs *or* alcohol swabs

10 or 20 ml syringe

25g or 23g butterfly (if no preexisting IV)

Normal saline (0.9% sodium chloride), 5 ml syringe, and needle, sterile

ESSENTIAL STEPS

1. Prepare the child and family. Refer to "Blood Administration: General Procedure."
2. Assemble the equipment.
3. Wash hands and put on gloves.
4. After the physician has ordered the *approximate* number of units needed, call the blood bank to determine the "units per vial" available. (Each lot number has varying units per vial.)
5. After receiving this information, the physician amends the order so that entire vials are given (such as PCC, 5 vials of 480 units per vial).
6. To reduce the child's risk/exposure to viral agents, request that the blood bank supply all vials from the same lot when ordering.

7. Keep PCC refrigerated until ready to use; warm to room temperature before reconstituting.

8. Check the vial label(s) and request form. Refer to "Blood Administration: General Procedure."

9. After removing the tops of the vials and cleaning with povidone-iodine or alcohol swabs, use the double-ended transfer needle to inject the diluent supplied with PCC into the vial using a sterile technique. Add diluent slowly to avoid foaming, which will inactivate PCC.

10. Roll the vial *gently* between the hands or gently swirl the vial until the PCC is dissolved. *Do not shake.*

11. Attach the supplied filter needle to the sterile syringe; withdraw PCC solution into the syringe. *Remove the filter needle.* (Do *not* administer PCC solution through this needle.)

12. Identify the child by checking the identification band.

13. Refer to "Blood Administration: General Procedure" for steps to initiate the administration of blood/blood products.

14. Establish an IV line with butterfly if there is no preexisting IV device. Flush with normal saline.

15. Administer PCC by direct IV push at a maximum rate of 10 ml per minute, by retrograde, or via metriset (buretrol). (Note: Direct IV push is the preferred method of administration.)

16. Follow PCC with a normal saline flush.

17. After PCC administration, observe for and record signs and symptoms of continued or decreased bleeding.

DOCUMENTATION

- Name of blood product.
- Start time.
- Vital signs.
- Lot number, volume (in milliliters), and number of units infused.
- Child's response.
- Amount of any normal saline flushes.
- Completion time.

Skills Checklist

☐ Prepare the child and family. Check for informed consent.
☐ Assemble the equipment.
☐ Wash hands and put on gloves.
☐ Obtain PCC.
☐ Verify that the blood product is correct.
☐ Reconstitute PCC.
☐ Identify the child by checking the identification band.
☐ Obtain baseline vital signs.
☐ Flush the IV line with normal saline.
☐ Administer PCC.
☐ Flush the IV line with normal saline.
☐ Document.

POTENTIAL RELATED NURSING DIAGNOSES

Fear

Anxiety

Infection: *high risk*

Tissue perfusion, altered, peripheral

POTENTIAL RELATED MEDICAL DIAGNOSES

Factor II, VII, IX, and/or X deficiencies

REFERENCES

Mott, S., James, S., and Sperhac, A. 1990. *Nursing care of children and families.* Redwood City, Calif.: Addison-Wesley.

National Blood Resource Education. 1991. Choosing blood components and equipment. *AJN* 91, no. 6: 42–52.

Lab Values

PROTHROMBIN TIME (PT)—NORMAL

Birth–1 month: <17 seconds
Other ages: 11–15 seconds

PARTIAL THROMBOPLASTIN TIME (PTT)—NORMAL

Birth–1 month: <90 seconds
Other ages: 60–85 seconds (nonactivated)
  25–35 seconds (activated)

12 Blood Administration: Transfusion Reaction

• Assess the patient frequently for
itching, rash, fever, or flushing of
the skin.

PSYCHOSOCIAL CONSIDERATIONS: Explain events in developmentally appropriate terms. Avoid using terms with mixed meanings, such as *reaction*. The child may be frightened by the reaction and fear dying. Do not leave the child until reaction subsides; provide support. Prevent the child from self-injury. Allow the family to remain in the room if possible.

TIME: Varies, usually within 1 hour of administration

PURPOSE

To assess the child for any reaction to blood/blood products.

To intervene appropriately, based on the type of reaction.

To decrease the possibility of further complications and adverse reactions related to blood or blood products.

OBJECTIVES

• To identify a reaction.
• To lessen the severity of a reaction.
• To prevent shock.

EQUIPMENT

Gloves, nonsterile

Normal saline (0.9% sodium chloride) and appropriate administration set

Blood/blood product bag(s) and administration set(s); for nonmild reactions, must be from transfusions receiving/received during the previous 24 hours

Needle to cap blood administration set, sterile

Two blood tubes

Urine specimen container

ESSENTIAL STEPS

1. Prepare the child and family throughout the following steps.

2. Assemble the equipment as needed throughout the following steps.

3. For a mild allergic reaction (mild rash, hives, and/or itching or fever; see Table 12.1):

   Stop the flow of blood/blood product immediately.

   Wash hands and put on gloves.

   Do not remove the IV needle or angiocatheter. Disconnect the transfusion set at the hub of the needle and hang normal saline at a keep-vein-open rate (KVO) to maintain the IV site. If the transfusion set is connected to a stopcock and saline is hanging to the second port, disconnect the transfusion set at the stopcock and run saline at a KVO rate. Maintain the sterility of the blood/blood product administration set by covering the hub with a sterile cap.

   Obtain vital signs.

   Contact the physician immediately.

   Monitor vital signs every 15 minutes or per the physician's plan of care.

   Obtain an order for the type and rate of IV solution.

If the physician orders the transfusion to be resumed:

Give the blood/blood product slowly over the next 15 minutes, observing the child continuously.

Assess the child every 15 to 30 minutes thereafter, taking vital signs.

If the child's allergic signs and symptoms increase, stop the flow rate, infuse normal saline at KVO, and contact the physician.

The physician may order Benadryl, another antihistamine, or epinephrine. If so, administer and monitor the response. An antihistamine may have been given as a premedication prior to the transfusion, especially if the child has a history of transfusion reaction.

4. For blood/blood product reactions other than mild allergic reactions (see Table 12.1):

Complete steps 1 through 7 as for a mild reaction.

Place the child on strict intake and output.

Skills Checklist

☐ Prepare the child and family throughout the steps.
☐ Assemble the equipment as needed throughout the steps.
☐ Stop the flow of blood/blood product.
☐ Wash hands and put on gloves.
☐ Disconnect the transfusion set; begin normal saline infusion at KVO rate.
☐ Monitor vital signs.
☐ Contact the physician.
☐ For a mild reaction
  • Obtain an order for the type and rate of IV solution.
  • Administer medications.
☐ For a nonmild reaction
  • Place the child on strict intake and output.
  • Obtain a 3 ml blood sample.
  • Collect the first postreaction urine sample.
  • Send the blood bag and administration set to the blood bank.
  • Obtain a blood sample 5 to 7 hours postreaction, if requested.
☐ Document.

Obtain a 3 ml blood sample from a site other than the transfusion site and place in a tube. (If the sample must be obtained from the transfusion site, flush with normal saline before drawing.)

If there is a problem in obtaining 3 ml, contact the blood bank for

TABLE 12.1 *Transfusion Reactions*

Allergy	Pyrogenic Febrile	Hemolytic	Electrolyte Imbalance	Cold Blood	Fluid Overload
Urticaria, Itching	Fever, Chills	Backache, Headache	Hypocalcemia	↓ Temperature	Dyspnea, Cough
Diffuse rash	Headache	Abdominal pain	Hyperkalemia	↑ Heart rate	Rales, Frothy sputum
Asthma, Wheezing	↑ Pulse rate	Chills			Hemoptysis
Anaphylaxis	Flushing	Dark urine	↑ BUN (Blood Urea Nitrogen)		↑ Heart rate
		Pallor			Cyanosis
Laryngeal edema		Shock Jaundice			Distended neck veins
		Nausea/ vomiting			
		Signs of renal failure, i.e., ↓ BUN (Blood Urea Nitrogen)			
		Oliguria			

recommendations regarding the volume of sample needed.

The person drawing this sample should label it with the child's name and medical record number, date, time, and initials of the person drawing the blood.

Mark the sample as "Post Transfusion #1."

Collect the *first urine sample* following the reaction.

The physician may order a catheterized urine sample.

Label and mark "Post Transfusion Urine."

Send immediately to the blood bank for analysis of hemoglobinuria.

Send the following to the blood bank immediately:

Post Transfusion Blood Sample #1.

Partially used unit of blood/blood product with the administration set still attached to the blood bag.

Any available used bags of blood/blood product given to the child during the past 24 hours.

The blood bank may request that 3 ml of blood be sent 5 to 7 hours following the reaction. Label as "Post Transfusion #2."

DOCUMENTATION

For Symptoms of a Mild Transfusion Reaction:

• Time and description of signs and symptoms noted.
• Time the blood/blood product was stopped; volume infused. Volume of normal saline hung and KVO rate.
• Time and name of the physician notified.
• Vital signs.
• Name of any medication(s) given, dose, route, and child's response.
• Time the transfusion was restarted, rate, and child's response.

For Symptoms of a Severe Transfusion Reaction:

- Assessment of child, including vital signs.
- Time transfusion was stopped; volume of blood/blood product infused. Volume of normal saline hung and KVO rate.
- Time and name of physician notified.
- Time of physician's arrival.
- Interventions and child's response(s).
- That blood bag(s) and administration set(s) were sent to the blood bank.
- Times blood samples #1 and #2 sent to the blood bank.
- Time catheterized or voided urine sample sent to the blood bank.
- Name of any medication given, dose, route, and child's response.
- Color of urine following any type of reaction (such as cola or tea colored, pink red, and so on).
- Intake and output.

POTENTIAL RELATED NURSING DIAGNOSES

Tissue perfusion, impaired, peripheral

Injury: *high risk*

Hyperthermia

Skin integrity, impaired: *high risk*

POTENTIAL RELATED MEDICAL DIAGNOSES

Transfusion reaction

Anaphylactic shock

Pruritis

Urticaria

Renal failure

REFERENCES

American Association of Blood Banks. 1989. *Circular of information for the use of human blood and blood components.* Arlington, Va.: American Association of Blood Banks.

Mott, S., James, S., and Sperhac, A. 1990. *Nursing care of children and families.* Redwood City, Calif.: Addison-Wesley.

National Blood Resource Education. 1991. Choosing blood components and equipment. *AJN* 91, no. 6: 42–52.

Pisciotto, P., ed. 1989. *Blood transfusion therapy.* Arlington, Va.: American Association of Blood Banks.

13 Blood Administration: Type and Cross-Match

S SAFETY ISSUES

• The sample and appropriate request form must be properly and clearly labeled.

PSYCHOSOCIAL CONSIDERATIONS: Explain the procedure in developmentally appropriate terms. Avoid using terms with mixed meanings, such as *stick, shot,* and *take your blood.* Children often fear having blood drawn. They may fear that all their blood will be removed. Bandage the puncture site, if the child desires. Children often do not want to see blood; position the child to reduce this possibility. Use therapeutic play or needle play to reduce anxiety after the procedure.

TIME: 10 to 15 minutes

PURPOSE

To provide ABO grouping, Rh typing, and antibody screening for optimal cross-matching of red blood cells (packed RBCs, whole blood, washed RBCs, leukocyte-poor RBCs).

OBJECTIVES

• To obtain a blood sample.
• To avoid injury.

EQUIPMENT

Collection tube

Gloves, nonsterile

Age-appropriate blood-drawing equipment: needle, syringe, povidone-iodine swabs *or* alcohol swabs, tourniquet, adhesive bandage

ESSENTIAL STEPS

1. Prepare the child and family.
2. Assemble the equipment.
3. Wash hands.
4. Label the collection tube(s) with the date, time, and initials of the person drawing the sample.
5. Identify the child by checking the identification band.
6. Put on gloves.
7. Select the site. Help the child to hold still, as necessary.
8. Prep the skin with povidone-iodine or alcohol swab.
9. Draw a blood sample and place it in a labeled tube. Apply bandage, if appropriate. Typing usually requires 2 to 3 ml of blood. Typing and cross-matching (T&C) usually require a 3 ml sample of blood when 1 to 4 units are ordered. For more than 4 units, a 7 ml sample is required. At least 10 ml of blood are usually necessary for T&C of children with cyanotic heart defects admitted for corrective surgery.

10. Complete a blood bank request card/form. The following is usually required:

    The child's name and medical record number.

    The name of the person drawing the sample(s).

    A signature verifying that:

        The child has been identified correctly.

        The tube label and card/form have been completed correctly.

    A note that the mother's blood has been sent, when appropriate.

    Specification if a split unit has been ordered. (When a physician has ordered a split unit, add 30 ml to that volume to purge the blood administration set.)

11. Place the labeled sample in a plastic bag and send to the blood bank.

12. Allow approximately 1 hour for the blood bank to complete a routine T&C before requesting a blood-product pickup.

DOCUMENTATION

- Time the sample was obtained.
- Name of the individual obtaining the sample.
- Amount of blood drawn, if appropriate (important in neonates).

Skills Checklist

- ☐ Prepare the child and family.
- ☐ Assemble the equipment.
- ☐ Wash hands.
- ☐ Label collection tube(s).
- ☐ Identify the child by checking the identification band.
- ☐ Put on gloves.
- ☐ Prepare skin.
- ☐ Obtain the sample.
- ☐ Place bandage, if appropriate.
- ☐ Send the specimen to the lab.
- ☐ Document.

POTENTIAL RELATED NURSING DIAGNOSES

Fear

Anxiety

Gas exchange, impaired

POTENTIAL RELATED MEDICAL DIAGNOSES

Preoperative measures

Hemorrhage

Gastrointestinal bleeding

Anemia

REFERENCES

National Blood Resource Education. 1991. Choosing blood components and equipment. *AJN* 91, no. 6: 42–52.

Pisciotto, P., ed. 1989. *Blood transfusion therapy*. Arlington, Va.: American Association of Blood Banks.

14 Blood Administration: Uncross-Matched Blood

 SAFETY ISSUES

• Check for informed consent.

PSYCHOSOCIAL CONSIDERATIONS: Explain the procedure in developmentally appropriate terms. Avoid using terms with mixed meanings, such as *take blood, stick,* and *shot.* Explain the screening procedure to detect the HIV virus, if appropriate; parents may fear AIDS. Also explain to parents that the procedure is being performed as a lifesaving method.

TIME: 30 minutes to 4 hours

PURPOSE

To provide for transfusion without compatibility testing in life-threatening situations.

OBJECTIVES

• To administer blood in emergency situations.
• To prevent injury.

EQUIPMENT

Blood/blood product

Gloves, nonsterile

Blood administration set

Normal saline (0.9% sodium chloride), 5 ml syringe, and needle, sterile

Stopcock and extension tubing, if appropriate

Infusion pump, as appropriate

Medication, if ordered

Needle to cap intravenous tubing, sterile

ESSENTIAL STEPS

1. Prepare the child and family. Refer to "Blood Administration: General Procedure."
2. If possible, obtain a 3 to 5 ml blood sample for blood typing. A cross-match can be done after the blood is released.
3. Assemble the equipment. Notify the blood bank of the need for uncross-matched blood.
4. Wash hands.
5. Obtain blood/blood product.
6. Check the blood bag label and blood request form. Refer to "Blood Administration: General Procedure."
7. Put on gloves and prime the blood administration set.
8. Identify the child by checking the identification band.
9. Refer to "Blood Administration: General Procedure" for steps to initiate the administration of blood/blood product.
10. Infuse blood/blood product. Refer to the procedure regarding the specific blood product for infusion steps.

11. Carefully observe for transfusion reaction. Refer to "Blood Administration: Transfusion-Reaction."

12. If a pretransfusion blood sample was not obtained, draw blood and send to the blood bank as soon as possible.

13. If the transfusion is canceled for any reason, return the blood immediately to the blood bank.

14. Discard the blood bag and administration set in an appropriate manner.

DOCUMENTATION

- Name of blood/blood product.
- Start time.
- Baseline and serial vital signs.
- Amount infused.
- Child's response.
- Amount of any normal saline flushes.
- Completion time.

POTENTIAL RELATED NURSING DIAGNOSES

Injury: *high risk*

Tissue perfusion, altered, cardiopulmonary

Fluid volume deficit

Cardiac output, decreased

Skills Checklist

- ☐ Prepare the child and family.
  - • Check for informed consent.
  - • Premedicate.
- ☐ Assemble the equipment.
- ☐ Notify the blood bank of the need for uncross-matched blood.
- ☐ Wash hands.
- ☐ Obtain blood/blood product.
- ☐ Verify that the blood product is correct.
- ☐ Put on gloves and prime the tubing.
- ☐ Identify the child by checking the identification band.
- ☐ Obtain baseline vital signs.
- ☐ Flush the IV line with normal saline.
- ☐ Administer blood/blood product.
- ☐ Monitor vital signs.
- ☐ Put on gloves and flush the IV line with normal saline.
- ☐ Disconnect the blood administration set and reconnect the IV.
- ☐ Discard the blood bag and administration set.
- ☐ Document.

POTENTIAL RELATED MEDICAL DIAGNOSES

Hemorrhage

Disseminated intravascular coagulopathy

Trauma

REFERENCES

Hahn, K. 1989. Monitoring a blood transfusion. *Nursing 89* 19, no. 10: 20–21.

National Blood Resource Education. 1991. Choosing blood components and equipment. *AJN* 91, no. 6: 42–52.

15 Blood Administration: Warmed Blood

PSYCHOSOCIAL CONSIDERATIONS: Explain the procedure in developmentally appropriate terms. Avoid using terms with mixed meanings, such as *stick*. Explain the screening process to detect the HIV virus, if appropriate; parents may fear AIDS.

TIME: 1 to 6 hours

PURPOSE

To prevent the myocardial temperature from falling during massive transfusion, which would increase the risk of ventricular fibrillation and impair the body's ability to withstand blood loss.

To prevent intravascular hemolysis when transfusing a child with a high titer of cold agglutinins.

OBJECTIVES

- To administer warmed blood safely.
- To prevent damage to the blood.

EQUIPMENT

Waterless blood-warming unit and 60-inch extension tubing *or*

Water-bath blood-warming unit:

    Blood coil for use with water-bath warmer

    Distilled water

Gloves, nonsterile

Blood/blood product and administration set

SAFETY ISSUES

- Warm blood only in a blood warmer.
- Use blood warmers during exchange transfusions.
- Warm all blood given in surgery and the recovery room (when body temperatures are low and cold blood could decrease temperature further).

ESSENTIAL STEPS

1. Prepare the child and family.
2. Assemble the equipment.
3. Wash hands.
4. Review "Blood Administration: General Procedure" and the procedure on administration of the specific type of blood product to be transfused.
5. If using a waterless blood warmer:

    Put on gloves and place the 60-inch extension tubing in the warmer. (See Fig. 15.1) Shut the warmer door and then attach the blood administration set and prime.

    Plug the warmer into a wall outlet.

    If the unit alarms because blood is too warm, unplug the machine.

6. If using a water-bath blood warmer:

    Fill the blood-warming unit with distilled water to the appropriate water-level mark on the inside of the unit. Maintain this water level.

    Plug the blood warmer in after water is in the machine. The thermostat on the blood warmer is preset by the manufacturer.

    Place the blood coil in the blood warmer.

    Put on gloves, attach the blood coil to the administration set, and prime.

7. Maintain the temperature of blood between 32.0°C and 37.0°C (89.6°F and 98.6°F) during administration as indicated by the unit's temperature gauge.

8. Administer the blood according to the procedure for the specific type of blood product to be administered.

DOCUMENTATION

- Use of the warmer.
- Temperature of the warming solution, if applicable.
- Temperature of blood.

POTENTIAL RELATED NURSING DIAGNOSES

Hypothermia

Hyperthermia

Gas exchange, impaired

Injury: *high risk*

Fluid volume deficit: *high risk*

POTENTIAL RELATED MEDICAL DIAGNOSES

Anemia

Surgery

Hemorrhage

Hyperbilirubinemia

REFERENCES

American Association of Blood Banks. 1989. *Circular of information for the use of human blood and blood components.* Arlington, Va.: American Association of Blood Banks.

Mott, S., James, S., and Sperhac, A. 1990. *Nursing care of children and families.* Redwood City, Calif.: Addison-Wesley.

National Blood Resource Education. 1991. Choosing blood components and equipment. *AJN* 91, no. 6: 42–52.

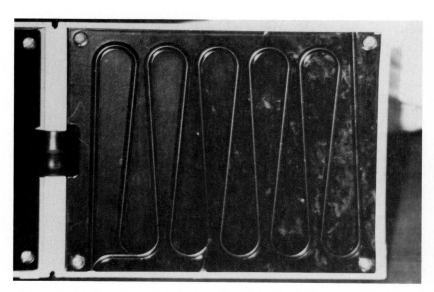

FIGURE 15.1 *Tubing placed in grooves; door closed.*

16 Blood Administration: Whole Blood and Others

PSYCHOSOCIAL CONSIDERATIONS: Explain the procedure in developmentally appropriate terms. Avoid using terms with mixed meanings, such as *shot* and *stick*. A child who has had a transfusion reaction may fear another such occurrence. Explain the screening process to detect the HIV virus, if appropriate; parents may be fearful of AIDS.

TIME: Up to 4 hours

PURPOSE

To correct red blood cell deficiency.

To improve the oxygen-carrying capacity of the blood.

To provide partial or complete exchange transfusions.

OBJECTIVES

- To administer blood product(s) safely.
- To prevent injury.

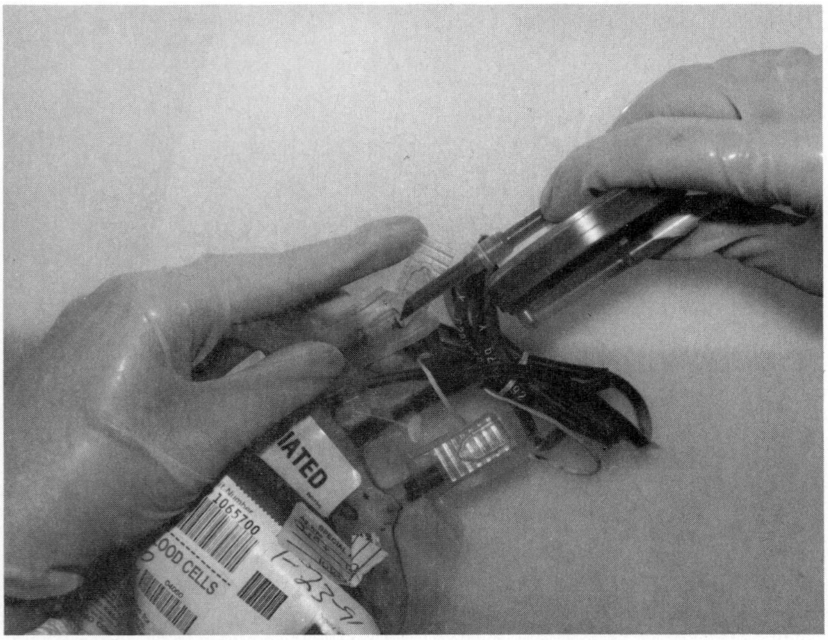

EQUIPMENT

Patent IV cannula with the largest bore possible (19g preferred; at least 21g for a child or 23g for an infant)

Blood/blood product

Gloves, nonsterile

Blood administration set

Leukocyte filter, if appropriate

Normal saline (0.9% sodium chloride), 5 ml syringe, and needle, sterile

Stopcock and extension tubing, if appropriate

Infusion pump, if appropriate

Medication, if ordered

Needle to cap IV tubing, sterile

S | SAFETY ISSUES

- **Check for informed consent.**
- **Always have a type and cross-match.**
- **Blood can hang a maximum of 4 hours after being removed from the refrigerator. If a volume of blood is to be administered over an interval of time greater than 4 hours, request that the volume be split into separate blood bags. Give split units sequentially.**
- **If the blood product is ordered "leukocyte poor," obtain a leukocyte filter. Change the filter after each 2 units.**

ESSENTIAL STEPS

1. Prepare the child and family. Refer to "Blood Administration: General Procedure."
2. Assemble the equipment.
3. Wash hands.

FIGURE 16.1 Spiking the blood bag with the filter and tubing.

4. Obtain blood/blood product.
5. Check the blood bag label and form. Refer to "Blood Administration: General Procedure."
6. Put on gloves and prime the blood administration set.

> Assemble the blood administration set with a filter for red blood cells (RBCs) in line.
>
> Open either outlet port on the plastic blood bag.
>
> Use aseptic technique to insert the spike of the blood administration set into the open bag port. If the spike punctures the bag, return the bag immediately to the blood bank. (See Figs. 16.1, 16.2, and 16.3.)
>
> Fill the blood administration set according to the manufacturer's directions.

Skills Checklist

- ☐ Prepare the child and family.
  - • Check for informed consent.
  - • Premedicate.
- ☐ Assemble the equipment.
- ☐ Wash hands.
- ☐ Obtain blood/blood product.
- ☐ Verify that the blood product is correct.
- ☐ Put on gloves and prime the tubing.
- ☐ Identify the child by checking the identification band.
- ☐ Obtain baseline vital signs.
- ☐ Flush the IV line with normal saline.
- ☐ Administer blood product(s).
- ☐ Monitor vital signs.
- ☐ Put on gloves.
- ☐ Flush the IV line with normal saline.
- ☐ Disconnect the blood administration set and reconnect the IV.
- ☐ Discard the blood bag and administration set.
- ☐ Document.

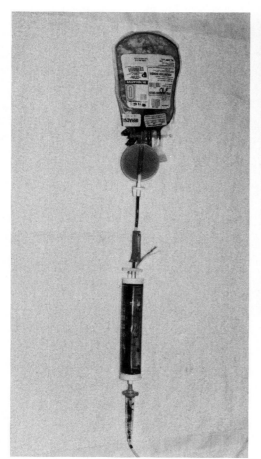

FIGURE 16.2 *Primed blood tubing and filter.*

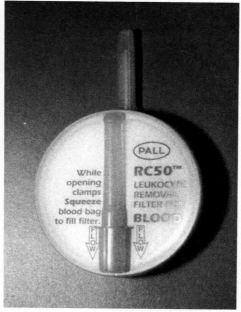

FIGURE 16.3 *Leukocyte filter.*

Lab Values

PLATELETS

Birth−1 month	$84–478 \times 10^9/L$
Other ages	$150–400 \times 10^9/L$

HEMOGLOBIN

1−3 days	14.5−22.5 g/dL
3 days−1 month	14.0−23.0 g/dL
1−2 months	9.0−14.0 g/dL
2−3 months	9.0−14.5 g/dL
3−4 months	9.0−14.0 g/dL
4 months−1 year	10.0−15.0 g/dL
1−6 years	10.0−16.0 g/dL
6−12 years	11.0−15.5 g/dL
12−18 years	
male	13.0−18.0 g/dL
female	11.5−16.0 g/dL

HEMATOCRIT

1−3 days	0.44−0.75 vol. fraction
3 days−2 months	0.43−0.75 vol. fraction
2 months−1 year	0.28−0.41 vol. fraction
1−6 years	0.31−0.435 vol. fraction
6−12 years	0.36−0.45 vol. fraction
12−18 years	
male	0.37−0.54 vol. fraction
female	0.36−0.47 vol. fraction

RED BLOOD CELL COUNT

1−3 days	$4.0–6.6 \times 10^{12}/L$
3 days−1 month	$3.0–6.3 \times 10^{12}/L$
1 month−2 years	$2.7–5.4 \times 10^{12}/L$
2−12 years	$3.9–5.3 \times 10^{12}/L$
12−18 years	
male	$4.5–5.3 \times 10^{12}/L$
female	$4.1–5.1 \times 10^{12}/L$

7. Identify the child by checking the identification band.

8. Refer to "Blood Administration: General Procedure" for steps to initiate the administration of blood/blood products.

9. Turn off the infusing IV solution and disconnect the tubing. Cap the IV tubing with a sterile needle.

10. Flush the IV with 3 to 5 ml of normal saline to clear any existing IV solution or medication.

11. Connect the blood administration set to the hub of the IV device or add extension tubing and a stopcock to the hub of the IV device prior to connecting the blood administration set. Use second port on the stopcock for a normal saline line or a normal saline syringe.

12. Begin the blood transfusion.

13. The physician usually orders RBCs to infuse over 2 to 4 hours, specifying the number of ml over a number of hours (for example, "Transfuse 100 ml PRBCs *over* 4 hours").

14. Contact the physician if the *ordered* flow rate cannot be maintained.

15. Observe for signs and symptoms of blood transfusion reaction. Refer to "Blood Administration: Transfusion Reaction."

16. If infusing more than 1 unit of blood, change the filter

After each 2 units, *or*

After each 4-hour interval.

17. Put on gloves and flush the extension tubing following the transfusion with normal saline. Replace the extension tubing and stopcock if unable to clear the blood from them. Blood is a medium for bacterial growth.

18. Disconnect the blood administration set and reconnect the IV. Discard the blood bag and administration set in the appropriate manner.

DOCUMENTATION

• Name of blood product.
• Start time.
• Baseline and serial vital signs.
• Amount infused.
• Child's response.
• Completion time.

POTENTIAL RELATED NURSING DIAGNOSES

Tissue perfusion, altered, peripheral

Fear

Anxiety

Injury: *high risk*

Fluid volume deficit

POTENTIAL RELATED MEDICAL DIAGNOSES

Hemorrhage

Anemia

REFERENCES

American Association of Blood Banks. 1989. *Circular of information for the use of human blood and blood components.* Arlington, Va.: American Association of Blood Banks.

Hahn, K. 1989. Monitoring a blood transfusion. *Nursing 89* 19, no. 10: 20–21.

Landier, W., Barrell, M., and Styffe, E. 1987. How to administer blood components to children. *MCN* (May/June): 178–84.

Mott, S., James, S., and Sperhac, A. 1990. *Nursing care of children and families.* Redwood City, Calif.: Addison-Wesley.

National Blood Resource Education. 1991. Choosing blood components and equipment. *AJN 91,* no. 6: 42–52.

Pisciotto, P., ed. 1989. *Blood transfusion therapy.* Arlington, Va.: American Association of Blood Banks.

17 Blood Drawing: Culture

EQUIPMENT

Appropriate blood culture tube(s)/bottle(s)

Povidone-iodine swabs/swab sticks *or* alcohol swabs

Rack for culture tube(s)/bottle(s)

Tourniquet

Gloves, nonsterile

Syringe with appropriate-size needle or butterfly needle (size of syringe will depend on the amount of blood needed)

2″ × 2″ gauze, sterile

Adhesive bandage, if appropriate

21g or 20g needle(s)

PSYCHOSOCIAL CONSIDERATIONS: Explain the procedure to the child in developmentally appropriate terms. Avoid using terms with mixed meanings, such as *stick, puncture,* and *remove blood.* Tell the child the procedure is to check for bacteria in blood. Allow the child to cry or scream, but not to move. Do not tell the child, "It won't hurt." Be honest. Allow the child to touch and play with equipment before the procedure. Ask if the child would like a bandage after the procedure; children sometimes fear losing all their blood. Hold and comfort the child following the procedure.

TIME: 5 to 10 minutes

PURPOSE

To obtain a blood sample via venipuncture for children requiring a blood culture.

OBJECTIVES

- To obtain a blood sample aseptically.
- To prevent injury.

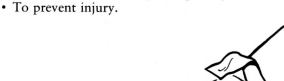

SAFETY ISSUES

- **Do not contaminate the needle.**
- **Clean the skin well.**

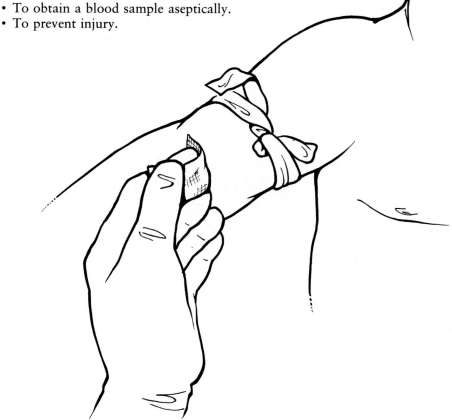

***FIGURE 17.1** Cleaning the antecubital area with a swab.*

ESSENTIAL STEPS

1. Prepare the child and family.

2. Assemble the equipment.

3. Wash hands.

4. Wipe off the top of each blood culture tube/bottle with a separate povidone-iodine or alcohol swab. *Allow to dry.* Place the culture tube(s)/bottle(s) in a rack to stabilize them.

5. Apply a tourniquet above the venous access site selected and palpate the vein.

6. Put on gloves.

7. Wipe the area with a povidone-iodine or alcohol swab in a circular motion, starting in the center and working outward. (See Figs. 17.1 and 17.2)

8. Using each swab only once, repeat step 7 with three povidone-iodine or alcohol swabs; then allow to dry for 30 seconds. Do not touch the site with a finger before venipuncture as this will contaminate the area.

Skills Checklist

☐ Prepare the child and family.

☐ Assemble the equipment.

☐ Wash hands.

☐ Wipe off the top(s) of culture tube(s)/bottle(s) and place in a rack.

☐ Apply a tourniquet.

☐ Put on gloves.

☐ Clean the site.

☐ Perform venipuncture.

☐ Remove the tourniquet.

☐ Withdraw the needle and apply pressure to the site.

☐ Apply a bandage if the child desires.

☐ Place the blood in tube(s)/bottle(s).

☐ Label the specimen. Place in a plastic bag and send to the lab.

☐ Document.

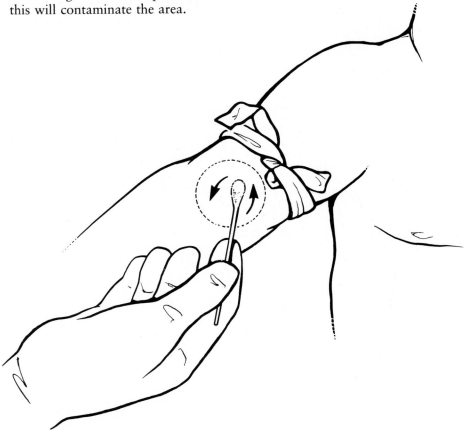

FIGURE 17.2 *Cleaning the antecubital area with a swab stick.*

9. Perform venipuncture. (See Figs. 17.3 and 17.4)

10. Remove the tourniquet.

11. Withdraw the needle and apply pressure to the site with a sterile gauze until the bleeding stops. Apply a bandage if the child desires.

12. Remove and discard the used needle using a passive recapping device (such as a hemostat) or a one-handed scoop technique.

13. Place a sterile 21g or 20g needle on the syringe containing the blood specimen.

14. Insert the needle into the top of the first blood culture tube/bottle while it remains stabilized in the rack. Allow the appropriate amount of blood to enter the tube.

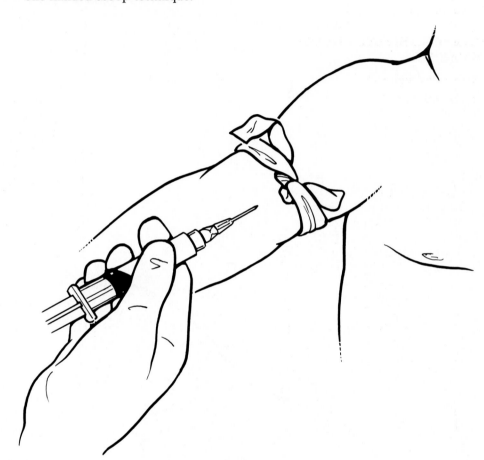

FIGURE 17.3 *Venipuncture using a syringe and needle.*

15. Repeat Step 14 for the second blood culture tube/bottle, when needed. Changing needles between each tube/bottle is not necessary.

16. Label the culture tube(s)/bottle(s) appropriately. Place in a plastic bag and send to the lab.

DOCUMENTATION

• Time.
• Site.
• Type of culture obtained.

POTENTIAL RELATED NURSING DIAGNOSES

Infection: *high risk*

Hyperthermia

Pain, acute

Anxiety

POTENTIAL RELATED MEDICAL DIAGNOSES

Sepsis

Meningitis

Hyperthermia

REFERENCES

Mott, S., James, S., and Sperhac, A. 1990. *Nursing care of children and families.* Redwood City, Calif.: Addison-Wesley.

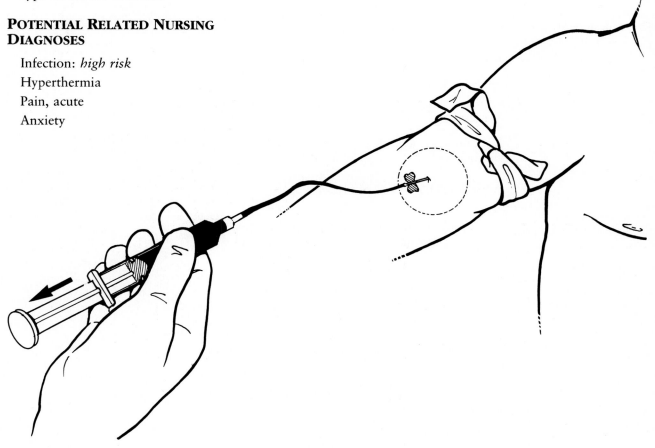

FIGURE 17.4 *Venipuncture using a butterfly needle and syringe.*

18

Blood Drawing: Heel and Finger Stick

EQUIPMENT

Washcloth and plastic bag for compress

Gloves, nonsterile

Povidone-iodine swabs *or* alcohol swabs

Lancet with 2.4 mm point *or* automatic lancet, sterile

2″ × 2″ gauze *or* cotton ball, sterile

Adhesive bandage, if appropriate

Appropriate sample container

S SAFETY ISSUES

- Alcohol used for skin preparation may cause rapid hemolysis.
- Use alcohol for chemstrips and dextrostix. Povidone-iodine interferes with interpretation of readings.
- Depth of puncture should not exceed 1.6 mm.
- Use bandages with caution on infants and young children. The child may swallow or aspirate the bandage.

PSYCHOSOCIAL CONSIDERATIONS: Explain the procedure in developmentally appropriate terms. Avoid using terms with mixed meanings, such as *stick*. Use words like *measure* or *check*. Ask if the child would like a bandage. Children may believe that they will lose all their blood and often want lesions or needle sites covered. Note, however, that bandages on the fingers or feet of infants or young children are potential safety hazards because the child might swallow or aspirate the bandage. Allow for therapeutic play when appropriate.

TIME: 3 to 5 minutes

PURPOSE

To obtain a small blood sample (≤1 ml) from an infant or child.

OBJECTIVES

- To obtain a blood sample.
- To perform the procedure quickly and accurately with minimal discomfort to the child.
- To prevent injury.

ESSENTIAL STEPS

1. Prepare the child and family.
2. Assemble the equipment.
3. Wash hands.
4. Select the site. Avoid previous puncture sites, area of bone injury, arteries, or edematous tissue.

   For a heel stick, choose a site on the plantar surface of the heel, beyond lateral and medial limits of the calcaneus.

   For a finger stick, choose a site on the side of the ball of the finger *across* the fingerprint. (If the stick is made along the lines of the fingerprint, the blood will stream down the finger.)

5. Moist compresses applied for up to 15 minutes may be used to facilitate blood supply to the area.
6. Put on gloves.
7. Clean the site thoroughly with a povidone-iodine or alcohol swab. Use alcohol if the child is iodine-sensitive or for chemstrips/dextrostix. *Allow to dry.*

8. Gently milk the extremity prior to puncture.
9. Puncture with a lancet. Never use a slashing technique to obtain blood. (See Fig. 18.1)

Skills Checklist

☐ Prepare the child and family.
☐ Assemble the equipment.
☐ Wash hands.
☐ Choose the site.
☐ Warm moist compresses, if appropriate.
☐ Put on gloves.
☐ Clean the site.
☐ Gently milk the extremity.
☐ Puncture with a lancet.
☐ Wipe away the first drop of blood.
☐ Hold the extremity downward.
☐ Obtain the blood needed.
☐ Apply pressure.
☐ Apply a bandage, if appropriate.
☐ Label the specimen. Place in a plastic bag and send to the lab.
☐ Document.

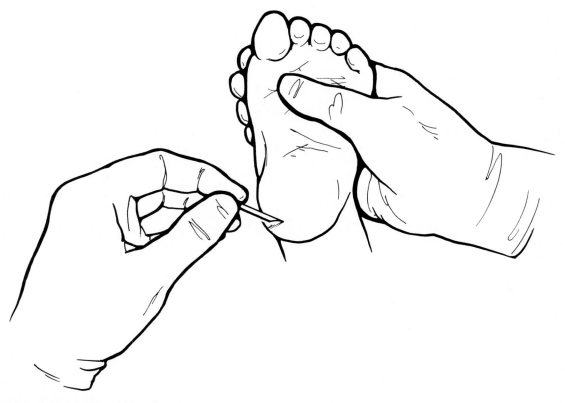

FIGURE 18.1 *Puncturing skin with a lancet.*

Lab Values

WHITE BLOOD CELL COUNT—NORMAL

Birth–1 month	$5.0–19.0 \times 10^9$ cells/L
1 month–1 year	$6.0–17.0 \times 10^9$ cells/L
1–3 years	$6.0–17.0 \times 10^9$ cells/L
3–4 years	$5.5–15.5 \times 10^9$ cells/L
4–13 years	$4.5–15.0 \times 10^9$ cells/L
13–14 years	$4.5–11.0 \times 10^9$ cells/L
14–18 years	$4.5–11.0 \times 10^9$ cells/L

RED BLOOD CELL COUNT—NORMAL

1–3 days	$4.0–6.6 \times 10^{12}$/L
3 days–1 month	$3.0–6.3 \times 10^{12}$/L
1 mo–2 years	$2.7–5.4 \times 10^{12}$/L
2–12 years	$3.9–5.3 \times 10^{12}$/L
12–18 years	
male	$4.5–5.3 \times 10^{12}$/L
female	$4.1–5.1 \times 10^{12}$/L

HEMOGLOBIN—NORMAL

1–3 days	14.5–22.5 g/dL
3 days–1 month	14.0–23.0 g/dL
1–2 months	9.0–14.0 g/dL
2–3 months	9.0–14.5 g/dL
3–4 months	9.0–14.0 g/dL
4 months–1 year	10.0–15.0 g/dL
1–6 years	10.0–16.0 g/dL
6–12 years	11.0–15.5 g/dL
12–18 years	
male	13.0–18.0 g/dL
female	11.5–16.0 g/dL

HEMATOCRIT—NORMAL

1–3 days	0.44–0.75 vol. fraction
3 days–2 mos	0.43–0.75 vol. fraction
2 months–1 year	0.28–0.41 vol. fraction
1–6 years	0.31–0.45 vol. fraction
6–12 years	0.36–0.45 vol. fraction
12–18 years	
male	0.37–0.54 vol. fraction
female	0.36–0.47 vol. fraction

10. Wipe the first drop of blood away with a sterile 2″ × 2″ gauze or cotton ball.

11. To obtain a sample that is not just plasma, hold the punctured extremity downward and avoid excessive squeezing. Obtain the amount of blood needed. (Note: excessive squeezing causes bruising and produces a sample that contains more plasma than cells.) (See Figs. 18.2 and 18.3)

12. Apply pressure with a sterile 2″ × 2″ gauze or cotton ball until bleeding stops.

13. Apply a bandage, if appropriate for the child.

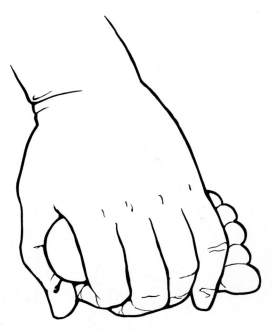

FIGURE 18.2 *Holding the heel to allow blood to drip.*

14. Label the specimen. Place in a plastic bag and send to the lab.

15. Observe the puncture site for adverse signs and symptoms, such as bleeding, bruising, or infection.

DOCUMENTATION

- Time.
- Site.
- That specimen was sent to lab.

POTENTIAL RELATED NURSING DIAGNOSES

Pain, acute

Infection: *high risk*

Skin integrity, impaired: *high risk*

Anxiety

POTENTIAL RELATED MEDICAL DIAGNOSES

Phenylketonuria (PKU) and other newborn screening, such as hypothyroidism or glucose-6-phosphate dehydrogenase deficiency

Preoperative workup

Juvenile diabetes mellitus or Type II diabetes

Hypoxemia

Universal application

REFERENCES

Meites, S. 1988. Skin-puncture and blood-collecting technique for infants: Update and problems. *Clinical Chemistry* 34, no. 9: 1890–94.

Mott, S., James, S., and Sperhac, A. 1990. *Nursing care of children and family.* Redwood City, Calif.: Addison-Wesley.

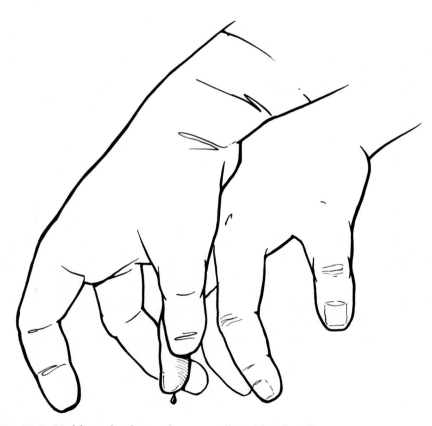

FIGURE 18.3 *Holding the finger down to allow blood to flow.*

19

Blood Drawing: Percutaneous Arterial Blood Sampling

1% xylocaine, if appropriate, *and* xylocaine gun *or* 3 ml syringe and 25g needle

Povidone-iodine swabs *or* alcohol swabs

25g needle or butterfly

2″ × 2″ gauze *or* cotton ball and tape, sterile

Syringe cap for arterial blood gases

Cup of ice, as needed

Appropriate lab tubes and/or heparin-coated syringe for arterial blood gas

PSYCHOSOCIAL CONSIDERATIONS: Explain the procedure in developmentally appropriate terms. Avoid using terms with mixed meanings, such as *stick*. Provide support and nurturing following the procedure.

TIME: 5 minutes

PURPOSE

To obtain percutaneous arterial blood sample(s).

OBJECTIVES

• To obtain an arterial blood sample.
• To prevent injury and trauma.

EQUIPMENT

Gloves, nonsterile

Blanket for mummy restraint *or* papoose board, if necessary

 SAFETY ISSUES

• **Do not use an extremity that is blanched, cold, swollen, or discolored.**
• **Keep pressure over the site for at least 5 minutes.**
• **Crying and/or hyperventilation during the procedure can alter blood gas values.**

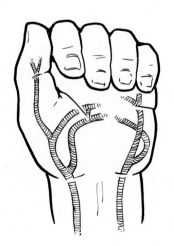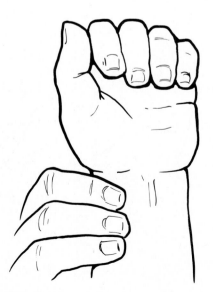

FIGURE 19.1 *Assessing the radial site for blood gases.*

ESSENTIAL STEPS

1. Prepare the child and family.

2. Assemble the equipment.

3. Wash hands and put on gloves.

4. Select a suitable artery and ascertain position. (See Fig. 19.1) The preferred order of choice is:

   Radial. (Ascertain the presence of a patent ulnar artery by conducting the Allen's test prior to radial puncture. To conduct the Allen's test, occlude the ulnar and radial arteries at the wrist. After the hand is blanched, release the ulnar artery. The hand should regain color.)

   Posterior tibial (inside ankle).

   Dorsalis pedis (top of foot).

   Femoral.

5. Have a second person restrain and provide support to the child. Use a mummy restraint or papoose board, if appropriate.

6. Anesthetize the area, as appropriate.

7. Prep the skin site with povidone-iodine or alcohol swabs. Apply povidone-iodine or alcohol vigorously and allow to dry for 30 seconds. (See Fig. 19.2)

8. Puncture the skin. Use the correct angle (15°–45°) of needle insertion with the needle bevel up. (See Fig. 19.3)

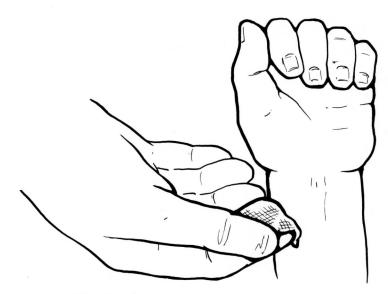

FIGURE 19.2 *Cleaning the site.*

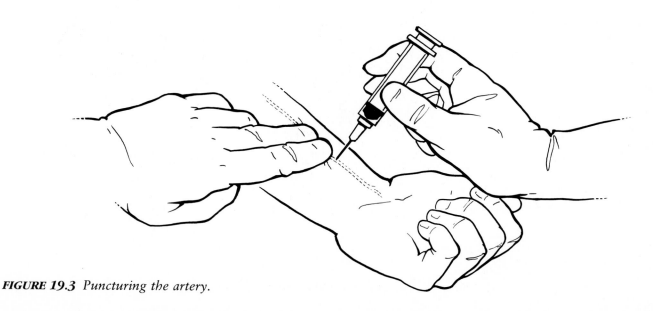

FIGURE 19.3 *Puncturing the artery.*

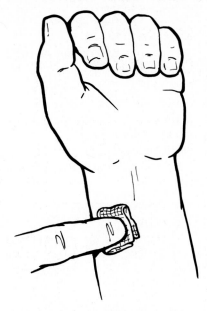

FIGURE 19.4 *Putting pressure on the artery site.*

9. Evaluate for blood return. Advance the needle until blood appears at the hub. Collect the amount of blood required for test(s).

10. Withdraw the needle slowly and hold pressure for a minimum of 5 minutes or until the bleeding stops. Apply a pressure dressing. (See Figs. 19.4 and 19.5)

11. Remove and discard the used needle using a passive recapping device (such as a hemostat) or a one-handed scoop technique.

12. For blood gases, remove air from the syringe, cap the syringe, and place it in ice. For other samples, inject the required amount of blood into the appropriate lab tube(s).

13. Label the specimen. Place in a plastic bag and send to the lab.

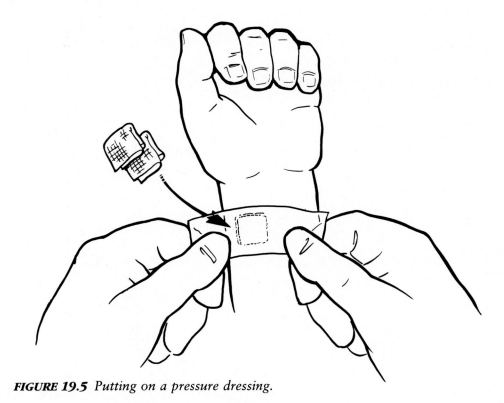

FIGURE 19.5 *Putting on a pressure dressing.*

DOCUMENTATION

- Site of puncture.
- Circulatory status distal to the extremity puncture site.
- For blood gases: if child cried or hyperventilated, child's temperature, and liters of oxygen if oxygen is in use.
- That specimen was sent to the lab.

POTENTIAL RELATED NURSING DIAGNOSES

Injury: *high risk*

Gas exchange, impaired

Anxiety

Fear

Pain, acute

POTENTIAL RELATED MEDICAL DIAGNOSES

Cardiovascular disorders

Respiratory disorders

Ventilator

Prematurity

Lab Values

PERIPHERAL OXYGEN LEVEL (PO$_2$)

Sea Level: 80%–100%

Altitude >5,000′: 65%–75%

PERIPHERAL CARBON DIOXIDE LEVEL (PCO$_2$)

Sea Level: 35%–45%

Altitude: >5,000′: 32%–38%

REFERENCES

Meites, S. 1988. Skin puncture and blood-collecting technique for infants: Update and problems. *Clinical Chemistry* 34, no. 9: 1890–94.

Millam, D. 1988. Arterial punctures. *American Journal of Nursing* 8, no. 9: 1213–24.

Mott, S., James, S., and Sperhac, A. 1990. *Nursing care of children and families.* Redwood City, Calif.: Addison-Wesley.

Suddaby, E., and Sourbeer, M. 1990. Drawing pediatric arterial blood gases. *Critical Care Nurse* 10, no. 7: 28–31.

20 Blood Drawing: Umbilical Artery/Vein Catheters

PSYCHOSOCIAL CONSIDERATIONS: Explain to parents the purpose and rationale of the procedure. Provide a supportive environment and encourage parents to ask questions.

TIME: 3 to 5 minutes

PURPOSE

To obtain blood sample(s) from an umbilical artery catheter (UAC) or umbilical vein catheter (UVC).

OBJECTIVES

- To obtain a blood sample.
- To prevent injury and trauma.

EQUIPMENT

Gloves, nonsterile

Injection cap

Povidone-iodine swabs *or* alcohol swabs

Syringe(s), appropriate size for discard and blood sample(s) (heparinized for arterial blood sample)

4″ × 4″ gauze, sterile

Heparin, of ordered concentration (usually 10 units/ml), with appropriate-size syringe and needle

Needle, if blood must be put in lab tube(s)

Appropriate lab tube(s) for lab test(s) other than blood gas

Syringe cap

S SAFETY ISSUES

- Readministering the blood/fluid sample drawn to clear the line is controversial. Some institutions do not readminister the blood/fluid sample because the blood may contain clots, plaques, and so on. The sample may be filtered prior to reinfusion. Some institutions require a physician's order to readminister the blood/fluid sample, especially into a UAC. If the blood/fluid sample is not reinfused, anemia and fluid volume depletion may result.

- Some institutions permit laboratory personnel to draw UAC/UVC samples.

- If the returned blood/fluid sample is heparinized, monitor bleeding times.

- If drawing frequent blood samples or not readministering the blood/fluid sample, monitor hemoglobin and hematocrit.

- Use different-size syringes for discard and blood sample to avoid potential mix-up.

ESSENTIAL STEPS

1. Prepare the child and family.

2. Assemble the equipment.

3. Wash hands and put on gloves.

4. Ensure that the stopcock is "off" to the sampling port.

5. Clean the injection cap/stopcock connection with povidone-iodine or alcohol swab.

6. Remove the injection cap from the stopcock sampling port.

7. Connect the empty syringe to the sampling port.

8. "Open" the stopcock to the empty syringe. The stopcock should be "off" to the IV line.

9. Withdraw the appropriate amount of blood to clear the catheter of heparin or IV fluids. (Note: Fluids in the line can alter lab levels. Therefore, the line must be cleared. The amount withdrawn will vary depending on the length and gauge of the line.) (See Fig. 20.1)

10. Turn the stopcock "off" to the sampling port and IV line.

11. Remove the syringe containing the blood/fluid sample. Place on a sterile 4″ × 4″ gauze.

Skills Checklist

☐ Prepare the child and family.

☐ Assemble the equipment.

☐ Wash hands and put on gloves.

☐ Open sterile 4″×4″ gauze.

☐ Make sure that stopcock is "off" to the sampling port.

☐ Clean the injection cap/stopcock connection.

☐ Remove the injection cap.

☐ Attach the empty syringe.

☐ "Open" the stopcock to the sampling port. The stopcock should be "off" to the IV line.

☐ Aspirate an appropriate amount to clear the line.

☐ Turn the stopcock "off" to the sampling port and IV line.

☐ Remove the syringe and place on a 4″×4″ gauze.

☐ Attach the syringe for a blood sample.

☐ "Open" the stopcock to the syringe. The stopcock remains "off" to the IV line.

☐ Aspirate a sample.

☐ Turn the stopcock "off" to the injection port and IV line.

☐ Remove the syringe with the blood sample and place on a 4″×4″ gauze.

☐ Attach the syringe with the blood/fluid sample, if applicable.

☐ "Open" the stopcock to the syringe. The stopcock remains "off" to the IV line.

☐ Aspirate .5 ml to clear air.

☐ Readminister the blood/fluid sample, if appropriate.

☐ Turn the stopcock "off" to the sampling port and IV line.

☐ Remove the syringe.

☐ Flush the line with heparin.

☐ Place the sterile injection cap on the sampling port.

☐ "Open" the stopcock to the IV line.

☐ Cap the blood sample syringe and place on ice or place the required amount of blood in the appropriate lab tube(s).

☐ Label the specimen(s). Place in a plastic bag, and send to the lab.

☐ Document.

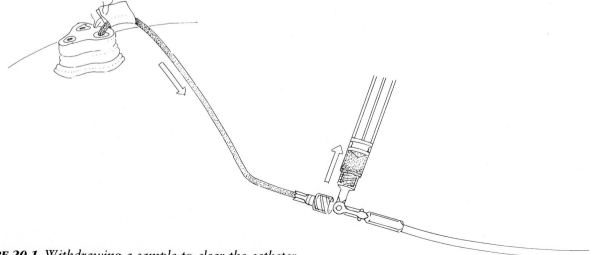

FIGURE 20.1 *Withdrawing a sample to clear the catheter.*

12. Connect a sterile syringe of the appropriate size for the blood sample(s), "open" the stopcock to the sampling port, and withdraw the amount of blood needed. Use a heparinized syringe to prevent clotting for all arterial blood samples. The stopcock remains "off" to the IV line. (See Fig. 20.2)

13. Turn the stopcock "off" to the sampling port and IV line.

14. Remove the syringe containing the sample and place on a sterile 4″ × 4″ gauze.

15. Attach the syringe with the blood/ fluid mixture to the sampling port, if applicable. All air must be removed from the syringe prior to attaching.

16. "Open" the stopcock to the syringe. The stopcock remains "off" to the IV line.

17. Aspirate .5 ml to clear air.

18. Readminister the blood/fluid sample, if appropriate.

19. Turn the stopcock "off" to the sampling port and IV line.

20. Remove the syringe.

21. Flush the line with heparin of ordered concentration. (See Fig. 20.3)

22. Place the sterile injection cap on the sampling port.

23. Turn the stopcock "open" to the IV fluid and "off" to the sampling port.

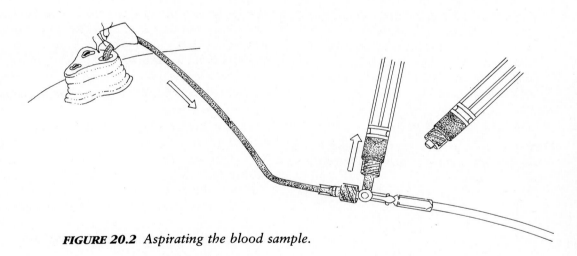

FIGURE 20.2 *Aspirating the blood sample.*

24. Cap the blood sample syringe and place on ice if for blood gas or place the required amount of blood in an appropriate lab tube(s).

25. Label the specimen(s). Place in a plastic bag and send to the lab.

DOCUMENTATION

* Time and date.
* That lab test(s) were drawn, specimen(s) sent to lab.
* Amount of blood drawn.
* Child's response.
* Readministeration of blood/fluid sample, if applicable.
* Heparin concentration and amount.

POTENTIAL RELATED NURSING DIAGNOSES

Fluid volume deficit: *high risk*

Infection: *high risk*

Tissue perfusion, altered, cardiopulmonary

Trauma: *high risk*

Skin integrity, impaired: *high risk*

POTENTIAL RELATED MEDICAL DIAGNOSES

Prematurity

Severely compromised neonate

Cardiac disorders

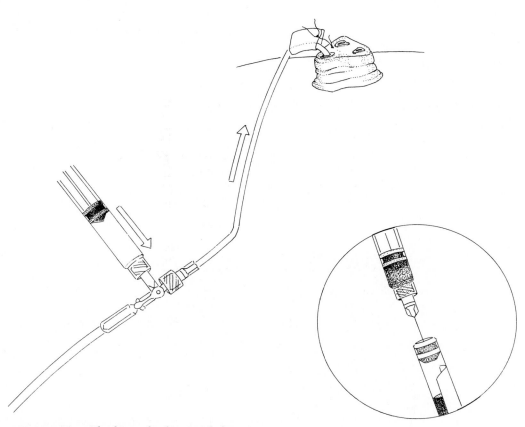

FIGURE 20.3 *Flushing the line with heparin.*

21 Blood Drawing: Venous

EQUIPMENT

Gloves, nonsterile

Tourniquet

Povidone-iodine swabs *or* alcohol swabs

Syringe (size depends on amount of blood needed) and appropriate-size needle/butterfly *or* vacuum collection system

Appropriate lab tube(s) if vacuum collection system not used

Cotton ball, sterile

Adhesive bandage, if appropriate

PSYCHOSOCIAL CONSIDERATIONS: Explain the procedure in developmentally appropriate terms. Avoid using terms with mixed meanings, such as *stick* and *bee sting*. Children are afraid of procedures that cause pain. Do not tell the child that the procedure will not hurt. Be honest. Younger children may benefit from therapeutic play with a doll or puppet.

TIME: 5 to 15 minutes

PURPOSE

To obtain a venous blood sample.

OBJECTIVES

- To obtain a blood sample.
- To prevent injury or trauma.

ESSENTIAL STEPS

1. Prepare the child and family.
2. Assemble the equipment.
3. Wash hands and put on gloves.

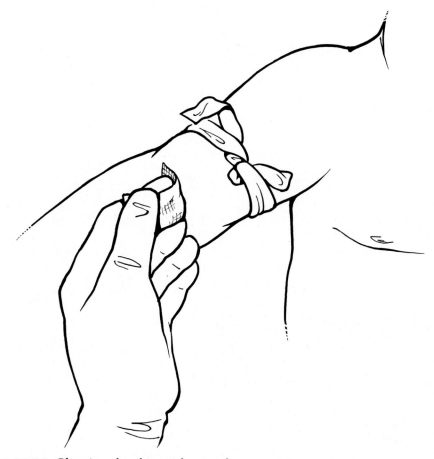

***FIGURE 21.1** Cleaning the skin with a swab.*

4. Select a site.

5. Apply a tourniquet above the venous access site and palpate the vein.

6. Prep the skin with povidone-iodine or alcohol swabs. (See Figs. 21.1 and 21.2)

7. Insert the needle, bevel up, into the vein. (See Fig. 21.3)

8. Connect the vacutainer or aspirate plunger of the syringe and obtain a specimen. (See Fig. 21.4)

9. Remove the tourniquet.

10. Remove the needle.

11. Apply pressure with a cotton ball.

12. Apply a bandage if the child desires.

13. Label the specimen(s). Place in a plastic bag and send to the lab.

Skills Checklist

☐ Prepare the child and family.
☐ Assemble the equipment.
☐ Wash hands and put on gloves.
☐ Select a site.
☐ Apply a tourniquet and palpate the vein.
☐ Prep skin.
☐ Perform venipuncture.
☐ Remove the tourniquet.
☐ Withdraw the needle and apply pressure.
☐ Apply a bandage if the child desires.
☐ Label the specimen. Place in a plastic bag and send to the lab.
☐ Document.

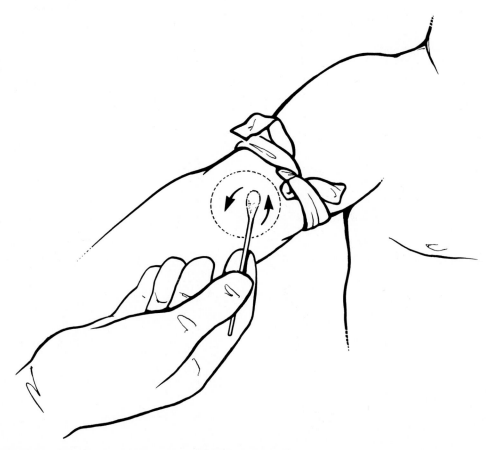

FIGURE 21.2 *Cleaning the skin with a swab stick.*

DOCUMENTATION

- Time.
- Site.
- Test(s) drawn and sent to the lab.
- Child's response and tolerance of procedure.

POTENTIAL RELATED NURSING DIAGNOSES

Pain, acute

Skin integrity, impaired: *high risk*

POTENTIAL RELATED MEDICAL DIAGNOSES

Universal application

REFERENCES

Swearingen, P. 1984. *Photo-atlas of nursing procedures 2E.* Redwood City, Calif.: Addison-Wesley.

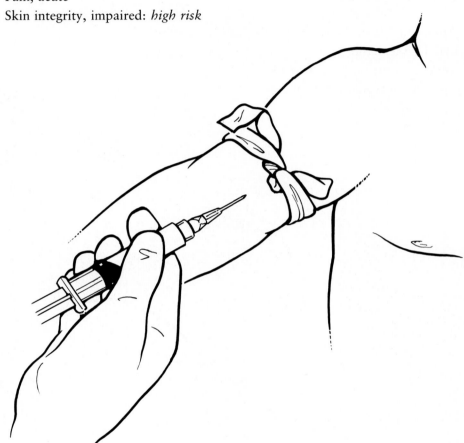

FIGURE 21.3 *Holding the syringe with the bevel of the needle up.*

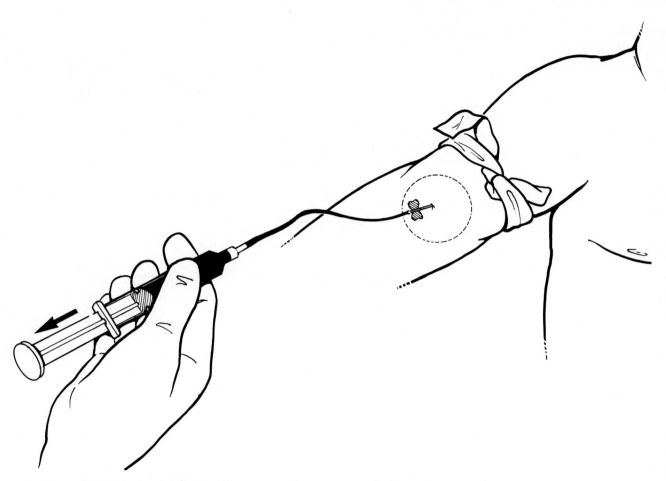

FIGURE 21.4 *Aspirating the blood sample.*

22 Body Substance Isolation

PSYCHOSOCIAL CONSIDERATIONS: Children may fear individuals in masks, gowns, and goggles. Be aware of what protection is required for each procedure. Explain the rationale for this protection to the child and/or parents. Practice good hand-washing techniques.

TIME: Varies

PURPOSE

To reduce the risk of transmitting infection. Wear protective clothing when anticipating direct contact with blood or other body fluids.

OBJECTIVES

- To prevent the spread of infection.
- To maintain a safe environment.

EQUIPMENT

Gloves, required when hand contact with blood or other body fluids is likely

Gowns, required when clothing may be soiled by blood or other body fluids

Masks and goggles, required when eyes, nose, or mouth may be splashed/sprayed with blood or other body fluids

Disposal container for all needles and sharps

Bags, isolation

ESSENTIAL STEPS

1. Prepare the child and family.
2. Assemble the equipment.
3. Wash hands.
4. Wear appropriate attire depending on the procedure and the likelihood of contact.
5. Place disposable needles and syringes in the disposal container in the child's room. Do not recap needles.
6. Bag trash and linen securely.

DOCUMENTATION

- Follow procedure with all patients. Procedure/protocol should be in an infection control manual. Therefore, documentation in the chart is not required.

POTENTIAL RELATED NURSING DIAGNOSES

Infection: *high risk*

Anxiety

Social isolation

Hyperthermia

POTENTIAL RELATED MEDICAL DIAGNOSES

Wound infection

AIDS

Hepatitis

Meningitis

Pneumonia

REFERENCES

Hammond, J., Eckes, J., Gomez, F., and Cunningham, D. 1990. HIV, trauma and infection control: Universal precautions are universally ignored. *The Journal of Trauma* 30, no. 5: 555–58.

Jackson, M., and Lynch, P. 1987. An alternative to isolating patients. *Geriatric Nursing* 8, no. 6: 308–11.

Skills Checklist

- ☐ Prepare the child and family.
- ☐ Assemble the equipment.
- ☐ Wash hands.
- ☐ Observe appropriate precautions.
- ☐ Dispose of needles and syringes.
- ☐ Bag trash and linen.

23 Bone Marrow Aspiration

PSYCHOSOCIAL CONSIDERATIONS: Explain the procedure in developmentally appropriate terms. Avoid using terms with mixed meanings, such as *taking out bone marrow* and *stick*. Restrain the child as necessary for safety. Allow the child to cry or scream. Describe the feeling of cold solutions used for cleaning prior to doing skin preparation. Be honest with the child and explain that the procedure may hurt, but only for a limited time. Comfort the child after the procedure.

TIME: 20 to 30 minutes

PURPOSE

To obtain a bone marrow specimen for diagnostic purposes.

OBJECTIVES

- To obtain a bone marrow specimen aseptically.
- To prevent injury.

EQUIPMENT

Sterile field

Medication, if ordered

Gloves, sterile, for individual performing bone marrow

Local anesthetic such as 1% xylocaine, if appropriate

Povidone-iodine solution *or,* if child is iodine-sensitive, Hibiclens

Bone marrow aspiration needle

Slip-tip syringe

Syringe and needle

Gloves, nonsterile

2″ × 2″ gauze

Tape or adhesive bandage

SAFETY ISSUES

- **Check for informed consent.**

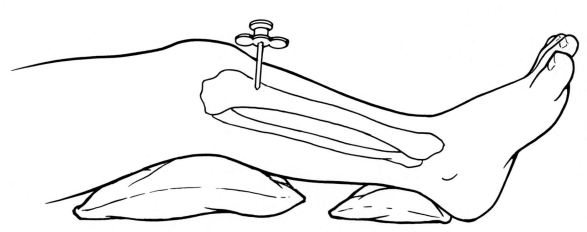

FIGURE 23.1 *Tibial site.*

ESSENTIAL STEPS

1. Prepare the child and family.

   Check for informed consent.

   Administer premedication, per physician's plan of care.

2. Assemble the equipment.

3. Wash hands and put on nonsterile gloves.

4. Check with the physician to determine whether laboratory personnel need to be present before the procedure begins.

5. Position and restrain the child, as necessary. Assist with local anesthetic, if appropriate. (See Figs. 23.1, 23.2, 23.3, and 23.4)

6. Postprocedure, place a 2″ × 2″ gauze over the aspiration site. Maintain pressure directly over the site for 3 minutes.

7. Apply a bandage. Apply a pressure dressing when indicated or requested by the physician (for example, when bleeding from the site might be anticipated because of low platelet count or other coagulation disorders). Check the site frequently for bleeding and/or a hematoma formation.

8. Label the specimen and send to the lab.

Skills Checklist

☐ Prepare the child and family.
  • Check for informed consent.
  • Premedicate.
☐ Assemble the equipment.
☐ Wash hands and put on gloves.
☐ Determine whether lab personnel need to be present.
☐ Position and restrain the child as necessary.
☐ Apply pressure postprocedure.
☐ Apply a bandage or pressure dressing.
☐ Check the site frequently for bleeding and/or hematoma formation.
☐ Label the specimen and send to the lab.
☐ Document.

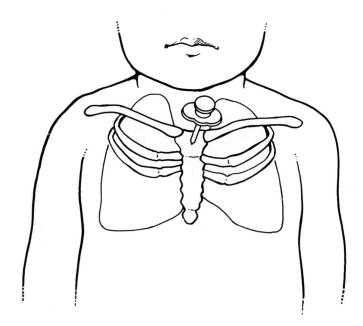

FIGURE 23.2 *Sternal site.*

DOCUMENTATION

- Date, time, and name of person performing procedure.
- Location of bone marrow aspiration site.
- Appearance of site.
- Type of dressing applied.
- That specimen was sent to the lab.
- Postprocedure checks.

POTENTIAL RELATED NURSING DIAGNOSES

Tissue perfusion, altered, peripheral

Anxiety

Pain, acute

POTENTIAL RELATED MEDICAL DIAGNOSES

Leukemia

Hodgkin's disease

Anemias

REFERENCES

Mott, S., James, S., and Sperhac, A. 1990. *Nursing care of children and families.* Redwood City, Calif.: Addison-Wesley.

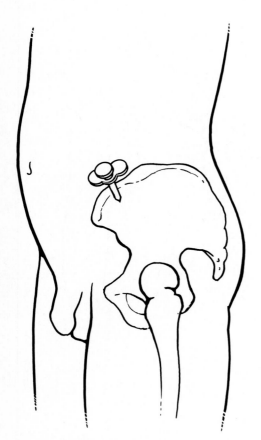

FIGURE 23.3 *Anterior iliac crest site (commonly used).*

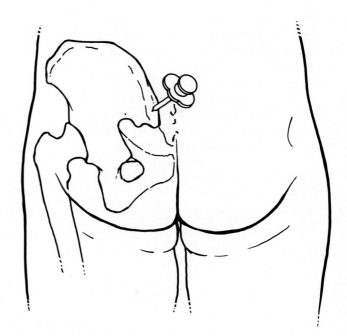

FIGURE 23.4 *Posterior iliac crest site (commonly used).*

24 Breast Pump: Electric

PSYCHOSOCIAL CONSIDERATIONS: Teach the mother about the electric breast pump; anxiety can inhibit the letdown reflex. Provide an atmosphere that facilitates relaxation with such things as a comfortable chair, privacy, and adequate time. Allow the mother to handle the equipment and ask questions. Breast massage and warm cloths may facilitate the letdown reflex.

TIME: 10 to 15 minutes

PURPOSE

To provide for safe and effective use of the electric breast pump.

OBJECTIVES

• To facilitate emptying the breasts.
• To provide breast milk for the infant.

EQUIPMENT

Electric breast pump
Accessory breast pump kit for use by one mother only (see Fig. 24.1)
Two towels
Plastic baby bottles with nipples and/or lids for milk storage
Label with the child's name

 SAFETY ISSUES

• **Explain to the mother that the breasts should be clean and that she should use only the equipment provided for her sole use.**

ESSENTIAL STEPS

1. Prepare the mother.
2. Assemble the equipment.
3. Wash hands and have the mother wash her hands.
4. Direct the mother to the electric breast pump.
5. Offer the mother any available information on breast-feeding.
6. Assist the mother in setting up the equipment. Share the manual regarding assembly of tubing and attaching the breast and collection receptacle with the mother, to facilitate instructions.
7. Assess for bleeding from or cracking of the nipples and share any information regarding this with the mother.
8. Provide the following information to the mother:

    Apply warm, moist cloths to the breast or use breast massage to help stimulate the letdown reflex.

    Pump for 10 to 15 minutes (no more) on each breast to decrease trauma to the nipples. (See Fig. 24.2)

    If the suction on the pump causes pain, decrease it.

    To release the pump from the breast, decrease the suction and gently release the nipple by using a finger pressed against the breast.

9. Label and store breast milk.

    Seal the bottle with a lid or a covered nipple.

    Write the date and time of collection on the child's name label and place on the bottle.

    Store the breast milk in the refrigerator for 48 hours or in the freezer for up to 6 months.

DOCUMENTATION

- Time.
- Amount of breast milk.
- Method of storage.
- Mother's response.

POTENTIAL RELATED NURSING DIAGNOSES

Nutrition, altered, less than body requirements

Swallowing, impaired

Growth and development, altered

POTENTIAL RELATED MEDICAL DIAGNOSES

Prematurity

Infection

Surgery

REFERENCES

Olds, S., London, M., and Ladewig, P. 1988. *Maternal-newborn nursing.* Menlo Park, Calif.: Addison-Wesley.

Skills Checklist

- ☐ Prepare the mother.
- ☐ Assemble the equipment.
- ☐ Wash hands.
- ☐ Set up the pump.
- ☐ Provide instructions to the mother.
- ☐ Store milk.
- ☐ Document.

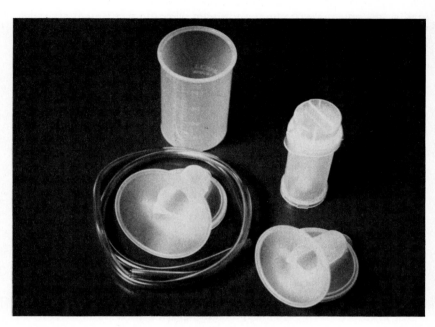

FIGURE 24.1 *Equipment for the breast pump.*

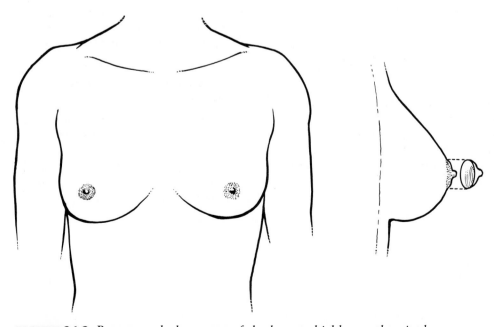

FIGURE 24.2 *Breasts and placement of the breast shield over the nipple.*

PSYCHOSOCIAL CONSIDERATIONS: Explain the procedure in developmentally appropriate terms. Avoid using terms with mixed meanings. If the child must remain bedridden, provide diversional activities. When removing the cast, avoid terms such as *saw*. Describe the warm feeling that a child may experience when a plaster cast is drying. Encourage therapeutic play.

TIME: 10 minutes

PURPOSE

To maintain the cast in good condition and prevent trauma or further injury.

OBJECTIVES

- To prevent skin breakdown.
- To maintain the cast's effectiveness.
- To prevent further injury.

EQUIPMENT

Ice packs (for immediate postcast application with a fracture or after surgery)

Plastic wrap, if appropriate

Sanitary napkin, if appropriate

Tape (for petaling), 1″, waterproof

Scissors

Plastic bag(s) for bathing, if appropriate

- Casts that cover the abdomen may alter elimination pattern(s). Monitor intake and output.
- Synthetic casts take approximately 30 minutes to dry. They can get wet without losing their integrity, but since it is difficult to dry the materials inside the cast, this is seldom desirable; allow only with a physician's permission and dry the cast thoroughly afterward. To keep the cast from becoming wet when bathing, cover with a plastic bag. Gently tape the bag to the skin above the level of the cast if possible. Plaster casts take 12 to 24 hours longer to dry than synthetic casts and will soften if they become wet, which would alter the support to the affected area. Do not immerse a plaster cast in water even if it is in a plastic bag.
- Petal the edges of a cast to reduce the risk of skin irritation, to prevent small plaster particles from falling down into the cast, and to waterproof the edges of the cast. (See Fig. 25.1)
- Teach the child and parents never to insert objects inside the cast.

ESSENTIAL STEPS

1. Prepare the child and family.

2. Assemble the equipment.

3. Wash hands.

4. Elevate the extremity: toes above the nose, hands above the heart.

5. Place ice packs along the sides of the cast for the first 48 hours after trauma or surgery, depending on the location of the affected area and the type of cast.

6. Use only palms to move an area in a cast. *Fingertips can cause indentations on wet casts and produce pressure points, especially with plaster casts.*

7. Reposition every 2 hours to prevent flattened area(s).

8. Check circulation every 30 to 60 minutes for 6 to 8 hours after trauma or surgery, then every 4 hours. Assess capillary refill, color, temperature, presence of edema, motion, sensation, and pulse(s). Inspect the skin at least once per day.

Skills Checklist

☐ Prepare the child and family.
☐ Assemble the equipment.
☐ Wash hands.
☐ Elevate the extremity.
☐ Place ice packs, if applicable.
☐ Reposition every 2 hours.
☐ Check circulation and inspect skin.
☐ Assess drainage.
☐ Protect the cast.
☐ Observe the cast for crack(s), dent(s), or foul odor.
☐ Petal the cast after it is dry.
☐ Document.

9. Circle any drainage on the cast with a pen and mark the date and time; note any increase in drainage. Monitor vital signs to assess bleeding status.

10. Use plastic wrap to protect the cast around the perineal area before and after petaling. If the child is young enough to be incontinent or wear diapers, consider placing a sanitary

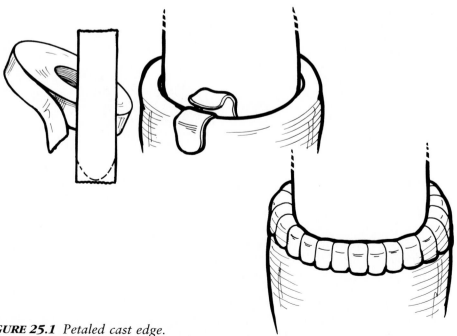

FIGURE 25.1 *Petaled cast edge.*

napkin in the diapers to absorb extra urine. Place the diaper between the child's skin and the cast. Position the child so gravity draws the urine away from the cast into the diaper or bedpan during voiding.

11. Observe the cast for crack(s), dent(s), or odor.

12. After the cast is dry, petal it.

   Prepare the child and family.

   Assemble the equipment.

   Wash hands.

   Ensure that the cast is dry.

   Cut strips of tape 2 to 3 inches long. Cut one end to a point.

   Insert the pointed end of adhesive inside the cast.

   Fold the other end of adhesive over the top edge of the cast.

   Continue to place pieces of tape in the above manner with the tape strips *overlapping*. Cover the entire edge.

DOCUMENTATION

- Type of cast. (See Fig. 25.2)
- Circulation checks of extremity.
- Presence of or increase in drainage.
- Comfort of the child.
- Petaling.

   That cast is dry.

   That petaling was performed.

   Comfort of the child.

POTENTIAL RELATED NURSING DIAGNOSES

Skin integrity, impaired: *high risk*

Tissue integrity, impaired

Infection: *high risk*

Mobility, impaired physical

Tissue perfusion, altered, peripheral

POTENTIAL RELATED MEDICAL DIAGNOSES

Trauma

Fracture

Congenital hip dysplasia

Clubfoot

REFERENCES

Mott, S., James, S., and Sperhac, A. 1990. *Nursing care of children and families.* Redwood City, Calif.: Addison-Wesley.

Shesser, L., and King, T. 1986. Practical considerations in caring for a child in a hip spica cast. *Orthopedic Nursing* 5, no. 3: 11–15.

Swearingen, P. 1984. *Photo-atlas of nursing procedures 2E.* Redwood City, Calif.: Addison-Wesley.

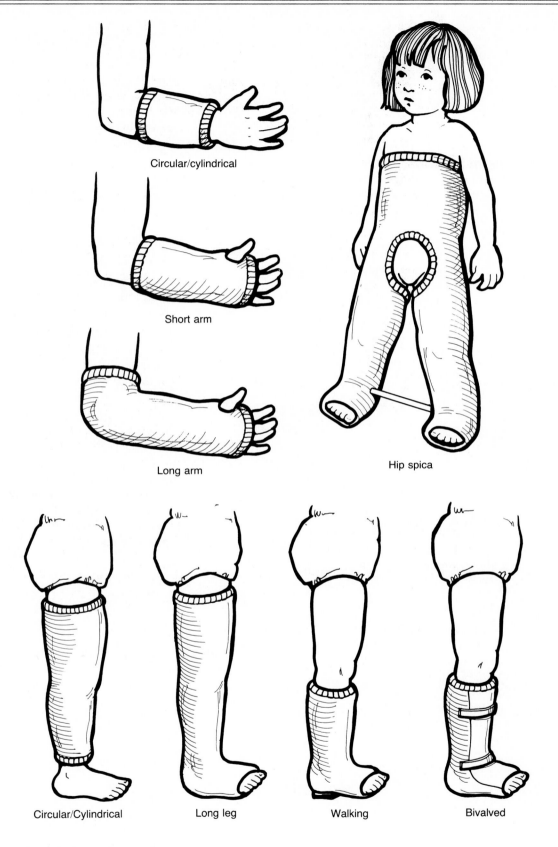

Circular/cylindrical

Short arm

Long arm

Hip spica

Circular/Cylindrical

Long leg

Walking

Bivalved

FIGURE 25.2 *Types of casts.*

26 Catheter: Care

- **Clean away from the meatus.**
- **Do not allow the urinary drainage bag to touch/lie on the floor or to be above the bladder level.**

PSYCHOSOCIAL CONSIDERATIONS: Explain the procedure in developmentally appropriate terms. Children may fear strangers touching their genitalia. Allow parents to provide support during the procedure if possible. Use therapeutic play with a doll to show what is going to happen.

TIME: 5 to 10 minutes, one time every 24 hours

PURPOSE

To prevent the complication of infection associated with an indwelling catheter.

To evaluate and clean the site of insertion.

OBJECTIVES

- To decrease the risk of urinary tract infection.
- To maintain a clean environment.

EQUIPMENT

Gloves, nonsterile

Soap, water, and washcloth

Irrigation tray and sterile water, if applicable

ESSENTIAL STEPS

1. Prepare the child and family.
2. Assemble the equipment.
3. Wash hands and put on gloves.
4. Clearly visualize the site of the catheter insertion and the surrounding skin area to be cleaned.
5. Clean the area with soap and water.

   For girls: Bathe as usual (shower or sponge-bathe); no special care needed.

   For boys: Gently retract the foreskin and clean the glans penis using a circular motion. Pull the foreskin back down.
6. Keep the drainage bag lower than the child's bladder to prevent retrograde flow toward the bladder. Teach parents and other care givers to correctly position the tubing and drainage bag.

7. Place excessive tubing on the bed to prevent a U-loop and to facilitate gravitational drainage. U-loops allow stasis of urine.

8. Support the drainage tube to prevent pull on the catheter. Always keep the bag lower than the child's bladder.

9. Consult with the physician about changing the catheter. Consider changing catheters if catheter concretions are felt or if urine contains gross precipitants. Silastic catheters may remain in place for prolonged periods of time.

10. Irrigate or remove an obstructed catheter per the physician's plan of care. Using sterile technique, irrigate the catheter with 5 to 10 ml of sterile water.

11. Change the drainage system and bag when changing the catheter.

12. Empty the bag, following the directions for that type of bag, at least once every 8 hours. Measure the urine. Always empty the bag using aseptic technique; avoid touching the drain to the cup.

DOCUMENTATION

- Time of catheter care.
- Secretion (color, consistency, amount), if applicable.
- Skin condition.
- Appearance of urine.
- Amount of urine when drainage bag emptied.
- That catheter was irrigated, if applicable.

Skills Checklist

- ☐ Prepare the child and family.
- ☐ Assemble the equipment.
- ☐ Wash hands and put on gloves.
- ☐ Clean the area.
- ☐ Check the level of the drainage bag. Place excessive tubing on the bed and check for tension on the catheter.
- ☐ Change the drainage system, if appropriate.
- ☐ Empty the bag and measure the urine at least once every 8 hours.
- ☐ Document.

POTENTIAL RELATED NURSING DIAGNOSES

Infection: *high risk*

Skin integrity, impaired: *high risk*

Anxiety

POTENTIAL RELATED MEDICAL DIAGNOSES

Universal application for all patients with indwelling urinary catheters

REFERENCES
Foley care. 1988. *Nursing 88* 18: 100.

Catheter: Insertion of Indwelling

Foley catheter of appropriate size, if not included in the tray (see Table 27.1)

Drainage system, if not included in the tray:

> Closed urine drainage bag *or*
>
> Urimeter drainage bag (for more accurate measurement of output)

PSYCHOSOCIAL CONSIDERATIONS: Explain the procedure in developmentally appropriate terms. Avoid using terms with mixed meanings, such as *stick into bladder* and *inflate a balloon*. The child may fear trauma to genitalia or fear a stranger touching genitalia. Provide reassurance and comfort. Allow parents to provide support during the procedure if possible.

TIME: 10 minutes

PURPOSE

To prevent or relieve urinary retention.

To facilitate frequent urine sampling.

To monitor urinary output accurately.

OBJECTIVES

- To facilitate drainage of urine.
- To prevent injury or trauma.

EQUIPMENT

Catheterization tray, including a sterile field, drape, sterile gloves, povidone-iodine solution, cotton balls, sterile lubricant, prefilled syringe, forceps, and a specimen cup; different trays available, some including catheter and/or drainage system

SAFETY ISSUES

- **Maintain sterility of the catheter. Do not use force when inserting the catheter into urinary meatus.**

ESSENTIAL STEPS

1. Prepare the child and family.
2. Assemble the equipment.
3. Wash hands.
4. Position and drape the child.
5. Put on gloves.
6. Check the balloon on the catheter by inflating and deflating it once before insertion.

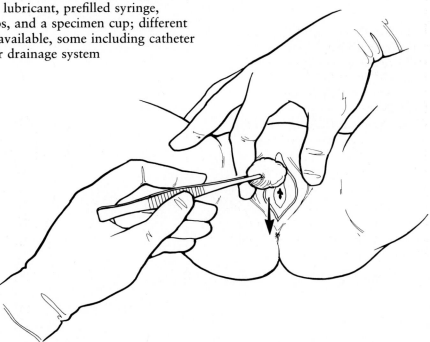

FIGURE 27.1 *Cleaning the labia using downward strokes.*

TABLE 27.1 *Urinary Catheter Sizes*

Premature	Not available
Newborn	6 french
Toddler	8 french
Preschooler	8 french
School-age child	10 french
Adolescent	10–12 french

NOTE: Use judgment regarding catheter sizes.

7. Clean genitalia for a girl:

   Gently separate the labia minora to visualize the meatus.

   Keep the meatus exposed until after insertion of the catheter.

   For each cleansing stroke, pick up a single povidone-iodine–soaked cotton ball with forceps. Clean from anterior to posterior, meatus toward rectum. (See Fig. 27.1)

   With the first stroke, clean down one side of the meatus, including the meatal opening. With the second stroke, clean down the opposite side, including the meatal opening. With the third stroke, wipe directly over the meatus.

8. To clean genitalia for a boy:

   If the child is not circumcised, gently retract the foreskin to expose the meatus.

   Pick up a povidone-iodine –soaked cotton ball with forceps and clean the glans penis, using a circular motion, from the meatus to the base of the glans penis.

   Clean the penis three times in this manner using a new povidone-iodine–soaked cotton ball for each stroke. *Do not contaminate sterile gloves.*

9. Lubricate the tip of the catheter with the lubricant contained in the tray. Do not plug the eye of the catheter with the lubricant.

Skills Checklist

- ☐ Prepare the child and family.
- ☐ Assemble the equipment.
- ☐ Wash hands.
- ☐ Position and drape the child.
- ☐ Put on gloves.
- ☐ Check the balloon.
- ☐ Clean genitalia.
- ☐ Lubricate the catheter tip.
- ☐ Insert the catheter.
- ☐ Inflate the balloon. Collect a urine sample, if ordered.
- ☐ Connect the catheter to the drainage system.
- ☐ Secure the catheter to the thigh.
- ☐ Secure the tubing to the bed.
- ☐ Wash povidone-iodine from the skin and dry genitalia.
- ☐ Label the specimen. Place in a plastic bag and send to the lab.
- ☐ Document.

10. Insert the catheter gently into the meatus, directing it downward until urine begins to flow. Continue to insert the catheter slightly past the point where urine begins to flow. (See Fig. 27.2) To facilitate insertion in the male, hold the penis stretched and in an upright position.

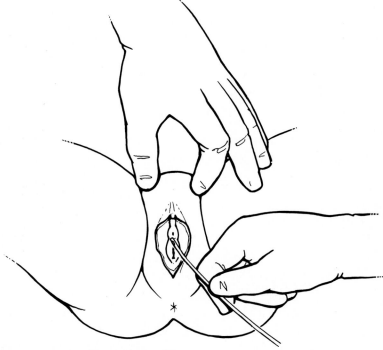

FIGURE 27.2 *Inserting the catheter.*

11. Never force the catheter when resistance is felt. Some resistance may be felt at the urethral sphincter; allow a moment for the sphincter to relax. Call the physician if unable to insert the catheter or if bleeding occurs.

12. Inflate the balloon with the recommended volume of sterile water. (See Fig. 27.3) If balloon inflation is painful to the child, the balloon could be in the urethra and not in the bladder. Deflate the balloon and try again. Reinflate. Pull the foreskin back down in the uncircumcised male.

13. Collect a sterile urine sample, if ordered.

14. Ensure that the catheter is connected to the drainage tube system.

15. Secure the catheter to the thigh with tape. (See Figs. 27.4 and 27.5)

16. Secure the tubing to the bed. Coil excess tubing in flat circles on the bed.

17. Hang the bag beneath the level of the child's bladder, preventing U-loops from forming in the drainage tubing.

18. Wash all povidone-iodine from the skin and dry genitalia.

19. Label the specimen. Place in a plastic bag and send to the lab.

20. Prior to removing a Foley catheter, *always* deflate the balloon.

    Wash hands and put on gloves.

    Aspirate air or water from the balloon with a syringe.

    Gently remove the catheter.

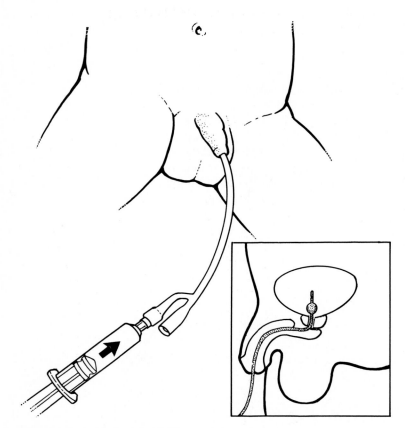

FIGURE 27.3 *Inflating the balloon.*

DOCUMENTATION

- Date and time.
- Size and type of catheter used.
- Amount and characteristics of urine obtained.
- Child's tolerance of procedure.
- That the specimen was sent to lab, if applicable.

POTENTIAL RELATED NURSING DIAGNOSES

Infection: *high risk*

Coping, ineffective individual

Urinary elimination, altered

POTENTIAL RELATED MEDICAL DIAGNOSES

Coma

Trauma

Postoperative procedure

Genitourinary surgery

Musculoskeletal diseases

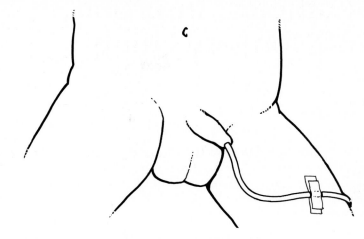

FIGURE 27.4 *Catheter tubing taped to the thigh.*

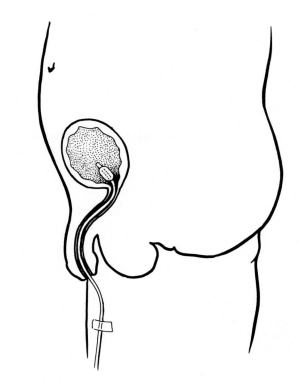

FIGURE 27.5 *Side view of catheter taped to the thigh.*

28 Catheter: Insertion of Nonindwelling

PSYCHOSOCIAL CONSIDERATIONS:
Explain the procedure in developmentally appropriate terms. Avoid using terms with mixed meanings, such as *insert, stick,* and *tube into your bladder.* The child may fear strangers seeing or touching genitalia. Allow parents to provide support during the procedure, if possible.

TIME: 10 minutes

PURPOSE

To obtain a sterile urine specimen for culture.

To intermittently relieve bladder distention.

To check for residual urine.

OBJECTIVES

• To obtain a sterile urine specimen.
• To prevent injury or trauma.

EQUIPMENT

Catheterization tray without drainage bag, including a sterile field, drape, sterile gloves, forceps, povidone-iodine solution, cotton balls, sterile lubricant, and specimen cup; different trays available, some including a catheter

Catheter of appropriate size, if not included in tray; straight catheter is usually used (see Table 28.1)

SAFETY ISSUES

• **Do not force when inserting the catheter into urinary meatus.**

ESSENTIAL STEPS

1. Prepare the child and family.
2. Assemble the equipment.
3. Wash hands.
4. Position and drape the child.
5. Put on gloves.
6. To clean genitalia for a girl:
    Gently separate the labia minora to visualize the meatus.

TABLE 28.1 *Urinary Catheter Sizes*

Premature	5 french feeding tube
Newborn	5 or 8 french feeding tube *or* 6 french
Toddler	8 french
Preschooler	8 french
School-age child	10 french
Adolescent	10–12 french

NOTE: Feeding tubes are often used as catheters because they are small and easy to insert. Use judgment regarding catheter sizes.

Keep the meatus exposed until after insertion of the catheter.

For each cleansing stroke, pick up a single povidone-iodine–soaked cotton ball with forceps. Clean from anterior to posterior, meatus toward rectum.

With the first stroke, clean down one side of the meatus, including the meatal opening. With the second stroke, clean down the opposite side, including the meatal opening. With the third stroke, wipe directly over the meatus. (See Fig. 28.1)

7. To clean genitalia for a boy:

If the child is not circumcised, gently retract the foreskin to expose the meatus.

Pick up a povidone-iodine–soaked cotton ball with forceps and clean the glans penis, using a circular motion, from the meatus to the base of the glans penis.

Clean the penis three times in this manner using a new povidone-iodine–soaked cotton ball for each stroke. Do not contaminate sterile glove.

8. Lubricate the tip of the catheter with the lubricant contained in the tray. Do not plug the eye of the catheter with the lubricant.

9. Insert the catheter gently into the meatus, directing it downward until urine begins to flow. (See Fig. 28.2) To facilitate insertion in the male, hold the penis stretched in an upright position.

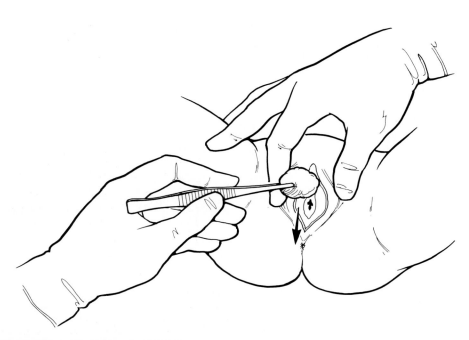

FIGURE 28.1 *Cleaning the labia.*

10. Never force the catheter when resistance is felt. Some resistance may be felt at the urethral sphincter; allow a moment for the sphincter to relax. Call the physician if unable to insert the catheter or if bleeding occurs.

11. Collect urine in a sterile container, if ordered.

12. Withdraw the catheter gently but firmly. Squeeze the catheter while withdrawing to prevent urine from backflowing. Pull foreskin back down in the uncircumcised male.

13. Wash all povidone-iodine from skin and dry genitalia.

14. Label the specimen. Place in a plastic bag and send to the lab.

DOCUMENTATION

- Date and time.
- Size of catheter used.
- Purpose of catheterization.
- Amount and characteristics of urine obtained.
- Time of last void prior to catheterization.
- Child's response to the procedure..
- That specimen was sent to the lab, if applicable.

POTENTIAL RELATED NURSING DIAGNOSES

Infection: *high risk*

Urinary elimination, altered

Anxiety

POTENTIAL RELATED MEDICAL DIAGNOSES

Universal application for all clients requiring catheterization

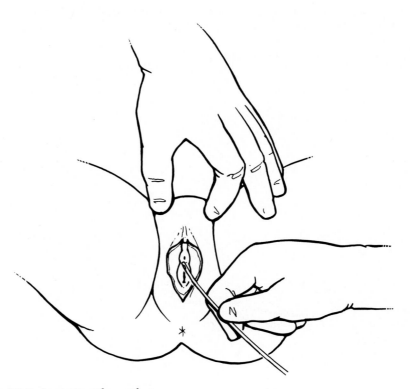

FIGURE 28.2 *Inserting the catheter.*

Central Venous Catheter: Blood Drawing

PSYCHOSOCIAL CONSIDERATIONS: Explain the procedure in developmentally appropriate terms. Allow the child to ventilate feelings. Some children fear that all of their blood will be removed. Younger children may benefit from therapeutic play with a doll or puppet.

TIME: 10 to 15 minutes

PURPOSE

To obtain a blood sample from the central venous catheter (CVC).

OBJECTIVES

• To obtain a blood sample.
• To prevent injury.

EQUIPMENT

10 ml vial of normal saline (0.9% sodium chloride)

10 ml syringe with 20g needle

Gloves, sterile

Povidone-iodine swabs *or* alcohol swabs

Smooth-edge clamps

3 ml syringe

Heparin (1,000 units/ml) to heparinize syringe (if blood is to be reinstilled)

5 ml syringe (or appropriate size for volume of blood required)

Lab tubes, as indicated

Tape

One or two needles, appropriate size

SAFETY ISSUES

• Do not reinstill blood withdrawn initially to clear the CVC unless the physician has specified to do so in the plan of care. A heparinized syringe is used to withdraw blood, if the blood is to be reinstilled.

• Draw blood through the largest lumen when using a multilumen catheter. Turn off infusions through other lumens during blood sampling.

• Minimize the number of times the catheter system is opened each day. If feasible, coordinate blood drawing with routine tubing or cap changes.

• Draw blood cultures directly from the catheter hub. Other blood samples may be drawn from the hub of the Luer-Lok extension tube.

ESSENTIAL STEPS

1. Prepare the child and family.
2. Assemble the equipment.
3. Wash hands.
4. Draw up 10 ml of normal saline into 10 ml syringe.
5. Remove the top layer of CVC dressing.
6. Remove the tape from the catheter hub/tubing connection.
7. Put on gloves.
8. Clean the hub/tubing connection for 30 seconds with povidone-iodine or alcohol swabs.
9. Clamp the catheter.
10. Turn off the infusions through all lumens except the largest, if applicable.
11. Disconnect the tubing or cap.
12. Connect 3 ml syringe to the catheter. If the physician has ordered that the blood be reinstilled, it may be drawn into a heparinized syringe.
13. Unclamp the catheter.

14. Withdraw blood to clear the catheter of heparin or IV fluid. The discard volume is equivalent to the filling volume of the catheter and the extension tube rounded to the nearest ml.

15. If unable to withdraw blood, reposition the child, flush the catheter with a small amount of normal saline, or have the patient do a Valsalva or cry. If blood withdrawal is still unsuccessful, notify the physician that the catheter is partially occluded. Refer to "Central Venous Catheter: Urokinase Irrigation for a Partial Occlusion."

16. After withdrawal of discard blood, clamp the catheter.

17. Disconnect the discard syringe and connect the 5 ml syringe to the catheter.

18. Unclamp the catheter.

19. Withdraw the appropriate volume of blood for the sample.

20. Clamp the catheter.

21. Disconnect the syringe.

22. After the procedure, place the blood sample in the appropriate lab tube(s).

23. Connect the normal-saline–filled syringe.

24. Unclamp the catheter.

25. Flush the catheter with normal saline.

26. Clamp the catheter.

27. Turn on any infusions through other lumens that have been turned off.

28. Connect the IV tubing or heparin-lock the catheter following the steps in "Central Venous Catheter: Priming and Changing IV Tubing" or "Central Venous Catheter: Heparin Lock/Cap Change."

29. Tape the connection.

30. Coil the catheter on top of the dressing and tape securely.

31. Label specimen(s). Place in a plastic bag and send to the lab.

Skills Checklist

☐ Prepare the child and family.
☐ Assemble the equipment.
☐ Wash hands.
☐ Draw up normal saline.
☐ Remove the top layer of dressing and tape from the catheter hub/tubing connection.
☐ Put on gloves.
☐ Prep the catheter hub/tubing connection.
☐ Disconnect the tubing or cap.
☐ Connect the syringe.
☐ Aspirate discard blood.
☐ Aspirate blood sample(s).
☐ Flush with normal saline.
☐ Connect the IV tubing or heparin lock.
☐ Document.

DOCUMENTATION

- Amount of blood withdrawn.
- Volume and concentration of any heparin administered.
- Amount of normal saline flush.

POTENTIAL RELATED NURSING DIAGNOSES

Injury: *high risk*

Infection: *high risk*

Fluid volume deficit: *high risk*

Anxiety

Fear

POTENTIAL RELATED MEDICAL DIAGNOSES

Universal application

30 Central Venous Catheter: Blunt Needle Repair

PSYCHOSOCIAL CONSIDERATIONS: Explain the procedure in developmentally appropriate terms.

TIME: 15 to 30 minutes

PURPOSE

To place a temporary hub for access into the central venous catheter (CVC) following damage to the catheter.

To avoid air emboli, blood loss, clotting of the catheter, and sepsis.

OBJECTIVES

- To repair a CVC temporarily.
- To prevent injury or trauma.

EQUIPMENT

Gloves, sterile

3 ml syringe with 25g 5/8″ needle

Normal saline (0.9% sodium chloride; 30 ml vial), sterile

Blunt needle, appropriate size, sterile

1 ml syringe

Heparin (volume dependent on the type and size of CVC; units/ml vary from 10 to 100, per institution policy)

Four povidone-iodine swabs *or* alcohol swabs

Smooth-edge clamps

Suture removal kit, sterile

Injection cap *or* new IV administration set

Nylon suture 4−0, sterile

Tongue blade, padded

Tape

Two 20g needles, sterile

 SAFETY ISSUES

- **Immediately clamp the CVC between the child and the damaged portion of the catheter.**
- **Place a blunt needle as a temporary hub until permanent repair can be performed, or until the CVC is removed or replaced.**

ESSENTIAL STEPS

1. Prepare the child and family.

2. Assemble the equipment.

3. Wash hands.

4. Disconnect the administration set from the CVC and turn off the infusion pump.

5. Open equipment packages and put on gloves.

6. Fill the 3 ml sterile syringe with 2.5 ml of normal saline and place the blunt needle on the end. Fill a sterile 1 ml syringe with heparin solution.

7. Hold the CVC with povidone-iodine swabs or alcohol swabs. Swab from the damaged area down the catheter for several inches toward the exit site. Repeat this sequence with a second set of povidone-iodine or alcohol swabs. (See Fig. 30.1)

8. Using scissors from the sterile suture removal kit, cut the end of the damaged catheter off, leaving a smooth edge (cut off no more than 1 inch of catheter).

Skills Checklist

☐ Prepare the child and family.
☐ Assemble the equipment.
☐ Wash hands.
☐ Disconnect the administration set and turn off the pump.
☐ Open the equipment packages and put on gloves.
☐ Draw up normal saline.
☐ Attach the blunt needle to the normal saline syringe.
☐ Draw up heparin.
☐ Prep the catheter with povidone-iodine or alcohol swabs.
☐ Cut off the damaged catheter.
☐ Insert the blunt needle into the CVC.
☐ Aspirate air.
☐ Irrigate the CVC.
☐ Attach the new administration set or heparin lock.
☐ Stabilize the CVC.
☐ Document.

9. Pick up the 3 ml normal saline –filled syringe and insert the blunt needle into the end of the CVC until the hub of the needle rests against the catheter. (See Fig. 30.2)

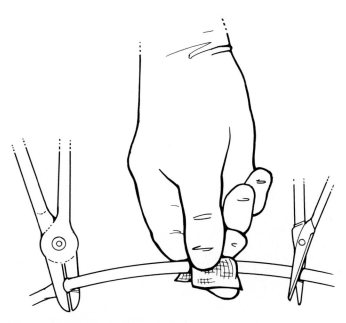

FIGURE 30.1 *Cleaning and trimming the catheter.*

10. Aspirate any remaining air from the catheter. (If air is suspected past the catheter clamp, remove the clamp and aspirate the catheter of any remaining air prior to irrigation.)

11. Release the clamp and gently irrigate the CVC.

12. If unable to irrigate with gentle, positive pressure, reclamp the CVC, disconnect the 3 ml syringe from the blunt needle, and attach the 1 ml syringe containing heparin solution. Unclamp the catheter and gently attempt irrigation. Do not use force to irrigate the CVC. If irrigation is still unsuccessful, complete the procedure and notify the physician. Completion of this procedure is necessary to allow access of the CVC for instillation of urokinase.

13. If the CVC is easily irrigated, reclamp it, remove the syringe, and connect the new administration set or heparin lock the CVC. Refer to "Central Venous Catheter: Priming and Changing IV Tubing" or "Central Venous Catheter: Heparin Lock/Cap Change."

14. Observe the connection for leaks and the CVC for air bubbles.

15. Stabilize the CVC blunt needle repair by tying two sutures over the blunt needle: one near the proximal end and one near the distal end. If necessary, remove gloves to tie the sutures securely. (See Fig. 30.3)

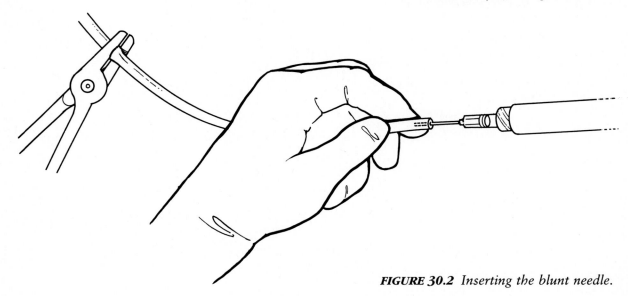

FIGURE 30.2 *Inserting the blunt needle.*

16. Protect the repair by bracing it on a padded tongue blade.

17. Tape the braced blunt needle repair to the CVC dressing (or near it) to prevent tension on the repair.

18. Inform the physician of the blunt needle repair.

DOCUMENTATION

- Placement of the blunt needle.
- Events leading to the catheter break.
- Nursing actions taken.

POTENTIAL RELATED NURSING DIAGNOSES

Injury: *high risk*

Infection: *high risk*

Anxiety

Fear

Fluid volume deficit: *high risk*

POTENTIAL RELATED MEDICAL DIAGNOSES

Universal application

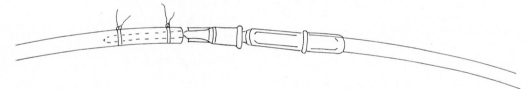

FIGURE 30.3 *Sutures tied around the catheter and needle.*

31 Central Venous Catheter: Care of the Child

PSYCHOSOCIAL CONSIDERATIONS: Explain the procedure in developmentally appropriate terms. Avoid using terms with mixed meanings, such as *into the heart, feed your body,* and *stick.* Allow the child to ventilate feelings. Explain to parents the purpose of the procedure. Encourage parents to ventilate fears and concerns. Younger children may benefit from therapeutic play with a doll or puppet.

TIME: Varies

PURPOSE

To ensure safe care of the child before and after insertion of a central venous catheter (CVC).

OBJECTIVES

- To establish venous access via a CVC.
- To prevent trauma and injury.
- To reduce the risk for infection.

EQUIPMENT

Dressing change kit or equivalent sterile supplies

Supplies for heparin lock or connection of IV tubing, as indicated (refer to "Central Venous Catheter: Priming and Changing IV Tubing" and "Central Venous Catheter: Heparin Lock/Cap Change")

Infusion pump, if indicated

SAFETY ISSUES

- Check for informed consent.
- Make sure that a chest x-ray or fluoroscopic exam has been done to verify the location of the catheter tip before beginning an infusion of IV fluid at other than a keep-vein-open (KVO) rate.
- After insertion of a central venous catheter, a procedure note including the location of the catheter tip should be placed on the chart. (See Fig. 31.1) For catheters placed in surgery, the catheter insertion and tip location may be documented in the operative note or on the anesthesia record.

ESSENTIAL STEPS

1. Prepare the child and family. Check for informed consent.
2. Assemble the equipment.
3. Wash hands.
4. To change the dressing postoperatively:

    Immediately following catheter insertion, apply a sterile dressing.

    Apply according to standard protocol. Refer to "Central Venous Catheter: Dressing Change."

    Generally, change the postoperative dressing 24 hours after CVC insertion. Change immediately if the dressing is noted to be wet, dirty, or loose or if excessive bleeding is noted.

5. For postinsertion infusion or heparin lock:

> If an infusion is to be started immediately postinsertion, the operating room nurse or technician will prime and connect the appropriate tubing. Refer to "Central Venous Catheter: Priming and Changing IV Tubing."

> Maintain the infusion at a KVO rate until the position of the catheter tip has been verified. The infusion should be monitored constantly.

> Upon arrival to the postanesthesia recovery area, connect the tubing to the pump and maintain the infusion at an appropriate rate.

> If the catheter is to be heparin-locked, the operating room nurse, technician, or surgeon will do so. Refer to "Central Venous Catheter: Heparin Lock/Cap Change."

DOCUMENTATION

- Preoperative checklist, if appropriate.
- That postinsertion infusion or heparin lock was done.
- That dressing was changed postoperatively.

POTENTIAL RELATED NURSING DIAGNOSES

Injury: *high risk*

Infection: *high risk*

Anxiety

Pain, acute

Fear

Skin integrity, impaired

Fluid volume excess

POTENTIAL RELATED MEDICAL DIAGNOSES

Any diagnoses requiring a CVC

REFERENCES

Whitney, R. 1991. Your guide to pediatric drug administration. *Nursing 91* 21, no. 8: 82–92.

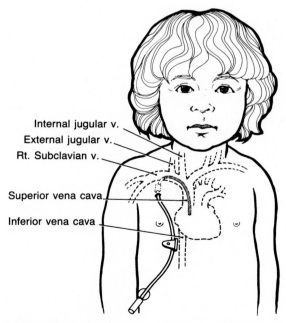

FIGURE 31.1 *Placement and position of a central venous catheter.*

32 | Central Venous Catheter: Thrombolytic Infusion

PSYCHOSOCIAL CONSIDERATIONS: Explain the procedure in developmentally appropriate terms. Reassure the child and family and encourage them to ventilate feelings. Explain to older children that the purpose of the procedure is to keep the catheter open. Younger children may benefit from therapeutic play with a doll or puppet.

TIME: Varies

PURPOSE

To provide for the safe administration of a continuous infusion of a thrombolytic agent (urokinase or streptokinase) in the treatment of a central venous catheter (CVC) occlusion that is unresponsive to bolus doses of thrombolytic agents.

OBJECTIVES

- To establish a patent line.
- To prevent injury.

EQUIPMENT

Thrombolytic agent (urokinase or streptokinase), prepared by a pharmacist

Infusion pump and tubing

Gloves, sterile

10 ml vial of normal saline (0.9% sodium chloride), sterile

10 ml syringe

3 ml syringe with needle

Povidone-iodine swabs *or* alcohol swabs

Smooth-edge clamps

20g or 22g needle

- This procedure may be contraindicated in children with active bleeding, cerebrovascular disease, surgery or an invasive procedure within the last 2 months, or other conditions associated with potential bleeding.
- A physician must specify the dose of thrombolytic agent and the duration of the infusion. The common dosages used for a continuous infusion are

    Loading dose: 4,400 units/kg over 10 minutes.

    Infusion dose: 4,400 units/kg/hour for 4 hours.

- A continuous infusion is indicated *only* if the catheter occlusion is unresponsive to bolus doses. Refer to "Central Venous Catheter: Urokinase Irrigation for a Partial Occlusion."
- Use this procedure only for partially occluded catheters that permit some flow, not for totally occluded catheters.
- A cardiac/apnea monitor is recommended during the infusion and for at least 1 hour following the infusion.
- The pharmacist should prepare the drug and dilute it in a compatible intravenous solution (5% dextrose in water or normal saline).

- Urokinase and streptokinase are not compatible with other medications. During the thrombolytic agent infusion, do not infuse any other medications into the same lumen of the catheter.
- This procedure is not universally used in all institutions. If a bolus injection does not clear a central line, the line may be pulled and a new one inserted.

ESSENTIAL STEPS

1. Prepare the child and family.

   Establish a baseline assessment of temperature, pulse rate, respiratory rate, and blood pressure. Assess skin and mucous membranes for petechiae, recent wounds, and any evidence of bleeding.

   Place the child on a cardiac/apnea monitor.

2. Assemble the equipment.

   Obtain the thrombolytic agent. Inspect the solution for any filaments.

   Prime tubing according to standard CVC procedure. Refer to "Central Venous Catheter: Priming and Changing IV Tubing."

3. Wash hands.

4. Open equipment packages and put on gloves.

5. Draw up normal saline into the 10 ml syringe.

6. Transfer a loading dose to the sterile 3 ml syringe.

7. Prep the catheter/tubing connection for 30 seconds with povidone-iodine swabs or alcohol swabs.

8. Clamp the catheter. Disconnect the old cap or tubing.

9. Attach the normal-saline–filled syringe and flush the catheter with 10 ml of normal saline after unclamping the catheter. (If the catheter is resistant to flushing with a 10 ml syringe, use a 3 ml syringe and flush with 3 ml of normal saline. Do not push against firm resistance.)

Skills Checklist

- ☐ Prepare the child and family. Do baseline assessment.
- ☐ Place child on a cardiac/apnea monitor.
- ☐ Assemble the equipment.
- ☐ Wash hands.
- ☐ Open equipment and put on gloves.
- ☐ Draw up normal saline. Place a loading dose of thrombolytic agent in a syringe.
- ☐ Prep the catheter/tubing connection.
- ☐ Flush with normal saline.
- ☐ Infuse the loading dose.
- ☐ Connect the continuous infusion.
- ☐ Set the rate.
- ☐ Monitor the child.
- ☐ Postinfusion, attempt to aspirate blood. Follow with normal saline flush.
- ☐ Heparin-lock or resume regular infusion.
- ☐ Document.

10. Clamp the catheter. Disconnect the flush syringe and attach the loading-dose syringe.

11. Unclamp the catheter. Infuse the loading dose gently over 10 minutes.

12. Clamp the catheter. Connect IV tubing and the bag containing the continuous infusion solution following standard CVC procedure.

13. Unclamp the catheter and set the rate on the infusion pump per the physician's plan of care.

14. Monitor the child during the procedure:

    Obtain hourly vital signs.

    Use a cardiac/apnea monitor.

    Observe hourly for evidence of bleeding, allergic reaction (such as skin rash or bronchospasm), or cardiac arrhythmia.

15. Report any adverse reaction to the physician immediately.

16. Following the infusion, attempt to aspirate 3 to 4 ml of blood from the catheter and flush with 10 ml of normal saline. If no blood return is obtained and/or resistance to flushing is present, complete the procedure and notify the physician.

17. Heparin-lock or resume regular infusion into the catheter according to standard CVC procedure. See "Central Venous Catheter: Heparin Lock/Cap Change."

18. Following the infusion, monitor the child closely for any adverse reaction:

    Obtain vital signs every 2 hours for the first 8 hours.

    Obtain vital signs every 4 hours for the next 16 hours.

Maintain a cardiac/apnea monitor for at least 1 hour after the infusion is complete.

Closely watch the child for signs of internal or superficial bleeding.

19. Notify the physician that the infusion is complete.

20. Notify the physician of the ease with which the catheter flushes and of the presence or absence of a blood return.

DOCUMENTATION

- Significant events leading to the catheter occlusion.
- Nursing assessment, including vital signs.
- Concentration and amount of loading dose and infusion.
- Results of the thrombolytic agent irrigation/infusion.
- Ease with which the catheter flushed.

POTENTIAL RELATED NURSING DIAGNOSES

Infection: *high risk*

Injury: *high risk*

Anxiety

Fear

Fluid volume deficit: *high risk*

POTENTIAL RELATED MEDICAL DIAGNOSES

Universal application

REFERENCES

Marcoux, C., Fisher, S., and Wong, D. 1990. Central venous access devices in children. *Pediatric Nursing* 16: 123–33.

33 Central Venous Catheter: Dressing Change

PSYCHOSOCIAL CONSIDERATIONS: Explain the procedure in developmentally appropriate terms. Allow the child to ventilate feelings. Younger children may benefit from therapeutic play with a doll or puppet. Older children may be able to assist with parts of the procedure.

TIME: 15 minutes

PURPOSE

To provide routine observation of the central venous catheter (CVC) exit site.

To provide protection for the catheter.

To reduce the risk of local or systemic catheter-related infection.

OBJECTIVES

- To clean the CVC site.
- To reduce risk for infection.

EQUIPMENT

Gloves, nonsterile

CVC dressing change kit, including three acetone/alcohol swabs (controversial, since acetone may promote skin breakdown), two povidone-iodine swabs, a benzoin swab, povidone-iodine ointment, 2″ × 2″ split gauze, 2″ × 2″ gauze, tape, and sterile gloves

If the child is iodine-sensitive: hibiclens, 10 ml of sterile water, 10 ml syringe, needle, other antimicrobial ointment, 2″ × 2″ gauze

Clear occlusive sterile dressing (such as Tegaderm), if applicable

SAFETY ISSUES

- Change the dressing immediately if it is noted to be wet, soiled, or loose. Also change immediately if the lower occlusive layer is disrupted.
- If the child has a fever greater than 38.5°C (101.3°F), change the CVC dressing and inspect the site for evidence of infection. Culture any drainage.
- Place a clear occlusive sterile dressing over the routine dressing if the dressing is likely to become wet or soiled (for example, if it is located near a tracheostomy or intestinal ostomy or in the diaper area).
- Use a clear occlusive sterile dressing instead of a gauze-and-tape dressing, if desired.
- If CVC occlusion arises, remove the CVC dressing to inspect for kinks.
- Change the dressing at least every 72 hours.

ESSENTIAL STEPS

1. Prepare the child and family.
   Determine if the child's skin is sensitive to povidone-iodine or benzoin.
2. Assemble the equipment.
3. Wash hands and put on clean gloves.
4. Remove the old dressing toward the exit site to avoid "pulling" on the catheter. Inspect the old dressing for drainage or odor. Inspect the CVC exit site for erythema, drainage, or swelling. Assess the integrity of the catheter and sutures.

5. If the child is iodine-sensitive, open a sterile 2" × 2" gauze and pour hibiclens onto it. Draw up 10 ml of sterile water and put 1 to 2 ml of sterile water from syringe on hibiclens gauze.

6. Open dressing kit and put on sterile gloves.

7. Hold the catheter up with the nondominant hand. With the dominant hand clean the exit site with an acetone/alcohol swab. Clean in a circular motion, beginning at the exit site and moving away from the catheter at least 3 to 4 inches. (See Fig. 33.1) *Avoid scrubbing the catheter with the acetone/alcohol swab.*

8. Repeat this step with the remaining two acetone/alcohol swabs.

9. Clean the exit site in the same circular fashion using a povidone-iodine swab. If the child is iodine-sensitive, clean with the hibiclens gauze for 1 minute. Rinse the skin with sterile water from the syringe to remove hibiclens.

10. Use the sides of the second povidone-iodine swab to clean the catheter from the exit site outward for several inches. (See Fig. 33.2)

Skills Checklist

☐ Prepare the child and family. Determine if the child is povidone-iodine- or benzoin-sensitive.
☐ Assemble the equipment.
☐ Wash hands.
☐ Put on clean gloves.
☐ Remove old dressing.
☐ Open the dressing kit and put on sterile gloves.
☐ Clean the site.
☐ Clean the catheter.
☐ Apply ointment.
☐ Apply dressing.
☐ Document.

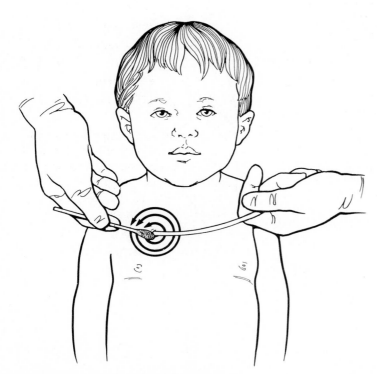

FIGURE 33.1 *Cleaning the catheter site.*

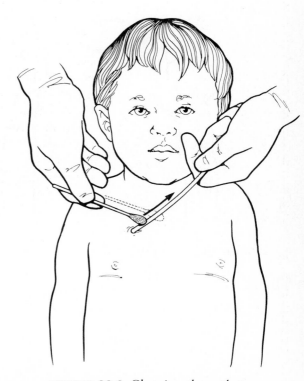

FIGURE 33.2 *Cleaning the catheter.*

11. Apply povidone-iodine (or other antimicrobial ointment if the child is iodine-sensitive) onto the exit site. (See Fig. 33.3) *Some institutions may omit ointment and use only povidone-iodine swabs.*

12. Apply the split 2″ × 2″ gauze around the catheter. (See Fig. 33.4)

13. Place a regular 2″ × 2″ gauze directly on top of the split 2″ × 2″ gauze.

14. Apply benzoin on the skin around the perimeter of the dressing, if appropriate. (Omit this step if the child's skin is sensitive to benzoin.) *Some institutions omit benzoin because of the drying and irritative effect on the skin.*

15. Apply one piece of tape on the top half of the dressing. (See Fig. 33.5)

16. Place a split piece of tape on the bottom half of the dressing to seal the opening around the catheter.

17. Coil and secure the catheter on top of the first layer of dressing using two pieces of tape; only the extension tubing should be visible. *Or* coil the catheter after cleaning and apply a clear occlusive dressing to the entire site. (See Fig. 33.6)

18. Write the date, the time, and your initials *on* the dressing.

19. Apply a clear occlusive sterile dressing if needed over the silk tape dressing.

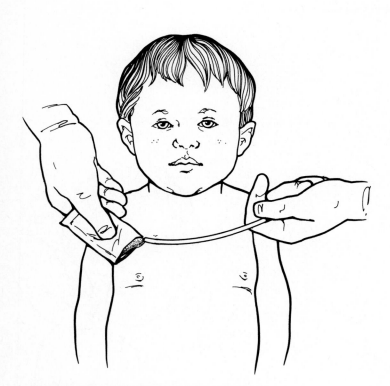

FIGURE 33.3 *Applying ointment to the site.*

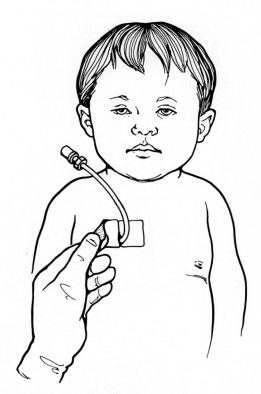

FIGURE 33.4 *Applying the split 2″ × 2″ gauze.*

DOCUMENTATION

- Drainage or odor on old dressing.
- That dressing was changed.
- Appearance of exit site and surrounding skin.
- Integrity of catheter and sutures.
- Child's response.

POTENTIAL RELATED NURSING DIAGNOSES

Infection: *high risk*

Injury: *high risk*

Anxiety

Fear

POTENTIAL RELATED MEDICAL DIAGNOSES

Universal application

REFERENCES

Newman, L. 1989. A side-by-side look, two venous access devices. *AJN* 89: 826–33.

Viall, C. 1990. Your complete guide to central venous catheters. *Nursing 90* 20: 34–41.

Whitney, R. 1991. Your guide to pediatric drug administration. *Nursing 91* 21, no. 8: 82–92.

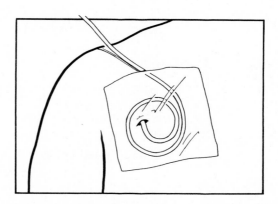

FIGURE 33.6 *Applying clear occlusive dressing.*

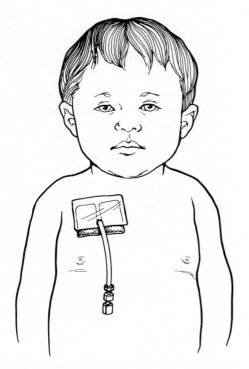

FIGURE 33.5 *Applying tape to the top of the dressing.*

34 Central Venous Catheter: Heparin Irrigation

PSYCHOSOCIAL CONSIDERATIONS: Explain the procedure in developmentally appropriate terms. Explain that the procedure will help the catheter stay open. Younger children may benefit from therapeutic play with a doll or puppet.

TIME: 5 minutes

PURPOSE

To maintain the patency of a heparin-locked central venous catheter (CVC).

OBJECTIVES

- To maintain CVC patency.
- To prevent injury.

EQUIPMENT

Heparin (the volume depends on filling volume of the CVC; units/ml vary from 10 to 100, per institution policy)

3 ml syringe with 25g 5/8″ needle, sterile

Povidone-iodine swab *or* alcohol swab

SAFETY ISSUES

- Base the volume of heparin on the filling volume of the catheter and extension tube (if used) rounded to the next highest ml.
- Irrigate the CVC any time blood is observed in or withdrawn from the catheter or after any infusion.
- If frequent flushes are required, heparin can affect bleeding times. Some institutions substitute normal saline as a flush in this situation.
- **The Groshong catheter *does not* need to be flushed with heparin. Flush with normal saline.**

ESSENTIAL STEPS

1. Prepare the child and family.
2. Assemble the equipment.
3. Wash hands.
4. Draw up the appropriate volume of heparin solution into the syringe. The type of catheter and extension tube will dictate the amount of heparin solution needed. Add the filling volumes together and round up to the next highest ml.
5. Prep the end of the infusion cap with a povidone-iodine swab or alcohol swab for 30 seconds to 1 minute.

6. Insert the needle of the 3 ml syringe into the center of the injection cap and infuse heparin solution, stopping when 0.1 ml of heparin remains in the syringe. Inject the remaining 0.1 ml of heparin while withdrawing the syringe from the injection cap. Maintain a positive pressure on the syringe plunger. (See Fig. 34.1)

7. Check institutional policies for frequency of irrigation: varies from twice per shift to once per week.

8. Notify a physician of any resistance during flushing.

DOCUMENTATION

- Concentration and volume of heparin solution used.
- Time of irrigation.
- Flushing of multiple lumens.
- Security of catheter under dressing.
- Ease with which catheter flushes.

POTENTIAL RELATED NURSING DIAGNOSES

Injury: *high risk*

Infection: *high risk*

Anxiety

Fear

Fluid volume deficit: *high risk*

Skills Checklist

- ☐ Prepare the child and family.
- ☐ Assemble the equipment.
- ☐ Wash hands.
- ☐ Draw up heparin.
- ☐ Prep the cap.
- ☐ Insert the needle.
- ☐ Flush with heparin.
- ☐ Document.

POTENTIAL RELATED MEDICAL DIAGNOSES

Universal application

REFERENCES

Viall, C. 1990. Your complete guide to central venous catheters. *Nursing 90* 20: 34–41.

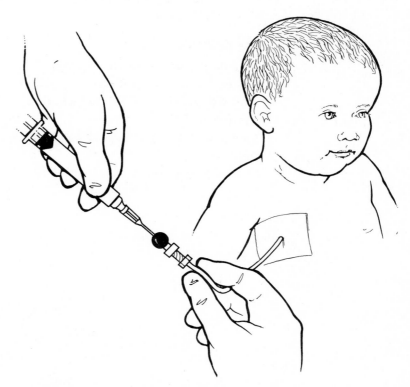

FIGURE 34.1 *Inserting a needle for injection of heparin into a central venous catheter.*

Central Venous Catheter: Heparin Lock/Cap Change

PSYCHOSOCIAL CONSIDERATIONS: Explain the procedure in developmentally appropriate terms. Allow the child to ventilate feelings. Younger children may benefit from therapeutic play with a doll or puppet.

TIME: 15 minutes

PURPOSE

To maintain catheter patency during intermittent IV therapy.

OBJECTIVES

• To maintain a patent catheter.
• To prevent injury.

EQUIPMENT

Heparin solution (units/ml vary from 10 to 100, per institution policy)

3 ml syringe with 25g 5/8″ needle, sterile

Gloves, sterile

Two povidone-iodine swabs *or* alcohol swabs

Smooth-edge clamps

Injection cap

Tape

• Base the volume of heparin on the filling volume of the catheter and/or extension tube rounded to the next highest ml.
• If the injection cap is removed, use a new cap as a replacement.
• Irrigate the heparin-locked catheter whenever blood is visible.
• Heparin-lock each lumen of a multi-lumen catheter not being used for continuous IV infusion.

ESSENTIAL STEPS

1. Prepare the child and family.
2. Assemble the equipment.
3. Wash hands.
4. Draw up heparinized solution with the sterile 3 ml syringe. The type of catheter and extension tube will dictate the amount of heparin solution needed. Add the filling

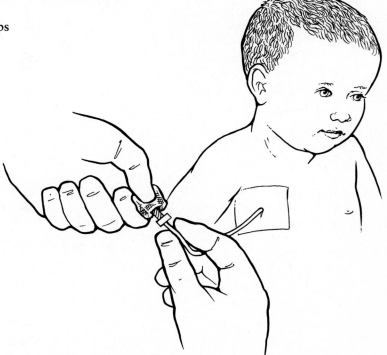

FIGURE 35.1 *Cleaning the connection site.*

volumes together and round up to the next highest ml.

5. Open the equipment packages and put on gloves.

6. Prep the catheter/tubing connection site for 30 seconds with povidone-iodine or alcohol swabs. (See Fig. 35.1)

7. Clamp the CVC or extension tubing.

8. Separate the CVC (or extension set) from the administration set tubing, or remove the old injection cap. (See Fig. 35.2)

9. Hold the catheter hub (or the extension set hub) and an injection cap in one hand while injecting some of the heparin solution from the syringe into both the inverted injection cap and the catheter hub (or extension set) to displace air. This step is institution-dependent.

10. Connect the injection cap to the catheter hub (or extension set).

11. Insert the needle of the heparin syringe into the cap and aspirate any remaining air from the catheter.

12. Unclamp the line.

13. Irrigate the catheter with heparin solution, stopping when 0.1 ml remains in the syringe. Inject the remaining 0.1 ml while withdrawing the needle from the injection cap and maintaining a positive pressure on the syringe plunger.

14. Tape the cap onto the catheter hub.

15. Coil the catheter and retape the top layer of dressing.

Skills Checklist

- ☐ Prepare the child and family.
- ☐ Assemble the equipment.
- ☐ Wash hands.
- ☐ Draw up heparin.
- ☐ Open equipment packages and put on gloves.
- ☐ Prep the catheter/tubing connection site.
- ☐ Fill the injection cap with heparin and connect the cap to the catheter hub.
- ☐ Insert the needle; aspirate air.
- ☐ Inject heparin. Tape the cap onto the catheter hub.
- ☐ Document.

DOCUMENTATION

- Date and time.
- Line heparin locked.
- Concentration and volume of heparin infused.

POTENTIAL RELATED NURSING DIAGNOSES

Infection: *high risk*

Injury: *high risk*

Anxiety

Fear

POTENTIAL RELATED MEDICAL DIAGNOSES

Universal application

REFERENCES

Viall, C. 1990. Your complete guide to central venous catheters. *Nursing '90* 20: 34–41.

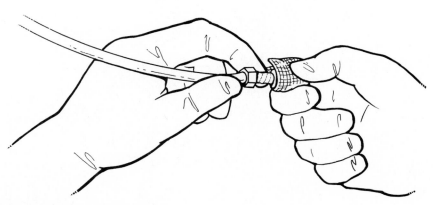

FIGURE 35.2 *Removing the old cap.*

36 Central Venous Catheter: Permanent Repair

PSYCHOSOCIAL CONSIDERATIONS: Explain the procedure in developmentally appropriate terms. Allow the child to ventilate feelings.

TIME: 15 to 30 minutes

PURPOSE

To repair a damaged central venous catheter (CVC).

OBJECTIVES

- To repair a CVC.
- To prevent injury.

EQUIPMENT

Permanent repair kit (specific to catheter type), including catheter segment, glue syringe, blunt needle, sterile field, and scissors

Gloves, sterile

3 ml syringe, 25g needle

Heparin (volume dependent on catheter size; units/ml vary from 10 to 100, per institution policy), syringe, 25g needle

Four povidone-iodine swabs *or* alcohol swabs

Smooth-edge clamps

Padded tongue blade

Injection cap

Medicine cup, cut to prevent contact with repair site until glue dries

SAFETY ISSUES

- **A physician or a nurse may perform this procedure. Check institution guidelines.**

ESSENTIAL STEPS

1. Prepare the child and family.
2. Assemble the equipment.
3. Wash hands.
4. Open the repair kit, put on gloves, and remove the catheter segment, scissors, glue syringe, and blunt needle. Place on a sterile field.
5. Connect the blunt needle to the empty 3 ml syringe. Remove the syringe plunger.
6. Load 1 ml of sterile glue into the syringe barrel and replace the plunger partially into the syringe.
7. Invert the syringe and displace air.
8. Draw up 2.5 ml plus the amount needed to heparin-lock of heparin solution.

9. Connect the heparin-filled syringe to the new segment of catheter tubing and flush.

10. Place sterile towels under the catheter.

11. Prep the remaining CVC segment with povidone-iodine or alcohol swabs for 30 seconds.

12. Clamp the CVC.

13. Remove the blunt needle from the damaged CVC and trim the end of the CVC with sterile scissors so the edge is smooth. (If there is enough catheter length, trim off the portion of CVC that held the blunt needle.)

14. Pick up the repair segment and thread the stint (already attached to the repair segment) into the trimmed catheter. If necessary, lubricate the stint with a small amount of heparin solution prior to threading. Thread very slowly to avoid tearing the catheter. (See Fig. 36.1)

15. Thread the stint into the end of the child's CVC until there is *no* gap between the new repair segment and the CVC. (The new and old ends must be evenly abutted.)

16. Unclamp the catheter.

17. Flush with a small amount of heparin to ensure patency.

18. Clamp the catheter.

19. Slide a protective sleeve down to cover the abutted ends and center the sleeve over the two ends of line. (It is sometimes necessary to carefully cut a small slit in the protective sleeve with the sterile scissors to allow it to slide over the two abutted ends.)

Skills Checklist

☐ Prepare the child and family.
☐ Assemble the equipment.
☐ Wash hands and open the repair kit.
☐ Put on sterile gloves.
☐ Connect the blunt needle to the syringe.
☐ Load sterile glue and displace air.
☐ Draw up heparin.
☐ Prep the CVC.
☐ Remove the blunt needle.
☐ Thread the stint.
☐ Flush with heparin.
☐ Place the protective sleeve.
☐ Inject glue.
☐ Heparin-lock.
☐ Secure.
☐ Document.

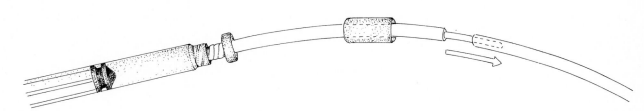

FIGURE 36.1 *Threading the stint into the catheter.*

20. Inject glue into and around the sleeve. (See Fig. 36.2)

21. Heparin-lock per standard CVC procedure.

22. Fasten the repaired joint to a padded tongue blade. (See Fig. 36.3)

23. Tape a plastic medicine cup over the repaired joint to vent air and protect the repair site.

24. Leave the repaired line heparin-locked for at least 1 hour following the repair procedure.

25. Fasten IV tubing with an attached Luer-Lok extension tube to the new CVC hub after the catheter has been heparin-locked for 1 hour, if appropriate.

26. Leave the line splinted with the tongue blade for 24 hours. The repaired joint will not achieve mechanical strength for 24 hours. Remove the splint after that time.

27. Do not use the catheter for infusions for 1 hour after repair to allow the glue to set.

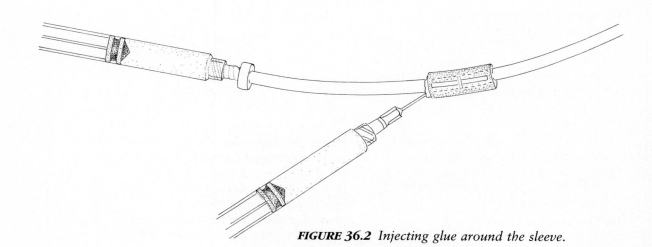

FIGURE 36.2 *Injecting glue around the sleeve.*

DOCUMENTATION

- That repair was completed.
- Length of time line was heparin-locked and stabilized.
- Cessation of IV fluid.
- Amount and concentration of heparin used.

POTENTIAL RELATED NURSING DIAGNOSES

Infection: *high risk*

Injury: *high risk*

Anxiety

Fear

POTENTIAL RELATED MEDICAL DIAGNOSES

Universal application

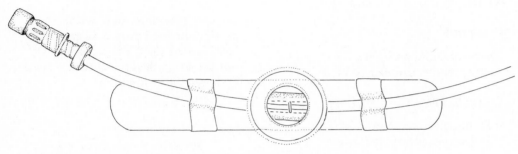

FIGURE 36.3 *Stabilizing the catheter on a tongue blade.*

37 Central Venous Catheter: Hydrochloric Acid Irrigation

PSYCHOSOCIAL CONSIDERATIONS: Explain the procedure in developmentally appropriate terms. Avoid using terms with mixed meanings, such as *stick* and *acid*. Explain to older children that the purpose of the procedure is to open the catheter. Allow the child to ventilate feelings. Younger children may benefit from therapeutic play with a doll or puppet.

TIME: 15 to 20 minutes

PURPOSE

To dissolve the precipitant occluding the central venous catheter (CVC).

OBJECTIVES

- To dissolve precipitant.
- To prevent injury and trauma.

EQUIPMENT

0.1 normal hydrochloric acid prepared aseptically by a pharmacist

1 ml syringe

Two 22g needles

Normal saline (0.9% sodium chloride; 1 vial), sterile

10 ml syringe

Heparin solution (units/ml varies per institution from 10 units/ml to 100 units/ml)

3 ml syringe with 25g 5/8″ needle

Gloves, sterile

Two povidone-iodine swabs *or* alcohol swabs

Smooth-edge clamps

2″ × 2″ gauze

Injection cap

5 ml syringe

SAFETY ISSUES

- **Use this procedure only when precipitant formation is suspected to have caused the CVC occlusion. Do *not* use for catheter occlusion caused by blood clot formation.**

ESSENTIAL STEPS

1. Prepare the child and family.
2. Assemble the equipment.
3. Wash hands.
4. Draw up

    0.5 ml of 0.1 normal hydrochloric acid into the 1 ml syringe.

    10 ml of normal saline into the 10 ml syringe.

    Heparin into the 3 ml syringe with 25g 5/8″ needle (volume dependent on filling volume of catheter).

5. Open equipment packages and put on gloves.

6. Prep the catheter hub/tubing connection site with povidone-iodine swabs or alcohol swabs for 30 seconds.

7. Clamp the catheter.

8. Disconnect the tubing or cap from the hub of the CVC using sterile 2″ × 2″ gauze.

9. Attach the 1 ml syringe with 0.1 normal hydrochloric acid to the hub of the catheter.

10. Alternate gently pushing and pulling on the plunger of the syringe for up to 5 minutes until a blood return is noted. If no blood return, place the injection cap on the catheter hub and notify the physician.

11. Once a blood return is visualized, clamp the CVC and remove the hydrochloric acid syringe.

12. Place the empty 5 ml syringe onto the CVC and aspirate at least 1 filling volume of blood after unclamping the CVC.

13. Reclamp the CVC. Remove the blood-filled syringe and replace it with the normal-saline–filled syringe.

14. Unclamp the CVC. Flush with 10 ml of normal saline. (Volume may be less if the child/infant is fluid restricted.)

15. Heparin-lock the CVC or reconnect it to the infusion. Refer to "Central Venous Catheter: Heparin Lock/Cap Change."

Skills Checklist

☐ Prepare the child and family.
☐ Assemble the equipment.
☐ Wash hands.
☐ Draw up hydrochloric acid, normal saline, and heparin.
☐ Open equipment packages and put on gloves.
☐ Prep the catheter hub/tubing connection.
☐ Disconnect the tubing or cap.
☐ Push and pull with the hydrochloric acid syringe.
☐ Aspirate blood.
☐ Flush with normal saline.
☐ Heparin-lock or reconnect to infusion.
☐ Document.

DOCUMENTATION

- Completion of hydrochloric acid irrigation of CVC.
- Any blood return obtained from the CVC.
- Ease with which normal saline infused after blood was obtained.
- Name of physician and time results of this procedure reported.
- Concentration and volume of heparin solution.

POTENTIAL RELATED NURSING DIAGNOSES

Injury: *high risk*

Infection: *high risk*

Anxiety

Tissue integrity, impaired

POTENTIAL RELATED MEDICAL DIAGNOSES

Universal application

Central Venous Catheter: Priming and Changing IV Tubing

PSYCHOSOCIAL CONSIDERATIONS: Explain the procedure in developmentally appropriate terms. Allow the child to ventilate feelings. Younger children may benefit from therapeutic play with a doll or puppet.

TIME: 15 to 20 minutes

PURPOSE

To aseptically change the IV tubing on a routine basis to reduce the risk of infection.

To remove air from tubing to prevent air embolism.

OBJECTIVES

• To change IV tubing.
• To prevent injury or trauma.

EQUIPMENT

Appropriate IV tubing

Tape

IV fluids

Smooth-edge clamps

Luer-Lok extension tube (if extension tube is due to be changed)

Povidone-iodine swabs *or* alcohol swabs

Alcohol swab

Gloves, sterile

SAFETY ISSUES

• Prevent air from entering the line.
• Clean catheter/tubing connection before disconnecting the IV tubing to decrease the risk of infection.
• Generally, change IV tubing used for infusions of total parenteral nutrition (TPN) and lipids every 24 hours (time varies with institutions).
• Generally, change IV tubing used for infusions of fluids or medications every 48 to 72 hours.
• Use an infusion pump for all infusions into CVCs except for the infusion of platelets.
• Change tubing using aseptic technique.

ESSENTIAL STEPS

1. Prepare the child and family.
2. Assemble the equipment.
3. Wash hands.
4. Prime IV tubing.

   Be sure to use appropriate tubing.

   Open the new tubing setup. Tighten and tape all connections.

   Insert the tubing spike into the IV bag/bottle and tape the spike securely.

   If using a metered chamber, fill with 40 ml of fluid. Fill the drip chamber to the appropriate level.

Prime the tubing.

If priming lipids and TPN, prime the lipid tubing *first,* then the TPN tubing.

Tap all injection ports to remove air.

Check the manufacturer's instructions as to priming any in-line filter.

Clamp each tubing.

5. To change tubing:

Remove the old tubing from the pump, place on gravity flow, and use the roller clamp to adjust the flow rate appropriately. Verify that gravity flow is present.

Insert the newly primed tubing into pump(s), per the manufacturer's instructions.

Open povidone-iodine swabs, alcohol swabs, and 2″ × 2″ gauze. Put on gloves.

Clean the catheter/tubing connection for 30 seconds with povidone-iodine swabs or alcohol swabs.

Clamp the catheter.

Disconnect old tubing from the catheter or extension tube.

Turn on the infusion pump, drip a small amount of fluid into the catheter hub to displace air, and then connect the new tubing.

Assure that the connection is tight and wipe away excess fluid with an alcohol swab.

Skills Checklist

☐ Prepare the child and family.
☐ Assemble the equipment.
☐ Wash hands.
☐ Open tubing, tape connections, and spike the bag/bottle.
☐ Prime lines.
☐ Clamp the tubing.
☐ Manage pumps.
☐ Put on gloves.
☐ Clean the connection.
☐ Attach the new tubing, adjust the pump, and tape the connection.
☐ Document.

Adjust the pump to the ordered rate of infusion and unclamp the catheter.

Tape the connection and evaluate for leaks.

DOCUMENTATION

• Volume and concentration of solutions.
• Tubing changeout.
• Rate of infusion.

POTENTIAL RELATED NURSING DIAGNOSES

Injury: *high risk*

Infection: *high risk*

Anxiety

Fear

POTENTIAL RELATED MEDICAL DIAGNOSES

Universal application

39 Central Venous Catheter: Urokinase— Partial Occlusion

PSYCHOSOCIAL CONSIDERATIONS: Explain the procedure in developmentally appropriate terms. Avoid using terms with mixed meanings, such as *clotted* or *blocked* catheter. Explain to older children that the purpose of the procedure is to open the catheter. Younger children may benefit from therapeutic play with a doll or puppet.

TIME: 20 to 30 minutes; up to 2 hours wait time

PURPOSE

To establish full patency of a partially occluded central venous catheter (CVC) when the cause is suspected to be a blood clot or fibrin deposit.

OBJECTIVES

- To establish a patent CVC.
- To prevent injury and trauma.

EQUIPMENT

Urokinase (5,000 units/ml, available in 1.0 and 1.8 ml vials; order appropriate size based on the filling volume of the catheter)

3 ml syringe

1 ml syringe (if unable to flush the catheter with 3 ml syringe)

10 ml vial of normal saline (0.9% sodium chloride), sterile

10 ml syringe with 20g needle

Gloves, sterile

Povidone-iodine swabs *or* alcohol swabs

Smooth-edge clamps

5 ml syringe

22g needle

To heparin-lock catheter following urokinase procedure:

    3 ml syringe with 25g 5/8″ needle

    Injection cap

    Heparin (volume dependent on catheter size; units/ml vary from 10 to 100, per institution policy)

SAFETY ISSUES

- Prior to performing this procedure, carefully assess the patency of the catheter. Gently flush the catheter with normal-saline–filled 3 ml and 1 ml syringes to assess the amount of resistance. *Do not apply excessive pressure as doing so may rupture the catheter.*

- This procedure is indicated only for partially occluded CVCs. A partially occluded CVC is defined as a CVC that permits some flow of infusates but

    In which mild to moderate resistance is encountered with instillation of heparin or saline.

    From which blood samples cannot be readily obtained.

- This procedure may be used to remove suspected fibrin deposits that may be seeding a catheter-associated infection.

- This procedure is *not* indicated for the following:

    External catheter occlusions (kinked or inadvertently clamped CVCs).

    Severe or total resistance present during flushing of the CVC.

    Occlusions caused by precipitant formation.

ESSENTIAL STEPS

1. Prepare the child and family.
2. Assemble the equipment.

    Determine the filling volume of the catheter. Assure that the appropriate-size vial of urokinase is available.

3. Wash hands.
4. Draw up urokinase into the 3 ml syringe (draw up into 1 ml syringe if previously unable to flush the catheter with a 3 ml syringe). Draw up a volume of urokinase equivalent to the filling volume of the catheter.
5. Draw up 10 ml of normal saline into the 10 ml syringe.

6. Remove the top layer of dressing and tape from the catheter/extension tube or catheter/cap connection.

7. Open the equipment packages and put on sterile gloves.

8. Prep the catheter/extension tube or catheter/infusion cap connection for 30 seconds with povidone-iodine swabs or alcohol swabs.

9. Clamp the catheter.

10. Disconnect and discard the cap, if applicable. If total parenteral nutrition (TPN) or other medications have been infusing into the CVC, flush with normal saline prior to instilling urokinase.

11. Connect the urokinase-filled syringe to the catheter hub.

12. Unclamp the catheter.

13. Instill urokinase into the catheter.

14. Clamp the catheter. If a 1 ml syringe has been used to instill urokinase, remove the 1 ml syringe and attach an empty 5 ml syringe.

15. Wait 5 minutes.

16. Unclamp the catheter.

17. Attempt to aspirate blood from the catheter.

18. If a free flow of blood returns:

    Aspirate 2 to 4 ml of blood from the catheter and clamp the catheter.

    Flush the catheter with 10 ml of normal saline.

    Heparin-lock the CVC or connect IV tubing following standard CVC procedures.

    Notify the physician that the irrigation is complete, of the presence of blood return, and of the ease with which the catheter was flushed.

19. *If unable to aspirate blood:*

    Wait an additional 5 minutes and reattempt aspiration every 5 minutes for up to a maximum of six tries (over 30 minutes).

    If still unsuccessful, wait a full 30 minutes and again attempt aspiration.

Skills Checklist

- ☐ Prepare the child and family.
- ☐ Assemble the equipment.
- ☐ Wash hands.
- ☐ Draw up urokinase.
- ☐ Draw up normal saline.
- ☐ Remove the top layer of dressing and tape from the catheter/extension tube or catheter/cap connection.
- ☐ Open equipment packages and put on gloves.
- ☐ Prep the catheter/cap connection.
- ☐ Discard the cap.
- ☐ Instill urokinase.
- ☐ Aspirate.
- ☐ Flush with normal saline.
- ☐ Heparin-lock.
- ☐ Document.

If still unsuccessful, repeat the procedure once using newly reconstituted urokinase. Instill urokinase for 30 to 60 minutes. Attempt aspiration. If blood is obtained, perform step 18.

If still unable to aspirate blood, heparin-lock the catheter and notify the physician.

DOCUMENTATION

- Events leading to catheter occlusion.
- Results of urokinase irrigation.
- Ease with which catheter flushes.
- Volume and concentration of urokinase.

POTENTIAL RELATED NURSING DIAGNOSES

Injury: *high risk*

Infection: *high risk*

Anxiety

Fear

Fluid volume deficit: *high risk*

POTENTIAL RELATED MEDICAL DIAGNOSES

Universal application

Central Venous Catheter: Urokinase— Total Occlusion

PSYCHOSOCIAL CONSIDERATIONS: Explain the procedure in developmentally appropriate terms. Avoid using terms with mixed meanings, such as *clotted off* and *stick*. Explain to older children that the purpose of the procedure is to open the catheter. Younger children may benefit from therapeutic play with a doll or puppet.

TIME: 20 to 30 minutes

PURPOSE

To restore full patency of a totally obstructed central venous catheter (CVC) when a blood clot or fibrin deposit is suspected as the cause of obstruction.

OBJECTIVES

- To establish a patent CVC.
- To prevent injury.

EQUIPMENT

Urokinase (5,000 units/ml; available in 1.0 and 1.8 ml vials; order appropriate size based on the filling volume of the catheter, plus extra in case the procedure must be repeated)

Two 3 ml syringes

Two 22g needles

22g cutdown catheter, sterile

Gloves, sterile

Three povidone-iodine swabs *or* alcohol swabs

Smooth-edge clamps

Two injection caps

Two 10 ml vials of normal saline (0.9% sodium chloride), sterile

5 ml syringe

10 ml syringe with 20g needle

Heparin (units/ml vary from 10 to 100, per institution policy)

 SAFETY ISSUES

- **Prior to performing this procedure, carefully assess the patency of the catheter. Gently flush the catheter with normal-saline–filled 1 and 3 ml syringes to assess the amount of resistance. *Do not apply excessive pressure as doing so may rupture the catheter.***
- **To keep the urokinase from entering the circulatory system, do not exceed the catheter's filling volume.**
- **Use this procedure only for totally occluded CVCs. A totally occluded CVC is defined as a CVC in which:**

  Severe to total resistance is encountered when heparin or normal saline is instilled into the catheter.

  The catheter balloons out when flushed.

- **Do *not* use this procedure for the following:**

  External catheter occlusions.

  Partial catheter occlusions. Refer to "Central Venous Catheter: Urokinase Irrigation for a Partial Occlusion."

  Occlusions caused by precipitant formation.

- **An upright chest x-ray should be taken to verify catheter placement.**
- **If the catheter has more than one lumen, instill urokinase in all lumens.**

ESSENTIAL STEPS

1. Prepare the child and family.

2. Assemble the equipment.

3. Wash hands.

4. Draw up urokinase into the 3 ml syringe. Draw up a volume of urokinase equivalent to the filling volume of the catheter.

5. Remove the needle from the syringe and attach the cutdown catheter to the urokinase syringe. Maintain sterility of the cutdown catheter.

6. Prime the catheter with urokinase.

7. Remove the top layer of dressing and tape from the catheter hub/cap junction.

8. Open equipment packages and put on gloves.

9. Prep the catheter hub/cap junction for 30 seconds with povidone-iodine swabs or alcohol swabs.

10. Clamp the catheter as close to the child as possible.

11. Disconnect and discard the cap.

12. Hold the CVC away from the child's body and estimate the length of cutdown catheter needed to reach the CVC exit site.

13. Thread the cutdown catheter into the CVC until resistance is met or until the estimated length is reached. Do not advance the catheter past the point where the CVC exits the skin.

14. Unclamp the catheter.

15. Instill urokinase until the urokinase solution is noted at the catheter hub.

16. Gradually withdraw the cutdown catheter while continuing to instill urokinase.

17. Clamp the catheter just before completely removing the cutdown catheter.

18. Place the injection cap on the catheter, leaving a urokinase-locked CVC.

19. Unclamp the catheter.

20. Optimally, allow the urokinase to dwell in the catheter for 60 minutes.

21. Assemble the sterile field. Have an additional cutdown catheter, urokinase, 3 ml syringe with needle, and injection cap readily available in case the procedure must be repeated.

Skills Checklist

☐ Prepare the child and family.
☐ Assemble the equipment.
☐ Wash hands.
☐ Draw up urokinase. Remove the needle from the syringe.
☐ Attach the cutdown catheter to the urokinase syringe. Prime the catheter.
☐ Remove the top layer of dressing and tape from the hub/cap junction.
☐ Open equipment packages and put on gloves.
☐ Prep the catheter hub/cap junction.
☐ Discard the cap.
☐ Thread the cutdown catheter.
☐ Instill urokinase.
☐ Remove the cutdown catheter.
☐ Place injection cap.
☐ Assemble the sterile field and draw up normal saline.
☐ Prep the catheter hub/cap connection.
☐ Discard the cap.
☐ Aspirate blood.
☐ Flush with normal saline.
☐ Heparin-lock the catheter.
☐ Document.

22. Draw up 2 ml of normal saline into a 5 ml syringe and 10 ml of normal saline into a 10 ml syringe.

23. Prep the catheter hub/cap connection for 30 seconds with a povidone-iodine swab or alcohol swab.

24. Clamp the catheter.

25. Disconnect and discard the cap.

26. Connect the 5 ml syringe to the catheter.

27. Unclamp the catheter.

28. Attempt to aspirate the catheter by gently pushing and pulling on the plunger of the syringe.

29. If blood return is obtained, aspirate 3 to 4 ml of blood and discard.

30. Clamp the catheter.

31. Attach the normal-saline–filled 10 ml syringe and flush the catheter.

32. Heparin-lock the catheter or connect IV tubing as indicated following CVC procedure. See "Central Venous Catheter: Heparin Lock/Cap Change."

33. Notify the physician that the irrigation is complete, of the presence or absence of blood return, and of the ease with which the catheter flushes.

34. If no blood return is obtained, notify the physician and repeat this procedure once using newly reconstituted urokinase. Leave the CVC urokinase locked for 1 to 3 hours.

DOCUMENTATION

- Significant events leading to the catheter occlusion.
- Results of urokinase irrigation.
- Ease with which the catheter flushes.
- Volume and concentration of urokinase.

POTENTIAL RELATED NURSING DIAGNOSES

Injury: *high risk*

Infection: *high risk*

Anxiety

Fear

Fluid volume deficit: *high risk*

POTENTIAL RELATED MEDICAL DIAGNOSES

Universal application

REFERENCES

Brown, L., Wantroba, I., and Simonson, G. 1989. Reestablishing patency in an occluded central venous device. *Critical Care Nurse* 9: 114–20.

Viall, C. 1990. Your complete guide to central venous catheters. *Nursing 90* 20: 34–41.

41 Chest Physiotherapy

Percussor (for a premature infant); a plastic medicine cup with the open end covered and padded with a 4″ × 4″ gauze may also work as a percussor

Wall or portable suction apparatus, as appropriate

Suction kit with catheter of appropriate size

Oxygen flowmeter with appropriate-size bag and mask

PSYCHOSOCIAL CONSIDERATIONS: Explain the procedure in developmentally appropriate terms. Avoid terms with mixed meanings, such as *beat* and *pound*. Use terms like *percussion* and *lightly pat*. The child may relax and fall asleep during treatments.

TIME: 15 to 20 minutes

PURPOSE

To facilitate drainage of secretions from the upper respiratory system. Chest physiotherapy (CPT) includes postural drainage, percussion, and vibration.

OBJECTIVES

- To maintain a patent airway.
- To facilitate drainage of secretions.
- To prevent further injury or trauma.

EQUIPMENT

Stethoscope

Mechanical vibrator *or,* for a premature infant, electric toothbrush

SAFETY ISSUES

- To perform percussion, use a cupped hand and clap over the specified area. Air should be trapped in the palm. The hand should make a popping sound when clapped over the skin.
- A padded electric toothbrush handle can be used to provide vibrations for a premature infant.
- CPT can increase intracranial pressure (ICP). Avoid trendelenburg positioning in children at risk for ICP.
- Avoid bare skin; the child should wear an undershirt or gown. (Note: Children in illustrations in this procedure have been drawn without shirts only to clarify positioning.)

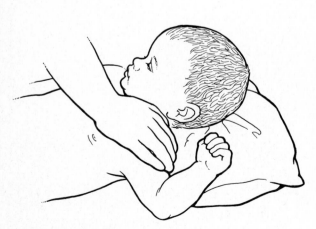

FIGURE 41.1 *Draining anterior segments of the upper lobe.*

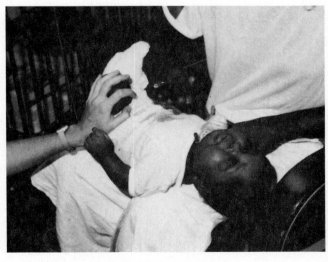

FIGURE 41.2 *Draining anterior segments of the upper lobe.*

ESSENTIAL STEPS

1. Prepare the child and family.

2. Assemble the equipment.

3. Wash hands and perform a respiratory assessment.

4. Position the child. To begin, have the child sit.

5. Percuss over the front apices for 1 to 2 minutes.

6. Vibrate over the front apices for at least 1 minute. Vibrate only during expiration.

7. Repeat Steps 5 and 6 over all areas.

   Child sitting—percuss/vibrate over front apices.

   Child lying supine—percuss/vibrate between the clavicles and the nipples. (See Figs. 41.1 and 41.2)

   Child propped at a 30° angle—percuss/vibrate on the upper back. (See Fig. 41.3)

   Child lying on the side, head down—percuss/vibrate over the nipple area. (See Figs. 41.4 and 41.5) Repeat on opposite side.

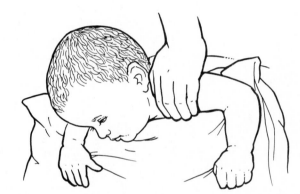

FIGURE 41.3 *Draining posterior segments of the upper lobe.*

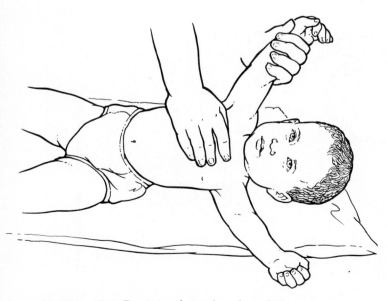

FIGURE 41.4 *Draining lateral and medial segments of the middle lobe.*

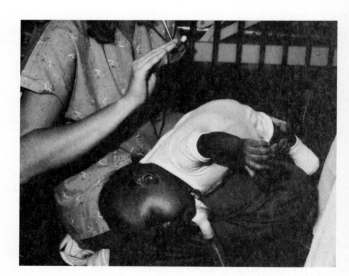

FIGURE 41.5 *Draining lateral and medial segments of the middle lobe.*

121

Child lying prone, head down—percuss/vibrate on both sides below the scapula. (See Fig. 41.6)

Child lying on the side, head down—percuss/vibrate over the lower ribs beneath the axilla. (See Fig. 41.7) Repeat on opposite side.

Child lying prone, head down—percuss/vibrate over the lower ribs. Repeat on opposite side.

Child lying prone, head down; turn body slightly—percuss/vibrate over the lower ribs. (See Fig. 41.8)

8. Ask the child to cough or suction as necessary to clear secretions.

9. Perform posttreatment respiratory assessment.

DOCUMENTATION

- Date and time.
- Length of treatment.
- Child's response.
- Respiratory assessment pre- and posttreatment.

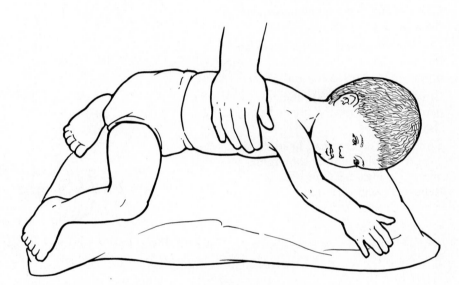

FIGURE 41.6 *Draining anterior basal segments of the lower lobe.*

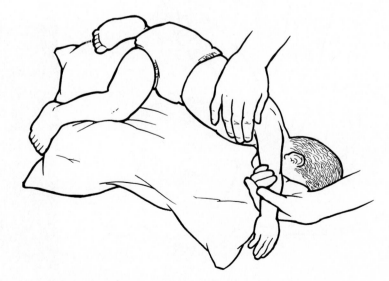

FIGURE 41.7 *Draining superior segments of the lower lobe.*

POTENTIAL RELATED NURSING DIAGNOSES

Airway clearance, ineffective

Gas exchange, impaired

Injury: *high risk*

POTENTIAL RELATED MEDICAL DIAGNOSES

Cystic fibrosis

Pneumonia

Bronchopulmonary dysplasia

Pneumocystis

REFERENCES

Fedorovich, C., and Littleton, M. 1990. Chest physiotherapy: Evaluating the effectiveness. *Dimensions of Critical Care Nursing* 9, no. 2: 68–74.

Mott, S., James, S., and Sperhac, A. 1990. *Nursing care of children and families.* Redwood City, Calif.: Addison-Wesley.

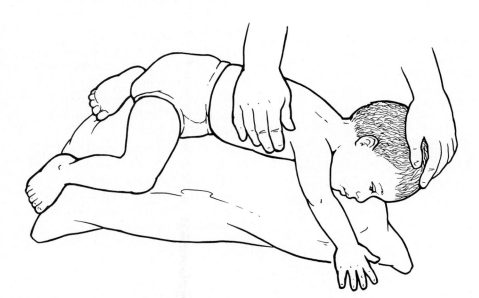

FIGURE 41.8 *Draining posterior basal segments of the lower lobe.*

Chest Tubes to Water-Seal Drainage Systems

Overview

PSYCHOSOCIAL CONSIDERATIONS: Explain the procedure in developmentally appropriate terms. Avoid using terms with mixed meanings, such as *suctioning out fluid or water*. The child may be afraid of losing all fluid from the body.

TIME: Varies

PURPOSE

To maintain proper functioning of chest tubes for optimal evacuation of air, fluid, and/or blood from the chest cavity.

OBJECTIVES

- To maintain inflation of the lungs.
- To prevent injury.

NOTE For Equipment, Essential Steps, Documentation, and Skills Checklists, see procedures (following) for Insertion, Culture Collection, Maintenance, and Removal.

- Check for informed consent.
- The physician should write "to water seal" or specify the amount of suction to apply in cm of water (for example, -20 cm H_2O).
- The physician should order a stat chest x-ray following insertion.
- The physician should order milking and/or stripping, and the frequency. Do not milk or strip the soft, silastic chest tube. Use the yellow latex drainage tubing for this purpose. This is a controversial procedure and should be done per the physician's plan of care.
- Keep vaseline gauze, tube occluding forceps, 4″ × 4″ gauze, and adhesive tape with the child.
- Do not elevate the drainage system above the level of the insertion site unless it is clamped.
- Clamp the chest tube only if raising the drainage system above the level of insertion or if there is a break or leak in the closed system. This is controversial and should be done only per the physician's plan of care.

- Do not allow the suction control tubing to be obstructed or occluded at any time.
- Monitor fluid movement in the drainage system.

POTENTIAL RELATED NURSING DIAGNOSES

Infection: *high risk*

Gas exchange, impaired

Breathing pattern, ineffective

Anxiety

Fear

Injury: *high risk*

POTENTIAL RELATED MEDICAL DIAGNOSES

Cardiothoracic surgery

Pneumothorax

Flail chest

Pneumonia

REFERENCES

Connor, P. 1987. When and how do you use a Heimlich flutter valve? *AJN* 87: 288–90.

Mott, S., James, S., and Sperhac, A. 1990. *Nursing care of children and families.* Redwood City, Calif.: Addison-Wesley.

Skills Checklist

Chest Tube Insertion

☐ Prepare the child and family. Check for informed consent.

☐ Premedicate, if applicable.

☐ Assemble the equipment.

☐ Wash hands.

☐ Assess the child's respiratory status.

☐ Prepare the drainage system.

☐ Assist the physician with insertion.

☐ Connect the drainage catheter to the collection system.

☐ Tape the tube connection.

☐ Assist the physician in dressing the site.

☐ Secure the chest drainage tube.

☐ Assess the child's respiratory status.

☐ Document

Culture Collection

☐ Prepare the child and family.

☐ Assemble the equipment.

☐ Wash hands.

☐ Clean the drainage tube with a povidone-iodine swab or alcohol swab.

☐ Obtain the sample.

☐ Send the specimen to the lab.

☐ Document.

Maintenance

☐ Prepare the child and family.

☐ Assemble the equipment.

☐ Wash hands.

☐ Assess the insertion site, connections, and water level.

☐ Add sterile H_2O to the water-seal container as needed.

☐ Empty or replace the collection system, as needed.

☐ Milk and/or strip the chest tube per the physician's plan of care.

☐ Assess breath sounds.

☐ Document.

Removal

☐ Prepare the child and family.

☐ Assemble the equipment.

☐ Wash hands and put on gloves.

☐ Position the child.

☐ Prepare petroleum gauze or povidone-iodine ointment on sterile gauze.

☐ Assist the physician in dressing the wound.

☐ Measure drainage.

☐ Assess the child's respiratory status.

☐ Document.

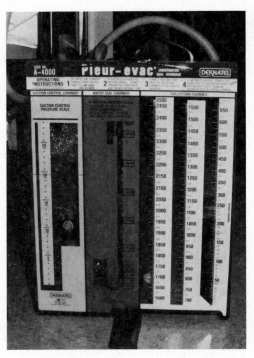

FIGURE 42.1 Pleur-evac drainage system.

Insertion

Also see Overview.

EQUIPMENT

Medication, if appropriate

One of the following chest tube drainage systems:

> Pleur-evac (neonatal or pedia/adult) (see Fig. 42.1)

> 90 ml one- to three-bottle underwater drainage set (see Figs. 42.2, 42.3, and 42.4)

> Emerson pump

Water (H_2O), sterile

Chest tube tray, including a trocar, suture scissors, hemostats, a needle holder, drapes, towels, syringes, needles of various sizes, a stopcock, a knife handle and blades, a 4″ × 4″ gauze, a medicine cup, a Y connector, and forceps

Radiopaque thoracic catheter (size designated by physician)

Povidone-iodine solution

Gloves, sterile

Gowns and masks (optional), sterile

1% xylocaine

Suture with needle

Cable tie gun (optional)

Tube occluding forceps

Safety pin and rubber band (optional)

Heimlich valve, used primarily for transporting a child (see Fig. 42.5)

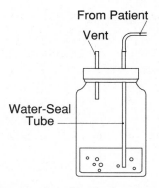

FIGURE 42.2 One-bottle drainage system.

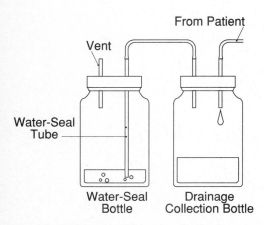

FIGURE 42.3 Two-bottle drainage system.

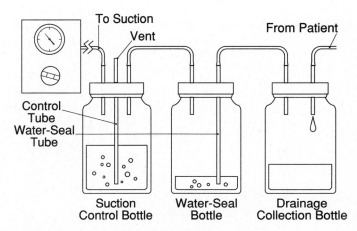

FIGURE 42.4 Three-bottle drainage system.

ESSENTIAL STEPS

1. Prepare the child and family. Administer premedication, as appropriate.

2. Assemble the equipment.

3. Wash hands and assess the child's respiratory status.

4. Prepare the drainage system.

   For Pleur-evac *or* a 90 ml one- to three-bottle underwater drainage set, refer to package insert instructions.

   For the Emerson pump:

   Fill the marked bottle to cover the ends of the tubes with sterile H_2O.

   Mark the initial fluid level on a piece of tape along the bottle.

   Attach packaged tubing.

   Apply 1″ tape to connections.

   If the child has one chest tube, place a stopper in one of the suction tubings on the Emerson.

5. Assist the physician with insertion of the chest tube: Open sterile packages, help the child remain still, comfort the child, and so on. (See Fig. 42.6)

6. Connect the drainage catheter to the water-seal collecting system or to the suction tubing on the Emerson.

7. Tape the tube connection or secure the connection using a cable tie gun (adjustable-tension installing tool).

8. Assist the physician with dressing the site.

9. Secure the chest drainage tube to a sheet or gown by using a tube occluding forceps or safety pin and rubber band.

10. Assess the child's respiratory status.

DOCUMENTATION

- Premedication given, if appropriate.
- Type of drainage system used.
- Size and location of tube.
- Amount, color, and consistency of any drainage.
- Functioning of drainage system:

  Emerson—presence of bubbling, which signifies air leak.

  Pleur-evac—presence of bubbling, which signifies proper functioning.

- Assessment of the child pre- and postprocedure, including vital signs, respiratory status, and color.

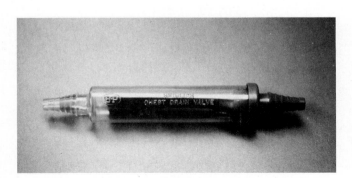

FIGURE 42.5 *Heimlich valve.*

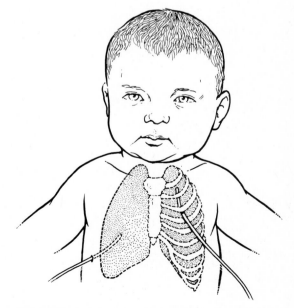

FIGURE 42.6 *Placement of chest tubes.*

Culture Collection

Also see Overview.

EQUIPMENT

Povidone-iodine swab *or* alcohol swab
25g needle
5 ml syringe

ESSENTIAL STEPS

1. Prepare the child and family.
2. Assemble the equipment.
3. Wash hands.
4. Clean the area of drainage tubing as close to the chest tube connection as possible with a povidone-iodine swab or alcohol swab. Allow to dry.
5. Pierce the prepped area with a needle and withdraw a sample (3 to 5 ml).
6. Remove the needle from the syringe using a passive technique, such as hemostat. Cap the syringe.
7. Label the specimen. Place it in a plastic bag and send it to the laboratory.

DOCUMENTATION

- Time specimen obtained.
- That specimen was sent to lab.

Maintenance

Also see Overview.

EQUIPMENT

Water (H_2O), sterile
Lubricant: alcohol wipe, antiseptic foam, or hand lotion (optional, to decrease friction when stripping the tube)

ESSENTIAL STEPS

1. Prepare the child and family.
2. Assemble the equipment.
3. Wash hands.
4. Check the insertion site, connections, and water level at least every 2 to 4 hours.
5. Add sterile water to water-seal container as needed. Clamp the chest tube (briefly) while refilling the water-seal bottle (not necessary with the Pleur-evac system).
6. Empty or replace the collection system per directions.
7. Milk and/or strip the chest tube per the physician's plan of care.

   Milk only the latex (yellow) portion of the tube by placing several fan folds (8″ to 12″) of the tubing in the palm of one hand *or* by alternating hand compressions down the length of the latex tubing. Repeat as necessary.

Strip the chest tube by using one hand to pinch the latex tube, holding the tube firmly, and using the other hand to firmly compress the tubing between the thumb and forefinger. Slide the thumb and finger 8″ to 12″ down the tube. A small amount of water-soluble lubricant (an alcohol wipe, antiseptic foam, or hand lotion) may be used to facilitate stripping. Repeat as necessary.

8. Assess breath sounds with each set of vital signs and after stripping and/or milking.

DOCUMENTATION

- Amount, color, and consistency of any drainage from the chest tube.
- Child's pulmonary status.
- Presence or absence of air leak. If possible, provide a rough estimation of leak (such as "4 to 5 bubbles per minute").
- Any milking and/or stripping performed.

Removal

Also see Overview.

EQUIPMENT

Gloves, nonsterile

Suture removal set

Petroleum gauze *or* povidone-iodine ointment

Gauze, sterile

2″ adhesive or microfoam tape

1. Prepare the child and family.
2. Assemble the equipment.
3. Wash hands and put on gloves.
4. Position the child with the chest tube site up or as directed by the physician.
5. Ask a child who is old enough to take a deep breath and hold it. Instruct the child to yell as loudly as possible while the physician simultaneously pulls out the chest tube. This prevents air from entering the pleural cavity. Prepare petroleum gauze or povidone-iodine ointment on a sterile gauze for the physician to place over the chest tube site as the tube is removed. (See Fig. 42.7)
6. Assist the physician in dressing the wound.
7. Measure the amount of drainage in the collection chamber or bottle.
8. Discard the disposable collection system.
9. Assess breath sounds immediately after removal and with each set of vital signs.
10. Chest x-ray per the physician's plan of care.

DOCUMENTATION

- Time chest tube removed.
- Dressing to site.
- Amount of drainage prior to discarding collection system.
- Assessment of child.

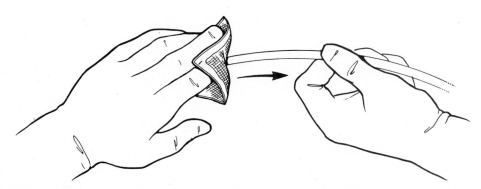

FIGURE 42.7 *Removing a chest tube and applying an occlusive dressing.*

43 Circumcision Care

1. Prepare the child and family.
2. Assemble the equipment.
3. Wash hands and put on gloves.
4. Inspect the site. A petroleum jelly gauze should be wrapped loosely around the penis to prevent the diaper from sticking.
5. Gently clean around glans with a 4″ × 4″ gauze moistened with sterile water or normal saline. (See Fig. 43.1)
6. Apply pressure to the site if excessive bleeding occurs.
7. Replace the petroleum jelly gauze if soiled with stool. (See Fig. 43.2)
8. Apply a diaper loosely and place the child on the side.
9. Monitor voiding, adequacy of stream.

PSYCHOSOCIAL CONSIDERATIONS: The neonatal response during this procedure is to pain and cold. Take the child to the parent for comforting following the procedure. If parents are not present, comfort the child.

TIME: 3 to 5 minutes

PURPOSE

To provide care to the circumcision site.

OBJECTIVES

• To reduce risk for infection.
• To prevent injury or trauma.

EQUIPMENT

Gloves, nonsterile

4″ × 4″ gauze *or* strip of gauze

Water or normal saline (0.9% sodium chloride)

Petroleum jelly gauze, if applicable

SAFETY ISSUES

• **Assess for bleeding from the penis.**
• **Do not use petroleum jelly if the circumcision was performed with a plastibell.**

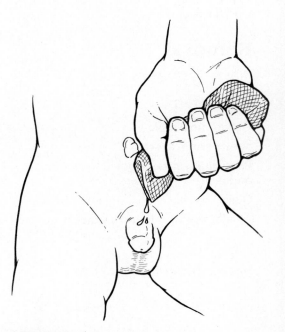

FIGURE 43.1 *Cleaning the penis.*

DOCUMENTATION

- Urine output.
- Description of urinary stream.
- Appearance of penis and any bleeding noted.
- That petroleum jelly gauze was applied, if appropriate.

POTENTIAL RELATED NURSING DIAGNOSES

Skin integrity, impaired

Pain, acute

POTENTIAL RELATED MEDICAL DIAGNOSES

Infection

Circumcision

REFERENCES

Olds, S., London, M., and Ladewig, P. 1988. *Maternal-newborn nursing.* Menlo Park, Calif.: Addison-Wesley.

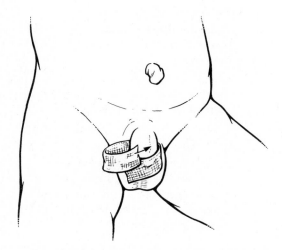

FIGURE 43.2 *Applying petroleum jelly to the penis.*

44 Cooling/Warming Blanket

PSYCHOSOCIAL CONSIDERATIONS: Explain the procedure in developmentally appropriate terms. Children with high fevers may be confused; therefore, explanations should be simple and clear. Children may fear that they may die if their fever becomes too high.

TIME: Varies

PURPOSE

To increase or decrease the body temperature.

OBJECTIVES

- To increase or decrease the body temperature.
- To prevent injury and trauma.

EQUIPMENT

Blanketrol machine (refer to machine instructions; see Figs. 44.1 and 44.2)
Distilled water
Blanketrol blanket

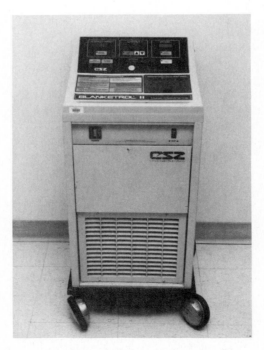

FIGURE 44.1 *Cooling/warming machine.*

- Record the temperature and skin condition before placing the child on Blanketrol, 30 minutes after starting Blanketrol, and at least every 2 hours during the procedure. Record temperature 30 minutes and again 1 hour after discontinuation of Blanketrol.
- The Blanketrol blanket may be disposable. If nondisposable, clean appropriately after use.

ESSENTIAL STEPS

1. Prepare the child and family.
2. Assemble the equipment.

   Ensure that the Blanketrol switch is in the off position.

   Fill the Blanketrol reservoir to the designated level with distilled water.

   Place the Blanketrol blanket on the bed. Connect the Blanketrol to the blanket.

   Check for water leaks in the blanket-hose-machine system by turning the switch to on.

   Cover the Blanketrol blanket with a bed sheet.

   Set the temperature of the circulating water and monitor the actual temperature indicated on the machine. (See the instructions for a particular model.)

3. To cool the child:

Assess the temperature and skin condition.

Protect the hands and feet to prevent peripheral vasoconstriction.

Turn the child frequently. Assess skin integrity and perfusion status.

If shivering occurs, turn the Blanketrol off, take the child's temperature, and contact the physician before resuming cooling.

Turn off the Blanketrol upon reaching the desired effect.

4. To warm the child:

Assess the temperature and skin condition.

Turn the child frequently. Assess skin integrity and perfusion status.

Turn the warming blanket off upon reaching the desired effect.

DOCUMENTATION

- Start time.
- Serial temperatures and skin condition.
- Child's response.
- Completion time.

POTENTIAL RELATED NURSING DIAGNOSES

Hyperthermia

Skin integrity, impaired: *high risk*

Injury: *high risk*

Hypothermia

POTENTIAL RELATED MEDICAL DIAGNOSES

Sepsis

Central nervous system disorder

Hypothermia

REFERENCES

Mott, S., James, S., and Sperhac, A. 1990. *Nursing care of children and families.* Redwood City, Calif.: Addison-Wesley.

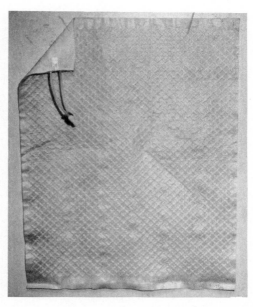

FIGURE 44.2 *Blanket for cooling/warming.*

45 Cord Care

Triple dye, alcohol swab, *or* povidone-iodine swab

Cotton-tip applicators (for use with triple dye only)

PSYCHOSOCIAL CONSIDERATIONS: The solution applied to the cord may feel cold to the infant. Comfort by cuddling after the procedure.

TIME: 2 to 3 minutes

PURPOSE

To provide care to the umbilical cord to reduce risk for infection.

OBJECTIVES

• To reduce risk for infection.

ESSENTIAL STEPS

1. Prepare the child and family. Inform parents that triple dye may stain the skin but will eventually fade.
2. Assemble the equipment.
3. Wash hands.
4. Inspect the area around the cord. Obtain a culture if drainage is present, per institution policy.
5. Clean the base of the cord with triple dye or alcohol or povidone-iodine at least two to three times per day. (See Fig. 45.1)
6. Keep diapers turned down off of the cord. (See Fig. 45.2)

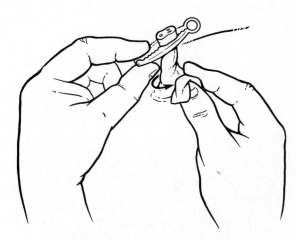

FIGURE 45.1 *Cleaning the umbilical cord.*

DOCUMENTATION

- Appearance of the cord and surrounding skin.
- Cord care given.

POTENTIAL RELATED NURSING DIAGNOSES

Infection: *high risk*

POTENTIAL RELATED MEDICAL DIAGNOSES

Infection

REFERENCES

Mott, S., James, S., and Sperhac, A. 1990. *Nursing care of children and families.* Redwood City, Calif.: Addison-Wesley.

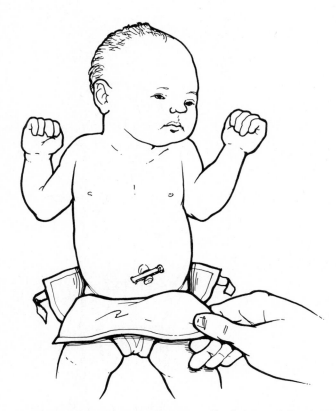

FIGURE 45.2 *Turning diapers off of the umbilical cord.*

46 Crutch Walking

PSYCHOSOCIAL CONSIDERATIONS: Explain the procedure in developmentally appropriate terms. Avoid terms with mixed meanings. Children range from being fearful of falling to having little sense of need for beginning cautiously. Provide safety during initial attempts. Decorating crutches can help the child feel less different, but make sure that decorations do not become a safety hazard.

TIME: Limit each session to 10 minutes and repeat several times if necessary

PURPOSE

To provide a means of walking without weight bearing.

OBJECTIVES

• To facilitate walking.
• To prevent trauma or injury.

EQUIPMENT

Crutches

ESSENTIAL STEPS

1. Prepare the child and family.
2. Assemble the equipment.
3. Fit the crutches.

   Measure the crutches with the child standing erect, elbows flexed 20° to 30° and crutches 15 cm anterolateral from the toes. Two fingers should insert easily between the axilla and the top of the crutch. (See Fig. 46.1)

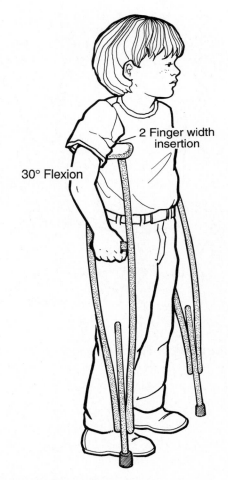

FIGURE 46.1 *Measuring crutches.*

If the child is in a supine position, measure from the anterior fold of the axilla to a point 10 cm lateral from the heel of the foot.

4. Teach the child to walk, using

A two-point gait. Move the right crutch and the left leg together, then the left crutch and the right leg together. (See Fig. 46.2)

A three-point gait. Move both crutches 6″ to 8″ with the affected leg and then bear weight on the crutches while moving the unaffected leg. (See Fig. 46.3)

Skills Checklist

☐ Prepare the child and family for each session.
☐ Assemble the equipment.
☐ Provide for safety.
☐ Fit the crutches.
☐ Teach the child to walk with crutches.
☐ Help the child learn to go upstairs.
☐ Help the child learn to go downstairs.
☐ Help the child sit in a chair.
☐ Help the child rise from a chair.
☐ Document.

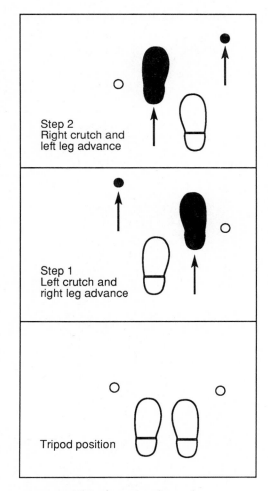

FIGURE 46.2 *A two-point gait.*

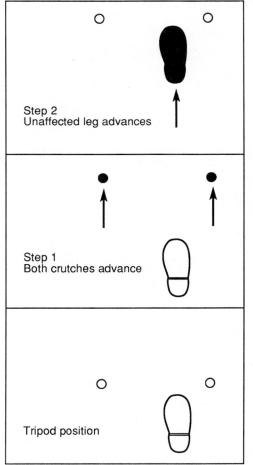

FIGURE 46.3 *A three-point gait.*

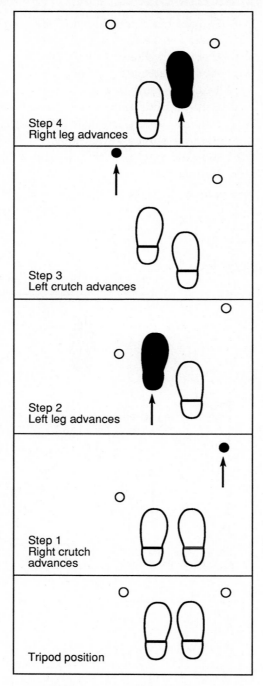

FIGURE 46.4 *A four-point gait.*

A four-point gait. Move the right crutch, the left foot, the left crutch, and the right foot. (See Fig. 46.4)

5. Teach the child to go upstairs.

Place the unaffected leg on the step.

Carefully raise the affected leg and crutches to that step.

6. Teach the child to go downstairs.

Place the crutches on the lower step.

Carefully bring the unaffected leg to the lower step, followed by the affected leg.

7. Teach the child to sit in a chair:

Brace the chair against the wall.

Place the unaffected leg against the seat of the chair.

Shift both crutches to the affected side and hold by the hand grips.

Grasp the arm of the chair with the hand on the unaffected side.

Lean forward, flex the knee on the unaffected side, and lower self into the chair.

8. To rise from a chair, the child should

Place the crutches on the outside of both feet.

Place hands on the hand grips of the crutches.

Push down on the hand grips while standing.

DOCUMENTATION

- Instructions given.
- Child's response.

POTENTIAL RELATED NURSING DIAGNOSES

Activity intolerance: *high risk*

Body image disturbance

Mobility, impaired physical

Injury: *high risk*

POTENTIAL RELATED MEDICAL DIAGNOSES

Fracture

Muscle weakness

Trauma

Cellulitis

REFERENCES

Mott, S., James, S., and Sperhac, A. 1990. *Nursing care of children and families.* Redwood City, Calif.: Addison-Wesley.

Swearingen, P. 1991. *Photo-atlas of nursing procedures 2E.* Redwood City, Calif.: Addison-Wesley.

Dialysis: Hemodialysis Accesses, Care, and Maintenance

PSYCHOSOCIAL CONSIDERATIONS: Explain the procedure in developmentally appropriate terms. Avoid using terms with mixed meanings, such as *stick* and *remove blood*. Answer questions honestly.

TIME: 10 minutes

PURPOSE

To ensure patency of the access.

To decrease the risk of infection and/or bleeding.

OBJECTIVES

- To maintain hemodialysis access.
- To prevent infection.

EQUIPMENT

For grafts and fistulas (see Figs. 47.1, 47.2, and 47.3):

Stethoscope

H_2O_2 *or* sterile normal saline (0.9% sodium chloride)

Tape and 4″ x 4″ gauze *or* clear occlusive dressing

Adhesive bandages (postdialysis)

Ice compress, if applicable

Gloves, nonsterile, if applicable

For femoral lines:

Central line dressing kit

½″ adhesive or foam tape

Heparin: 1 unit/ml for continuous drip *or* 10 units/ml for manual flush (units/ml for manual flush vary from 10 to 100, per institution policy)

Smooth-edge clamps

S SAFETY ISSUES

- Assess fistulas and grafts every 1 to 2 hours during the first 24 hours after surgery and every 2 to 4 hours thereafter, or per the physician's plan of care.
- Blood drawing or IV starts should be restricted from the fistula or graft extremity.

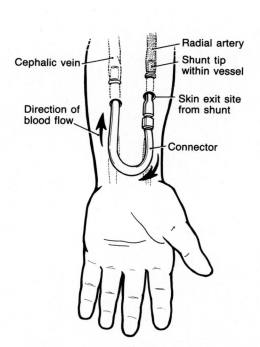

FIGURE 47.1 *Looped graft.*

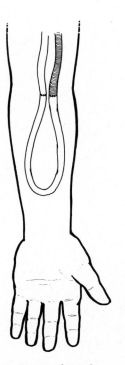

FIGURE 47.2 *Looped graft.*

- Generally, do not take blood pressures on the graft/fistula extremity.
- Generally, change the dressing on all new accesses *(first 7 postop days)* daily, except when a clear occlusive dressing has been used. Thereafter, change the dressings three times per week.
- Normal saline may be used instead of hydrogen peroxide (H_2O_2) because H_2O_2 may damage tissue.

ESSENTIAL STEPS

1. Prepare the child and family.
2. Assemble the equipment.
3. Wash hands.
4. For grafts and fistulas,

   Perform immediate postoperative care.

   Check for the presence of a palpable thrill and an audible bruit.

   Notify the physician if a thrill or bruit is not present.

   Clean the suture line with H_2O_2.

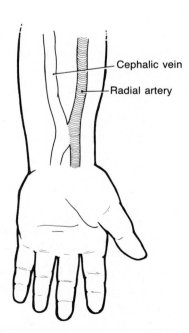

FIGURE 47.3 *Arteriovenous fistula.*

Cephalic vein

Radial artery

Skills Checklist

Grafts and Fistulas: Immediate Postoperative Care
☐ Prepare the child and family.
☐ Assemble the equipment.
☐ Wash hands.
☐ Check for a thrill and bruit.
☐ Clean the suture line.
☐ Wrap a loose dressing around the extremity.
☐ Elevate the graft/fistula extremity above heart level.
☐ Instruct the child in exercise techniques for fistulas, if applicable.
☐ Document.

Grafts and Fistulas: Routine Care
☐ Prepare the child and family.
☐ Assemble the equipment.
☐ Wash hands.
☐ Check for a thrill and bruit.
☐ Keep the graft/fistula site clean.
☐ Position the child to avoid lying on or exerting pressure on the extremity with the graft or fistula.
☐ Document.

Grafts and Fistulas: Postdialysis Care
☐ Prepare the child and family.
☐ Assemble the equipment.
☐ Wash hands.
☐ Place and maintain a bandage over venipuncture sites for a minimum of 4 hours after dialysis.
☐ Control mild pain and hematoma with an ice compress.
☐ Check thrill and bruit.
☐ Document.

Femoral Lines
☐ Prepare the child and family.
☐ Assemble the equipment.
☐ Wash hands.
☐ Change the dressing, if applicable.
☐ Flush the line with a heparin IV infusion or manual heparin flush, whichever is applicable.
☐ Instruct the child.
☐ Document.

Apply gauze and tape or a clear occlusive dressing over the site.

Elevate gortex grafts and fistulas above the child's heart level until the postop edema subsides.

Instruct a child with a fistula that exercise may be required for the development of a mature access. (See "Exercise Schedule for Arteriovenous Fistulas," following.)

When mature, routinely:

Check for the presence of a thrill and bruit every shift.

Notify the physician immediately if either is unobtainable. (The graft may be declotted if the problem is identified early.)

Keep the graft/fistula site clean.

Do not allow the child to lie on the graft or fistula. Avoid positions that exert pressure on the extremity with the graft or fistula.

Postdialysis:

Keep venipuncture sites bandaged for a minimum of 4 hours after dialysis.

Use an ice compress to alleviate mild pain and for immediate control of a hematoma at the puncture site(s).

Check thrill and bruit every 1 to 2 hours two times after each dialysis treatment.

If bleeding from the puncture site occurs, put on gloves and apply firm, direct pressure with a 4″ × 4″ gauze. While applying pressure, be sure that the thrill can be palpated and the bruit can be auscultated. The graft may clot if pressure is too constricting. If bleeding persists for more than 15 minutes, call the physician.

Notify the physician if any redness, heat, or swelling develops along the graft or fistula.

5. For femoral lines (Shaldon Catheter—9¾″ in length):

Change the dressing. (Refer to "Central Venous Catheter: Dressing Change.")

Take care not to accidentally remove or dislodge the catheter. It may *not* be sutured in place.

Using ½″ adhesive or foam tape, secure the catheter to the skin distal to the dressing. Take care not to tape across or to obstruct the 1″ clamping area.

Flush the line.

For a continuous IV drip,

The usual concentration of heparin used is 1 unit/ml added to the solution of choice per the physician's plan of care.

Run the drip at a keep-vein-open (KVO) rate or per the physician's plan of care.

For a manual flush,

Femoral lines hold 5 to 6 ml. Flush with 10 ml of heparinized solution.

The usual concentration of heparin is 10 units/ml.

Perform every 8 hours if no continuous drip is infusing.

Instruct the child/family on the following:

The child will be restricted to bedrest while this catheter is in place.

The child must keep the leg straight.

The child may not raise the head of the bed above 30°.

DOCUMENTATION

- Type, location, and appearance of access site.
- Presence of thrill and bruit, if applicable.
- If access is a femoral line:

Fluid infusing and rate of infusion.

Heparin concentration and amount each time a flush done.

Client Teaching

Exercise Schedule for Arteriovenous Fistulas

To make sure that a new arteriovenous (A.V.) fistula works well and to make veins bigger, stronger, and easier to find, exercise the fistula as described here unless it hurts a lot or unless a doctor says to stop.

1. *Days 5, 6, and 7* after the operation: Place a heating pad on the new fistula for 10 minutes before beginning each exercise. With the heating pad still on, start squeezing a rubber ball or tennis ball for 15 minutes four times each day. *Always* use the heating pad before and during exercises.

2. *Day 8:* Tie a tourniquet *above* the fistula for 1 minute. With the tourniquet on, squeeze the ball for 1 minute. Remove the tourniquet and continue to squeeze the ball for 14 more minutes. Do this exercise four times today. (The tourniquet should *not* be so tight that it stops the pulse in the fistula. A tight feeling or redness of the skin below the tourniquet may occur.)

3. *Day 9:* Exercise for 3 minutes with the tourniquet on and 12 minutes without the tourniquet. Do this four times today.

4. *Day 10:* Exercise for 5 minutes with the tourniquet on and 10 minutes without the tourniquet. Do this four times today.

5. *Day 11:* Continue to exercise as on Day 10 four times each day, until the nurse or doctor tells you to stop.

Cleaning the Fistula

1. Once home, clean the fistula every day. Clean with 4″ × 4″ gauzes and peroxide until old blood is gone. The doctor or nurse will remove the stitches when the fistula is healed.

2. After the fistula has healed, no special cleaning is needed. Wash the arm or leg well when taking a bath or shower.

Remember

1. Do not wear tight clothes on an arm or leg with a fistula.

2. No blood pressures can be taken on an arm or leg with a fistula except by dialysis staff.

3. No blood is to be drawn from the arm or leg with the fistula except by dialysis staff.

SOURCE: Children's Medical Center of Dallas, 1990, *Policy and procedures manual* (Dallas, Tex.: Children's Medical Center).

- Signs of redness, swelling, drainage, or tenderness along graft or fistula or at exit sites, and the name of the physician notified.
- Dressing change or if the dressing is reinforced.

POTENTIAL RELATED NURSING DIAGNOSES

Skin integrity, impaired

Infection: *high risk*

Trauma: *high risk*

POTENTIAL RELATED MEDICAL DIAGNOSES

Infection

Hemorrhage

Shunt malfunction

REFERENCES

Mott, S., James, S., and Sperhac, A. 1990. *Nursing care of children and families.* Redwood City, Calif.: Addison-Wesley.

48 Dialysis: Peritoneal

PSYCHOSOCIAL CONSIDERATIONS: Explain the procedure in developmentally appropriate terms. Avoid using terms with mixed meanings, such as *put water or fluid into your stomach*. Children sometimes fear that they will "explode." Provide appropriate activities when the child must remain quiet for long periods of time.

TIME: Varies

PURPOSE

To remove waste products using the peritoneum as the filtering membrane and to restore homeostasis.

OBJECTIVES

- To filter waste products from the body.
- To prevent injury and trauma.

EQUIPMENT

Manual Peritoneal Dialysis

Warming pad

Tubing (may need volumetric set if exchange volume is small)

Dialysate

Clamps

Drainage bag

Timer

Continuous Cycling Peritoneal Dialysis (CCPD)

Dialysate

Dialysis cycler

Tubing

Drainage bag(s)

Continuous Ambulatory Peritoneal Dialysis (CAPD)

Warming pad

Dialysate

Tubing

Clamp

 SAFETY ISSUES

- **Monitor the child for signs and symptoms of peritonitis.**
- **Dialysate must be warmed. Cold fluid can cause hypothermia and cramping.**
- **Do not use a microwave to warm dialysate as the fluid temperature can get too hot and the chemical composition of the dialysate may change.**

ESSENTIAL STEPS

Manual Peritoneal Dialysis (see Fig. 48.1)

1. Prepare the child and family.
2. Obtain weight.
3. Assemble the equipment.
4. Warm the dialysate to body temperature (may use a warming pad).
5. Wash hands.
6. Obtain baseline vital signs.
7. Attach tubing to dialysate and prime the line. Clamp the tubing.
8. Connect the tubing to the dialysis catheter using sterile technique.
9. Connect the drainage bag to the outflow circuit, maintaining sterile technique. Clamp the tubing. The drainage bag should be approximately 36″ below the child.
10. For inflow:

    Open the inflow tubing.

    Infuse dialysate into the abdomen. (The process takes 5 to 15 minutes.)

    Clamp the inflow tubing after infusing dialysate.

    Normally, infuse 15 to 30 ml/kg of dialysate per cycle.
11. For dwell time:

    The dialysate remains in the abdomen approximately 30 minutes.

    Set the timer.
12. Outflow:

    Unclamp the drainage tubing.

    Allow drainage. (The process takes 10 to 15 minutes.)

    The amount of drainage should at least equal the amount of inflow. The child may need to be repositioned several times to facilitate drainage of dialysate.
13. The process may be continued.
14. Monitor vital signs and weight per the physician's plan of care.

Skills Checklist

- ☐ Prepare the child and family. Obtain weight.
- ☐ Assemble the equipment. Warm the dialysate if not using a cycler.
- ☐ Wash hands.
- ☐ Obtain baseline vital signs.
- ☐ Attach tubing to the dialysate and prime the line. Clamp the tubing.
- ☐ Connect tubing to the dialysis catheter using sterile technique.
- ☐ Connect the drainage bag to the outflow circuit, using sterile technique (except in CAPD). Clamp the tubing.
- ☐ Infuse dialysate.
- ☐ Dwell.
- ☐ Drain dialysate.
- ☐ Monitor vital signs and weight.
- ☐ Document.

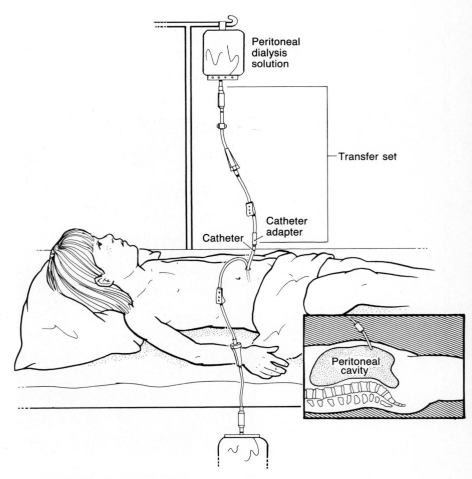

FIGURE 48.1 *Manual peritoneal dialysis.*

Continuous Cycling Peritoneal Dialysis

1. Prepare the child and family. Typically, this procedure is done at night.
2. Obtain weight.
3. Assemble the equipment.
4. Wash hands.
5. Obtain baseline vital signs.
6. Connect bags of dialysate to dialysis cycler, following manufacturer's instructions. (See Fig. 48.2)
7. Connect tubing to dialysis catheter using sterile technique.
8. Connect drainage bag(s) to outflow tubing using sterile technique.
9. Set the machine for appropriate inflow amount and dwell and outflow times.
10. Monitor vital signs and weight, per the physician's plan of care.

Continuous Ambulatory Peritoneal Dialysis

1. Prepare the child and family.
2. Obtain weight.
3. Assemble the equipment.
4. Warm the dialysate to body temperature (may use warming pad).
5. Wash hands.
6. Obtain baseline vital signs.
7. Attach tubing to dialysate and prime the line. Clamp the tubing.
8. Connect the tubing to the dialysis catheter using sterile technique.
9. Infuse dialysate. Clamp the tubing. Roll up the bag and attach to the abdomen or place in a pocket. (See Fig. 48.3)
10. Allow dialysate to remain in the peritoneal cavity for at least 4 to 6 hours.
11. Unroll the bag and place approximately 36″ below the child. (See Fig. 48.4)

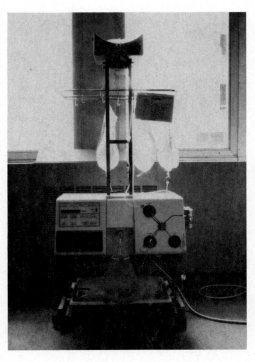

FIGURE 48.2 *Continuous cycling peritoneal dialysis machine.*

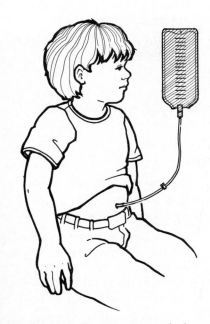

FIGURE 48.3 *Continuous ambulatory peritoneal dialysis: inflow.*

12. Unclamp the tubing and drain the dialysate.

13. Monitor vital signs and weight per the physician's plan of care.

DOCUMENTATION

- Date and time.
- Weight and vital signs.
- Amount and type of dialysate.
- Amount of dwell time.
- Color and amount of outflow.

POTENTIAL RELATED NURSING DIAGNOSES

Infection: *high risk*

Injury: *high risk*

Tissue perfusion, altered, renal

Skin integrity, impaired: *high risk*

Anxiety

Fear

Fluid volume deficit: *high risk*

Fluid volume excess

Pain, acute

POTENTIAL RELATED MEDICAL DIAGNOSES

Glomerulonephritis

Nephrosis

Renal failure, acute

Renal failure, chronic

REFERENCES

Mott, S., James, S., and Sperhac, A. 1990.
Nursing care of children and families.
Redwood City, Calif.: Addison-Wesley.

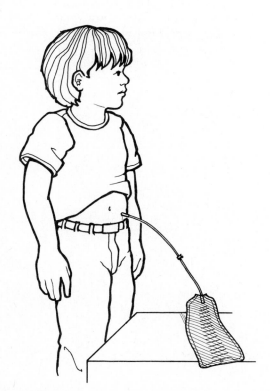

FIGURE 48.4 *Continuous ambulatory peritoneal dialysis: outflow.*

49 Dialysis: Peritoneal Catheter Care

- Monitor the child for signs and symptoms of peritonitis.

PSYCHOSOCIAL CONSIDERATIONS: Explain the procedure in developmentally appropriate terms, such as *this helps to clean the area around your tube.* Allow the child to vent feelings.

TIME: 5 to 10 minutes

PURPOSE

To reduce the risk for local infection at the exit site.

OBJECTIVES

- To clean the catheter site.
- To reduce the risk for infection at the catheter site.

EQUIPMENT

Gloves, sterile

Three povidone-iodine swabs *or* alcohol swabs

Hydrogen peroxide (H_2O_2) *or* normal saline (0.9% sodium chloride), sterile, if needed

Povidone-iodine ointment, if needed

Alcohol swab, if needed

Split 2″ × 2″ gauze *or* folded 4″ × 4″ gauze

Tape

Applicators, sterile, if needed

ESSENTIAL STEPS

1. Prepare the child and family.
2. Assemble the equipment.
3. Wash hands.
4. Remove the old dressing.
5. Examine the exit site for redness, swelling, tenderness, or drainage. Gently palpate the area where the catheter "tunnels" under the skin and examine for swelling or tenderness. Do not touch the exit site without sterile gloves.
6. Put on gloves.
7. Using aseptic technique, clean the exit site well with povidone-iodine or alcohol swabs. Clean from the exit site outward, using circles around the site, one way only. Do not go back over a previously cleaned area with the same swab. Allow povidone-iodine to dry. For well-healed catheter exit sites, use H_2O_2 to

remove any crusting before cleaning with povidone-iodine swabs. (See Fig. 49.1) (Note: Some institutions may apply povidone-iodine ointment to the exit site and clean the catheter with an alcohol swab, from skin to distal end, prior to applying 2″ × 2″ gauze.)

8. Cover with split 2″ × 2″ or folded 4″ × 4″ gauze and tape. The dressing need not be occlusive. (See Fig. 49.2)

DOCUMENTATION

• Drainage noted on old dressing.
• Condition of exit and "tunnel" sites.

POTENTIAL RELATED NURSING DIAGNOSES

Infection: *high risk*

Tissue integrity, impaired

POTENTIAL RELATED MEDICAL DIAGNOSES

Catheter infection

Renal failure, acute

Renal failure, chronic

Glomerulonephritis

Nephrosis

REFERENCES

Mott, S., Jones, S., and Sperhac, A. 1990. *Nursing care of children and families.* Redwood City, Calif.: Addison-Wesley.

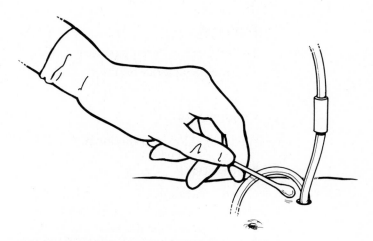

Skills Checklist

- ☐ Prepare the child and family.
- ☐ Assemble the equipment.
- ☐ Wash hands.
- ☐ Remove the old dressing.
- ☐ Examine exit and tunnel sites.
- ☐ Put on gloves.
- ☐ Clean the site.
- ☐ Apply a new dressing.
- ☐ Document.

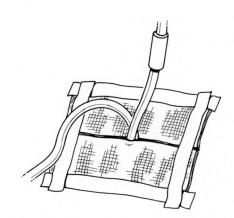

FIGURE 49.1 *Cleaning the catheter site.*

FIGURE 49.2 *Dressing over the catheter site.*

50 Diapering

PSYCHOSOCIAL CONSIDERATIONS: An infant may touch his or her genitalia, a normal developmental response. Males may have erections, also normal. Discuss these issues with parents and explain that these are natural behaviors.

TIME: 3 to 5 minutes

PURPOSE

To place dry material against the skin.

To provide material to absorb urine and/or stool.

OBJECTIVES

• To prevent skin breakdown.

EQUIPMENT

Gloves, nonsterile

Diapers, disposable *or* cloth (from an infection-control standpoint, disposables are preferable in the hospital setting, but they may increase skin irritation)

Washcloth, towel, and soap *or* disposable wipes

Ointment, if needed

Pins, if applicable

SAFETY ISSUES

• Avoid the use of powder; inhalation of powder can cause aspiration pneumonia.
• Cornstarch can increase the risk of fungal infections.
• The use of plastic pants with cloth diapers is controversial. The plastic retains moisture and heat and can increase the risk of skin breakdown.
• Diapers need to be changed frequently.

ESSENTIAL STEPS

1. Prepare the child and family.
2. Assemble the equipment.
3. Wash hands and put on gloves.
4. If using disposable diapers:

   Remove the old diaper.

   Clean the diaper area thoroughly, removing any ointment residue. Pat dry.

   Apply ointment if the diaper area is reddened.

   Apply the diaper and secure with adhesive strips.

   Dispose of the soiled diaper as appropriate.

5. If using cloth diapers:

   Fold the clean diaper according to the infant's shape.

   Remove the old diaper.

   Clean the diaper area thoroughly, removing any ointment residue. Pat dry.

   Apply ointment if the diaper area is reddened.

Apply the diaper. (See Fig. 50.1) When pinning, keep fingers between the pin and the child. (See Fig. 50.2) To protect the bed, use disposable pads or a rubber draw sheet covered by a sheet.

Dispose of the soiled diaper as appropriate.

DOCUMENTATION

- Intake and output (may weigh the diaper).
- Any abnormal color, odor, or consistency of urine and/or stool.
- Skin assessment and application of ointment, as appropriate.

POTENTIAL RELATED NURSING DIAGNOSES

Skin integrity, impaired: *high risk*

Urinary incontinence, functional

Skills Checklist

- ☐ Prepare the child and family.
- ☐ Assemble the equipment.
- ☐ Wash hands and put on gloves.
- ☐ Remove the old diaper.
- ☐ Clean the diaper area and, if needed, apply ointment.
- ☐ Apply the new diaper.
- ☐ Dispose of the soiled diaper.
- ☐ Document.

POTENTIAL RELATED MEDICAL DIAGNOSES

Universal application for infants and children who wear diapers

REFERENCES

Olds, S., London, M., and Ladewig, P. 1988. *Maternal-newborn nursing*. Redwood City, Calif.: Addison-Wesley.

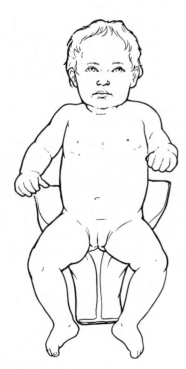

FIGURE 50.1 *Placing the child on the diaper.*

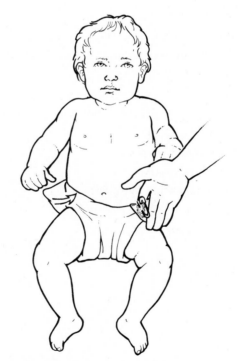

FIGURE 50.2 *Protecting the child from pin sticks.*

51 Drains: Care

- Some institutions use povidone-iodine instead of hydrogen peroxide (H_2O_2) because H_2O_2 may damage tissue.

PSYCHOSOCIAL CONSIDERATIONS: Explain the procedure in developmentally appropriate terms. Avoid using terms with mixed meanings. Children may become frightened at the sight of bloody drainage. Avoid bringing soiled dressings or drains within the child's field of vision if possible.

TIME: 3 to 5 minutes

PURPOSE

To facilitate drainage of fluids from an area of the body.

OBJECTIVES

- To monitor drainage.
- To assess for complications.

EQUIPMENT

H_2O_2 *or* povidone-iodine solution or swabs *or* normal saline

Cotton-tip applicators

Gloves, sterile, if applicable

To advance a penrose drain:

Forceps, sterile

Safety pin, sterile

Scissors, sterile

Povidone-iodine ointment

Split 4″ × 4″ gauze, if applicable

4″ × 4″ gauze, if applicable

Tape

ESSENTIAL STEPS

1. Prepare the child and family.
2. Assemble the equipment.
3. Wash hands.
4. Remove the old dressing, if applicable.
5. Clean around the insertion site of the drain with povidone-iodine solution/swabs *or* H_2O_2. Use cotton-tip applicators to apply H_2O_2 or povidone-iodine solution, or put on sterile gloves and clean with povidone-iodine swabs.
6. To advance a penrose drain:

    Put on gloves.

    Grasp the end of the penrose with forceps and gently pull out the amount specified by the physician.

    Insert a safety pin larger than the incision into the rubber drain at the level of the skin.

    Cut the end of the penrose to keep it from being too long, if appropriate. The drain should extend ½″ to 1″ beyond the skin level. (Note: Do not cut the drain too short. This might cause it to recede into the incision or to be difficult to grasp.)

7. Apply povidone-iodine or other antibacterial ointment and a split 4″ × 4″ gauze around the drain insertion site, if applicable. Apply a gauze dressing.

8. To empty the vacuum container (see Fig. 51.1):

   Put on gloves.

   Open the plug to empty the contents of the container.

   Clean the port with a povidone-iodine swab or alcohol.

   Compress the container with hands and, while compressing, recap the plug. (Note: Not all vacuum containers are emptied; check the manufacturer's instructions.)

DOCUMENTATION

- Site of drain.
- Type of drain.
- Skin integrity.
- Care given.
- Color, odor, amount, and consistency of drainage.

POTENTIAL RELATED NURSING DIAGNOSES

Infection: *high risk*

Tissue integrity, impaired

Skin integrity, impaired

POTENTIAL RELATED MEDICAL DIAGNOSES

Abscess

Peritonitis

Surgical procedures

REFERENCES

Lineaweaver, W., McMorris, S., Soucy, D., and Howard, R. 1985. Cellular and bacterial toxicities of topical antimicrobials. *Plastic and Reconstructive Surgery* 75, no. 3: 394–96.

Swearingen, P. 1991. *Photo-atlas of nursing procedures 2E.* Redwood City, Calif.: Addison-Wesley.

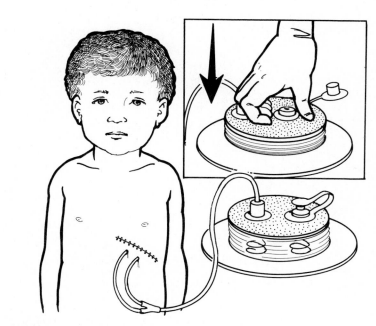

FIGURE 51.1 *Vacuum container drain.*

Dressing Change: Sterile

PSYCHOSOCIAL CONSIDERATIONS: Explain the procedure in developmentally appropriate terms.

TIME: 10 to 20 minutes

PURPOSE

To maintain a clean environment and to protect a wound.

OBJECTIVES

- To keep the dressing clean and dry.
- To reduce risks of infection.
- To monitor drainage.
- To evaluate wound healing.

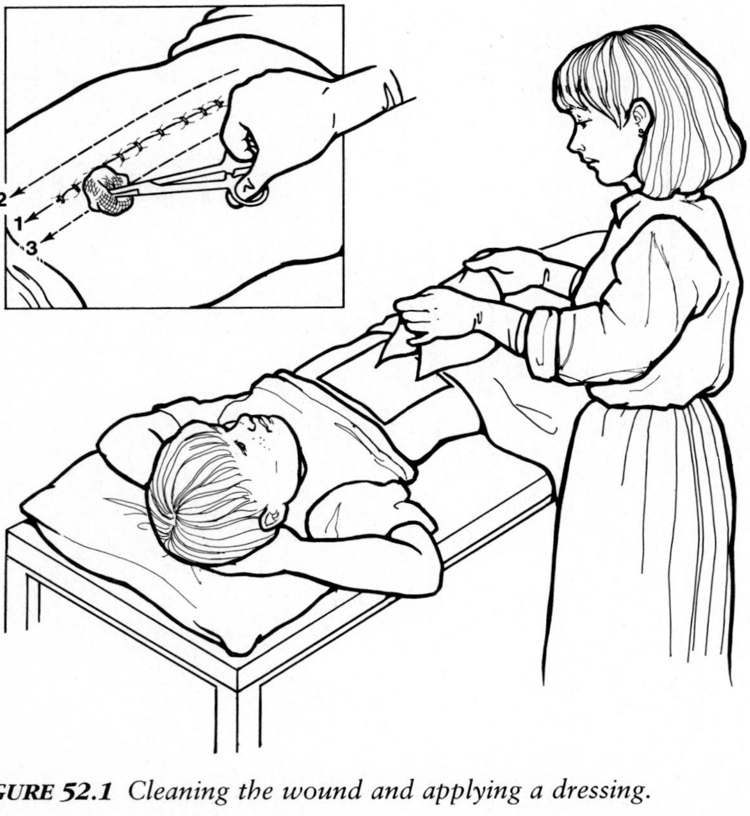

EQUIPMENT

Gloves, nonsterile, if applicable

Gloves, sterile

Cotton-tip applicators *or* gauze sponges, sterile

Povidone-iodine solution *or* H_2O_2 *or* hibiclens

Povidone-iodine ointment, per institution policy

Gauze pads, sterile, of appropriate size and number based on the size of the wound and the amount of drainage

Tape

Scissors, sterile, if dressings need to be adapted

SAFETY ISSUES

- **Some institutions use povidone-iodine instead of hydrogen peroxide (H_2O_2) because H_2O_2 may damage tissue.**

ESSENTIAL STEPS

1. Prepare the child and family.
2. Assemble the equipment.
3. Wash hands.
4. Remove the old dressing. Use nonsterile gloves if the dressing is moist. Note the amount, color, and odor of drainage. Dispose of the soiled dressing in an appropriate manner.
5. Assess skin integrity to determine any reactions to tape. Assess the wound.
6. Put on sterile gloves.

FIGURE 52.1 *Cleaning the wound and applying a dressing.*

7. Clean the wound area, using sterile applicators or gauze sponges, with povidone-iodine solution, H_2O_2, or hibiclens. Clean down the middle and then down each side of the wound using a new sterile applicator or gauze each time. Do not go back over any area with the same applicator or gauze. Use one stroke over each area. (See Fig. 52.1)

8. Apply povidone-iodine ointment, per institution policy.

9. Apply a sterile dressing; may apply a clear occlusive sterile dressing (such as Op-site or Tegaderm) directly over the wound. (See Figs. 52.1 and 52.2)

10. Change the dressing at least once every 24 hours, more often if drainage appears through the dressing.

DOCUMENTATION

- Description of drainage on the old dressing.
- Wound assessment.
- Care given.
- Ointment applied, if applicable.
- Dressing application.
- Child's response.

POTENTIAL RELATED NURSING DIAGNOSES

Infection: *high risk*

Skin integrity, impaired

POTENTIAL RELATED MEDICAL DIAGNOSES

Any surgical procedure with an external incision

Wounds

Trauma

Skills Checklist

☐ Prepare the child and family.
☐ Assemble the equipment.
☐ Wash hands.
☐ Remove the old dressing.
☐ Assess drainage on the dressing and wound.
☐ Put on sterile gloves.
☐ Clean the wound.
☐ Apply ointment, if applicable.
☐ Apply dressing.
☐ Document

REFERENCES

Lineaweaver, W., McMorris, S., Soucy, D., and Howard, R. 1985. Cellular and bacterial toxicities of topical antimicrobials. *Plastic and Reconstructive Surgery* 75, no. 3: 394–96.

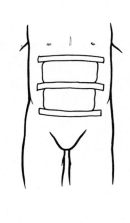
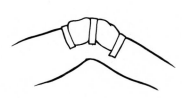
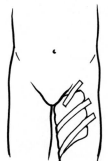
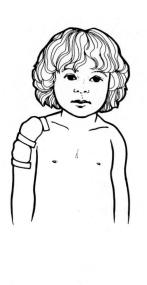

FIGURE 52.2 *Dressing types.*

53 Dying Child: After-Death Care

PSYCHOSOCIAL CONSIDERATIONS: Allow parents and family members to spend time alone with the child. Remove IV lines and tubes (if not a medical examiner's or coroner's case) and clean the body. Answer all questions, and provide a chaplain, if requested. Ensure that the eyes are closed. Be aware of own feelings concerning death. Family members may be in various stages of grief.

• Be aware of any applicable state laws or institution regulations. For example:

Telephone consent may not be acceptable for an autopsy. A telegram is usually acceptable when the family is not present.

Tubes and IVs are usually left in place for medical examiners' and coroners' cases.

There may be specifications related to reportable diseases.

TIME: 15 to 20 minutes

PURPOSE

To document the child's death.

To assist the family during the grieving process.

To prepare the body to be taken to the morgue.

OBJECTIVES

• To provide emotional support to the family.
• To prepare the body after death.

EQUIPMENT

Identification tags

Gloves, nonsterile, if applicable

Wash cloths and towels, as appropriate

Plastic bag, as needed

Tape, as needed

Clean dressings, as needed

Diaper or disposable pad

Body bag or wrap and safety pins

Permit for postmortem examination, if applicable

ESSENTIAL STEPS

1. Notify the following people and departments:

Physician.

Appropriate nursing supervisor.

Social worker.

Chaplain.

Admitting Department.

Morgue.

2. Assemble the equipment.
3. Provide privacy.
4. Complete the information on all identification tags.
5. Put on gloves if there is a chance of contact with blood or other body fluids.
6. Wash the body, as needed. Allow family members to participate if they wish. Preserve hair if it has been shaved or cut. Place the hair in a plastic bag and tape to the body.

7. Close the mouth and eyes and align the body with the head straight and elevated on a pillow.

8. Apply clean dressings and/or reinforce dressings, as needed.

9. Apply a diaper or disposable pad to contain excreta.

10. Dress the child appropriately if the family wishes to view the body. Drape the child with a blanket or sheet prior to the family's arrival.

11. Remove all unnecessary equipment from the room.

12. Provide emotional support for the family.

    Prepare the family for any tubes left in place and for possible body discoloration.

    Provide privacy for the family. The family may want to hold the child.

    Assist with gathering the child's belongings for the parents to take home.

    Remove all jewelry and give directly to the family.

13. After the family has left the child, attach the appropriate tag(s) to an extremity, leaving the hospital identification band in place.

14. Wrap the body (including any prostheses) in a sheet, pin securely, and attach a tag to the outside of the sheet.

15. Clear the hallway as much as possible.

16. Carry the body to the morgue, or transport by wagon or stretcher.

17. Place a door identification tag on the appropriate vault to identify the child as required in the morgue.

Skills Checklist

- ☐ Notify the appropriate people and departments.
- ☐ Assemble the equipment.
- ☐ Put on gloves, if appropriate.
- ☐ Prepare the body.
- ☐ Prepare the family; provide emotional support.
- ☐ Attach identification tags. Wrap the body.
- ☐ Transport to the morgue.
- ☐ Document.

DOCUMENTATION

- Time of death and name of physician who pronounced the child.
- Jewelry and other belongings given to the family.

POTENTIAL RELATED NURSING DIAGNOSES

Coping, ineffective family, compromised

Hopelessness

Spiritual distress

Powerlessness

POTENTIAL RELATED MEDICAL DIAGNOSES

Universal application

REFERENCES

Mott, S., James, S., and Sperhac, A. 1990. *Nursing care of children and families.* Redwood City, Calif.: Addison-Wesley.

54

Dying Child: Comfort Care

OBJECTIVES

- To provide nursing care for the dying child.
- To provide psychological support for the child and family.

EQUIPMENT

Varies with the individual case

ESSENTIAL STEPS

1. Prepare the child and family.
2. Assemble any needed equipment for comfort care.
3. Wash hands.
4. Take measures to provide physical and emotional comfort. These may include caring for the skin and/or a wound; managing pain, the temperature, the oxygen supply, and nutrition; nurturing the child and encouraging the family to nurture the child; and supporting and respecting a family's grieving processes.
5. Use the child's response to the comfort measures as a guide for obtaining additional physician orders for oxygen, nourishment, temperature control, pain medication, and/or a private room when feasible.
6. Advise the chaplain and/or social worker of the child's terminal status.

PSYCHOSOCIAL CONSIDERATIONS: Caring for the dying child and the child's family is as important as caring for the child who will regain health. The child may be afraid of dying and ask very direct questions. Be honest and straightforward without taking away hope. Encourage the child to draw pictures or write to describe fears. Use open-ended questions to ascertain feelings. Allow the child *not* to talk about death or dying if he or she indicates an unwillingness to do so. Allow parents to stay with the child as much as possible. Listen to the parents' fears and concerns. Allow them time alone with the child and with each other—but if death is imminent, a staff member should remain in the room.

TIME: Varies

PURPOSE

To facilitate optimum nursing care for the dying child and to provide psychological support to the child's family.

DOCUMENTATION

- Physical and emotional care given.
- Child's reaction(s).
- Family's reaction(s).

POTENTIAL RELATED NURSING DIAGNOSES

Anxiety

Fear

Hopelessness

Powerlessness

Grieving, anticipatory

Parenting, altered: *high risk*

Spiritual distress

Pain, acute

Pain, chronic

POTENTIAL RELATED MEDICAL DIAGNOSES

Universal application

REFERENCES

Mott, S., James, S., and Sperhac, A. 1990. *Nursing care of children and families.* Redwood City, Calif.: Addison-Wesley.

Skills Checklist

- ☐ Prepare the child and family.
- ☐ Assemble any needed equipment.
- ☐ Wash hands, if applicable.
- ☐ Provide comfort measures.
- ☐ Contact a chaplain and/or a social worker.
- ☐ Document.

55

Enema Administration

PSYCHOSOCIAL CONSIDERATIONS: Explain the procedure in developmentally appropriate terms. The child may fear having genitalia exposed to strangers. Perform this procedure with caution if sexual abuse is suspected; the child may require a longer period of preparation. Provide diversional activities during the procedure, such as conversation, singing, or television.

TIME: 5 to 20 minutes

PURPOSE

To promote expulsion of feces.

To clean the colon in preparation for diagnostic or surgical procedures.

To soothe colonic mucous membranes.

To instill medication.

OBJECTIVES

- To clear the bowel.
- To prevent constipation.
- To prevent injury.

EQUIPMENT

Gloves, nonsterile

Enema bag (sometimes a catheter and a syringe for an infant)

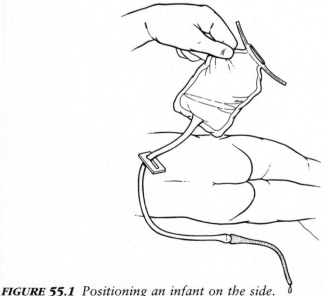

FIGURE 55.1 *Positioning an infant on the side.*

Water-soluble lubricant

Bedpan and protective pads

One of the following solutions, per the physician's plan of care; temperature should be tepid (body temperature):

Soapsuds: 1 tsp castile soap to 1 pt water

Normal saline (0.9% sodium chloride)

Fleets enema: infant, pediatric, or adult

Mucomyst

S SAFETY ISSUES

- **To determine volumes, consider the size and condition of the child. (See Table 55.1)**
- **Do not use plain tap water unless specified in the physician's plan of care.**

ESSENTIAL STEPS

1. Prepare the child and family.
2. Assemble the equipment.
3. Wash hands and put on gloves.
4. Expel air from the tubing or catheter and lubricate the tip of the tubing or catheter.
5. Place the older child in the left lateral Sims' position (lying on the side). Use Sims' position for the infant, if possible, or place the infant on his or her back or on pillows with buttocks over the edge of a bedpan. (See Fig. 55.1)
6. Insert the tip of the tube into the rectum, directing the tube toward the middle of the back for a distance of 2″ to 3″ (1½″ for an infant). Do not force the catheter. (See Figs. 55.2 and 55.3)
7. Anticipate that the infant or young child will be unable to hold the enema fluid volume well and may begin expelling the fluid after 30 to 50 ml have been administered.

TABLE 55.1 *Maximum Amounts of Enema Solutions*

Age of Child	Maximum Amount
Premature	5–20 ml
<1 year	50–100 ml
<2 years	100–150 ml
2–5 years	200–250 ml
5–10 years	300–500 ml
>10 years	500–750 ml

8. Lift the bag only enough to allow flow, not above 18″ for a large child or 6″ to 8″ for an infant. If the child is unable to hold the fluid, try holding the buttocks together with one hand while giving the enema.

9. Assist the child for elimination—in a diaper, bedpan, or bathroom.

10. When the physician does not specify an amount and orders "enemas until clear," give no more than two enemas to a child under 2 years of age and no more than three enemas to an older child. If the returned solution is still not clear, contact the physician before giving more fluids. An electrolyte imbalance may occur with excessive volumes of hypo/hypertonic fluids.

DOCUMENTATION

- Date and time.
- Type and amount of enema solution administered.
- Results (color, consistency, presence of mucus and amount).
- Child's response.

Skills Checklist

☐ Prepare the child and family.
☐ Assemble the equipment.
☐ Wash hands and put on gloves.
☐ Expel air from the tubing or catheter and lubricate the tip of the tubing or catheter.
☐ Position the child.
☐ Administer the enema.
☐ Document.

POTENTIAL RELATED NURSING DIAGNOSES

Constipation

Anxiety

POTENTIAL RELATED MEDICAL DIAGNOSES

Constipation

X-ray procedure

Preoperative preparation

Hirschsprung's disease

REFERENCES

Mott, S., James, S., and Sperhac, A. 1990. *Nursing care of children and families.* Redwood City, Calif.: Addison-Wesley.

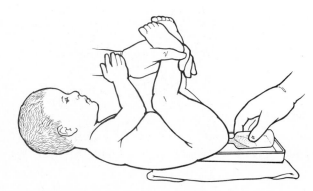

FIGURE 55.2 *Administering a Fleets enema.*

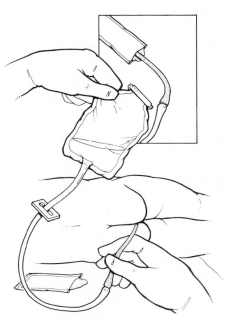

FIGURE 55.3 *Administering an enema from a bag.*

56 Enteral Feedings: Continuous

PSYCHOSOCIAL CONSIDERATIONS: Explain the procedure in developmentally appropriate terms. The child may feel anxiety related to having a feeding tube in the back of the throat. Explain that the feeling of gagging or choking is uncomfortable but will gradually diminish. The child may need restraints to prevent accidental removal of tube. Remove the restraints periodically when the child is supervised. Give infants a pacifier to maintain sucking strength. Nonnutritive sucking in conjunction with continuous feeding has been shown to increase weight gain.

TIME: Varies

PURPOSE

To deliver safe and accurate continuous enteral feedings.

OBJECTIVES

- To deliver continuous feedings.
- To prevent overdistention of the stomach.
- To prevent aspiration.

EQUIPMENT

N/G *or* N/D tube, appropriate size (see Figs. 56.1 and 56.2)

Syringe to check tube placement

Formula, as ordered

Feeding set and tubing

Pump

Stethoscope

Tap *or* sterile water

SAFETY ISSUES

- **A nasogastric (N/G) or nasoduodenal (N/D) tube in a child who has had gastric or esophageal surgery must not be removed or moved except by the surgeon, unless otherwise ordered.**

- **Single-lumen N/G tubes such as Argyle may be used on infants weighing more than 5 kg and on other patients needing short-term therapy. Change these tubes every 3 days, inserting the new tube in alternate naris.**

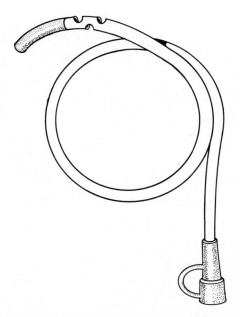

FIGURE 56.1 *Weighted feeding tube.*

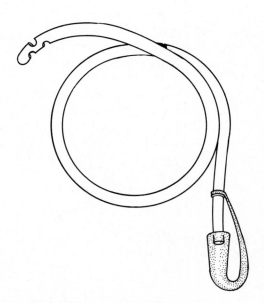

FIGURE 56.2 *Argyle feeding tube.*

- Use prelubricated silicone indwelling N/G or N/D tubes such as Corpak on infants weighing less than 5 kg and on patients receiving long-term therapy. Remove the indwelling tube to clean and replace it in the opposite naris monthly, or sooner if it malfunctions or if complications occur.
- Check N/G or N/D tube placement at least every 8 hours.
- Check residuals every 4 hours. The physician may specify the amount of residual for which he or she should be notified. If there is no specification, stop the feeding and notify the physician when a residual is one to one-and-one-half times the hourly rate. Return residual volumes to the child to decrease the possibility of electrolyte imbalance and digestive enzyme deficits.
- Ready-to-feed formula may hang for up to 12 hours, depending on the manufacturer.
- Date, time, and refrigerate ready-to-feed formula after opening. Discard after 24 hours.
- Use sterile water as an irrigant or flush for infants younger than 6 months. Tap water may be used for older children.
- Change continuous feeding tubing sets, including stopcocks and catheter adapters, every 24 hours. Rinse the bag every 4 to 8 hours, if specified.
- A nurse or a physician may place weighted N/D tubes. Save the stylet at the bedside so that the tube may be replaced if necessary. Use opposite naris when replacing the tube.
- Notify the physician of any residual obtained from an N/D tube. This may indicate displacement of the tube or a bowel obstruction.

Skills Checklist

☐ Prepare the child and family.
☐ Assemble the equipment.
☐ Position the child.
☐ Insert an N/G or N/D tube, if applicable.
☐ Check placement of the N/G or N/D tube.
☐ Add formula to the feeding set and prime the tubing.
☐ Connect the tube to the feeding set, set the pump, and start feeding.
☐ Monitor residual and placement.
☐ Document.

ESSENTIAL STEPS

1. Prepare the child and family.
2. Assemble the equipment.
3. Elevate the head of the bed 30° and assist the child to a sitting position if possible. If not possible, place the child supine on the right or left side or in a prone position with the head to one side.
4. Insert an N/G or N/D tube, if necessary. Refer to "Nasogastric Tube Insertion." (See Fig. 56.3)

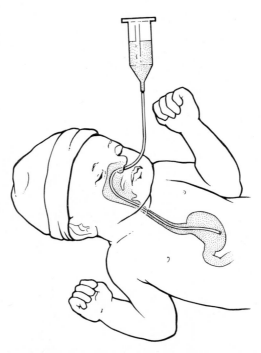

FIGURE 56.3 *Placement of an N/G feeding tube.*

5. Check tube placement by aspirating residual. If no residual is obtained, check by auscultating over the stomach while injecting a small amount of air into the tube (3 to 5 ml).

6. Add the appropriate amount of formula to the feeding set. Prime the tubing and connect to an N/G or N/D tube.

7. When changing the set and tubing, label the new feeding set with the date and time.

8. Set the pump rate and start the infusion. (See Fig. 56.4)

9. Allow infants to suck a pacifier at frequent intervals.

DOCUMENTATION

- Type and size of tube inserted, if applicable.
- Type of feeding.
- Each time tube placement was checked.
- Amount and appearance of residual.
- Reason feeding stopped and name of physician notified, if appropriate.
- Amount infused every hour.

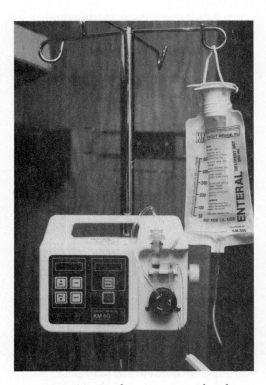

FIGURE 56.4 *Feeding pump with a bag.*

POTENTIAL RELATED NURSING DIAGNOSES

Aspiration: *high risk*

Fluid volume excess: *high risk*

Nutrition, altered, less than body requirements

Activity intolerance

Alteration in bowel elimination

Fluid volume deficit: *high risk*

POTENTIAL RELATED MEDICAL DIAGNOSES

Short bowel syndrome

Neuromuscular disorders

Unconsciousness

Dental problems

Paralysis

Prematurity

Anorexia nervosa

Head injury

REFERENCES

Anderson, K., Norris, D., and Godfrey, L. 1984. Bacterial contamination of tube-feeding formulas. *JPEN* 8: 673.

Eisenberg, P. 1989. Enteral nutrition. *Nursing Clinics of North America* 24: 315–37.

Mott, S., James, S., and Sperhac, A. 1990. *Nursing care of children and families.* Redwood City, Calif.: Addison-Wesley.

Swearingen, P. 1991. *Photo-atlas of nursing procedures 2E.* Redwood City, Calif.: Addison-Wesley.

Fecal Fat Collection: Timed

1. Prepare the child and family.
2. Assemble the equipment.
3. Wash hands.
4. Give first charcoal marker.
5. Record all liquid and solid food intake. This step is optional in some settings.
6. Put on gloves and collect a stool specimen. Record on the specimen container the time the first charcoal marker is passed and discard this stool. Begin the collection with the next stool. If charcoal is not used, discard one stool and then begin the collection.
7. Place each stool into the collection container. Urine mixed with stool does not affect test results.
8. Store the collection container on ice in the child's room or in the specimen refrigerator.
9. Give the second marker, per the physician's plan of care (for example, after 24 or 72 hours).

PSYCHOSOCIAL CONSIDERATIONS: Explain the procedure in developmentally appropriate terms. Avoid using terms with mixed meanings. Tell the child and parents about the markers and what the markers will look like. Markers may be easier to swallow if placed in food, such as applesauce.

TIME: 2 to 5 days

PURPOSE

To obtain stool specimens for determination of fat absorption.

OBJECTIVES

- To collect stool specimens.
- To document the time of administration of and excretion of markers.

EQUIPMENT

Charcoal markers (optional in some settings)

Gloves, nonsterile

Specimen collection container

Specipan or bedpan

Tongue blades (to facilitate the transfer of stool into the collection container)

10. Continue to save all stools until the child passes the second charcoal marker; record the time on the container. Save this stool as the last stool. If charcoal is not used, collect the last stool passed during the time period for collection.

11. Label the container and send it to the lab.

DOCUMENTATION

- Time first marker given.
- Time first marker appeared in stool.
- Time second marker given.
- Time second marker appeared in stool.
- If no charcoal used, collection time period.
- Description of stools.
- Diet (liquid and solid food intake).
- That specimen was sent to the lab.

POTENTIAL RELATED NURSING DIAGNOSES

Bowel incontinence

Diarrhea

POTENTIAL RELATED MEDICAL DIAGNOSES

Weight loss

Failure to thrive

Steatorrhea

Cystic fibrosis

Skills Checklist

☐ Prepare the child and family.
☐ Assemble the equipment.
☐ Wash hands.
☐ Give the first charcoal marker.
☐ Record liquid and solid food intake.
☐ Put on gloves and collect a stool specimen.
☐ Note the time the first charcoal marker passes. Discard this stool.
☐ Save all following stool.
☐ Give the second marker.
☐ Continue saving all stool until the second marker passes. Save this stool as the last stool. Note the time.
☐ End collection with excretion of the second marker.
☐ Label the specimen and send it to the lab.
☐ Document.

Lab Values

Fatty Acid Globules: 1–4 μ in diameter

58 Feeding: General

PSYCHOSOCIAL CONSIDERATIONS: Children often lack control in the hospital, and eating may be one of the few times when they can assert themselves. It is important, therefore, to avoid turning mealtimes into battles. Unless the child is on a restricted diet, allow foods that the child likes. Find out what foods the child would choose. Young infants should be held close during feeding—ideally by a parent or significant other. Allow older infants to eat in a high chair. Offer finger foods to promote growth and development activities. Permit adolescents to say when and where they would like to eat if possible; availability of a microwave allows food to be heated as needed.

TIME: Varies

PURPOSE

To promote appropriate nutrition.

OBJECTIVES

- To promote ingestion of nutrients.
- To prevent trauma or injury.

EQUIPMENT

Bottle and formula, if applicable
Feeding utensils
Meal tray, if applicable

ESSENTIAL STEPS

1. Prepare the child and family.
2. Assemble the equipment.
3. Wash hands.
4. For a bottle-fed infant:

   Hold in a supine position with the head elevated at least 30° (except for infants not to be held, such as those with myelomeningocele, premature infants with severe apnea or bradycardia, and infants who do not tolerate extra stimulation physiologically).

   Hold the bottle inverted, higher than the nipple, so no air can enter the nipple. Do not prop the bottle; the infant may aspirate. Avoid

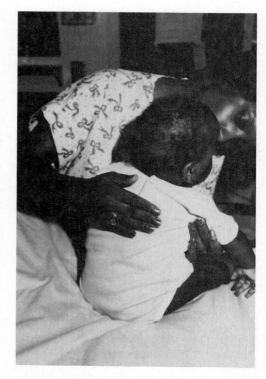

FIGURE 58.1 *Burping a baby from a sitting position.*

putting a child or infant to bed with a bottle, as this can cause tooth decay or aspiration.

Bubble or burp the infant after every 2 oz. To do this, hold the infant in an upright position and support the head and neck while gently patting or rubbing the back. Or place in a sitting position with a hand supporting the neck and chest. It is not necessary to vigorously pat the child's back. (See Figs. 58.1 and 58.2)

Place the infant in a crib on the side or abdomen. Or place in an infant seat with the head elevated. (See Fig. 58.3) If an infant has had problems with vomiting, do not place on the abdomen; pressure on the stomach can aggravate vomiting. Infants known to have gastroesophageal reflux (GER), however, may be positioned prone in a GER harness with the head of the bed elevated 30°. Do not leave an infant on his or her back immediately after a feeding.

Skills Checklist

Infant
- [ ] Prepare the child and family.
- [ ] Assemble the equipment.
- [ ] Wash hands.
- [ ] Position the infant.
- [ ] Feed the infant.
- [ ] Bubble or burp.
- [ ] Document.

Older Infant or Child
- [ ] Prepare the child and family.
- [ ] Assemble the equipment.
- [ ] Wash hands.
- [ ] Secure in a high chair, if appropriate.
- [ ] Assist the child as necessary with a meal tray.
- [ ] Observe eating.
- [ ] Document.

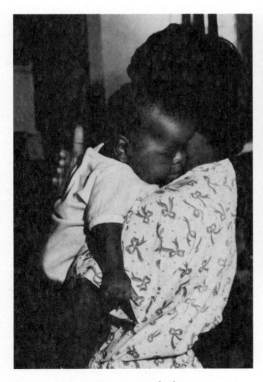

FIGURE 58.2 *Burping a baby over the shoulder.*

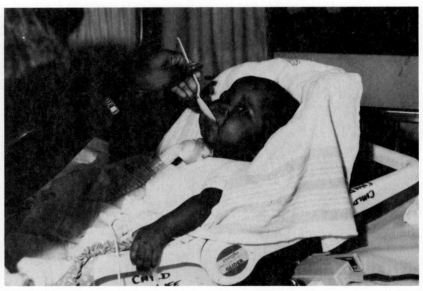

FIGURE 58.3 *Feeding an infant in an infant seat.*

5. For older infants and children:

Secure the child in a high chair with a safety strap if more than 5 months of age and if appropriate. Allow to feed self as much as possible. Do not leave a young child alone during a meal. (See Figs. 58.4 and 58.5) Seeing other children eat may encourage the individual child to eat. Do not threaten a child with punishment or an action that will not occur. Be honest. If a child cannot go home unless eating improves, tell the child.

Allow consumption of most fluids only after eating.

Make meals look fun and interesting. Ensure that meats (such as hot dogs) and hard foods (such as carrots) are cut lengthwise first, then into small pieces so that large pieces do not lodge in the throat.

Encourage a family member to feed or remain with the child during meals.

Offer small portions.

Remove candy and junk food from the room.

Make sure that the child is served foods that he or she can recognize.

DOCUMENTATION

- Date and time.
- Type of diet.
- Amount, in percent of total intake for solid food, in ml for liquids.
- Child's response.

POTENTIAL RELATED NURSING DIAGNOSES

Aspiration: *high risk*

Constipation

Diarrhea

Fluid volume deficit: *high risk*

Nutrition, altered: less than body requirements

Self-care deficit, feeding

POTENTIAL RELATED MEDICAL DIAGNOSES

Universal application

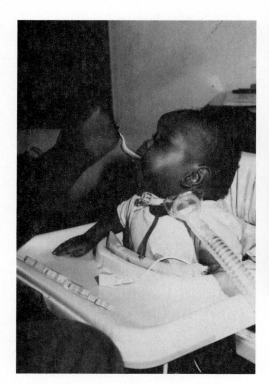

FIGURE 58.4 *Feeding an infant in a high chair.*

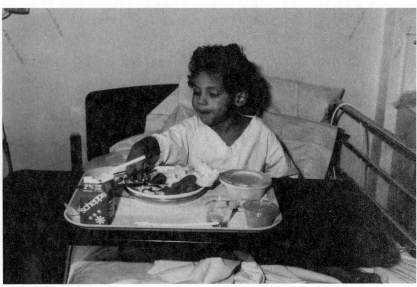

FIGURE 58.5 *An older child eating.*

PSYCHOSOCIAL CONSIDERATIONS: Explain the procedure in developmentally appropriate terms. Avoid using terms with mixed meanings, such as *tube into stomach* and *suctioning out*. Provide comfort to the child. Explain noises from the machine. The child may need to wear restraints to prevent accidental removal of the tube. Remove the restraints periodically when the child is supervised. Encourage therapeutic play.

TIME: Varies

PURPOSE

To decompress the stomach with a double-lumen nasogastric (N/G) tube with gravity drainage or connected to suction.

OBJECTIVES

- To decompress the stomach.
- To prevent injury or trauma.

EQUIPMENT

For insertion of an N/G tube:

Gloves, nonsterile

Double-lumen N/G tube (Salem Sump, Argyle, or Anderson Sump), appropriate size

Syringe with adapter

Emesis basin

Stethoscope

Water-soluble lubricant

Tape

Blanket for mummy restraint, if appropriate

For gravity drainage:

Gloves, nonsterile

Plastic container with lid or drainage bag *or* exam glove and rubber band

For suction:

Wall suction setup *or* intermittent suction equipment, such as Gomco

To irrigate:

Gloves, nonsterile

Normal saline (0.9% sodium chloride) irrigation solution *or* other solution, as ordered

Irrigation tray, including a 60 ml syringe, receptacle, and plastic bottle

Stethoscope

 SAFETY ISSUES

- **The N/G tube in a child who has had esophageal or gastric surgery must not be removed or moved except by the physician, unless otherwise indicated.**

- **The physician specifies the type of suction (constant or intermittent) and the amount. Intermittent is preferred as it is less damaging to tubes and does not increase the chance of electrolyte imbalances.**

- **The physician specifies the type, frequency, and amount of irrigation. Use normal saline unless the physician orders another solution.**

- **Do not clamp the air vent tubing as this will render the sump action inoperative. A vented plug is available commercially to prevent leakage.**

- When ambulating or transporting a child with a double-lumen tube, do not clamp or plug the tube; instead attach an exam glove with a rubber band to collect any drainage. Pin the tube to the child's gown to ensure comfort and prevent accidental pulling out of the tube.

ESSENTIAL STEPS

1. Prepare the child and family.

2. Assemble the equipment.

3. Wash hands and put on gloves.

4. For an N/G insertion, refer to "Nasogastric Tube Insertion."

5. For gravity drainage:

    Insert the end of the N/G tube into a hole cut in the lid of a plastic container or drainage bag *or* secure an exam glove over the end of the tube with a rubber band. (The glove is used less commonly and only until a container or bag can be obtained.)

    Position the collection container below the child's stomach.

6. For suction:

    Test suction equipment to ensure that it is functioning.

    Connect the N/G tube to the suction device, per manufacturer's instructions.

    Set the appropriate amount of suction, per physician's order. (See Fig. 59.1)

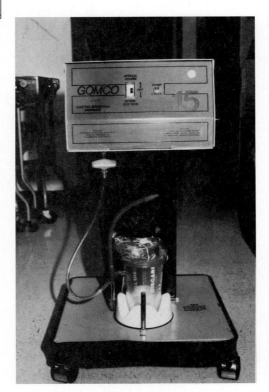

FIGURE 59.1 *Gomco suction.*

7. To irrigate:

> Pour irrigation solution into a plastic bottle from the irrigation tray.
>
> Check tube placement by aspirating gastric contents and/or ascultating over the epigastric region while injecting a small amount of air through the N/G tube. (See Figs. 59.2 and 59.3)

Draw irrigation solution up from the plastic bottle into the syringe and gently instill into the N/G tube.

Aspirate gently to obtain the amount of fluid instilled.

Inject 10 ml of air into the air vent after irrigating tube.

Should reflux of solution and/or gastric contents into the air vent occur, disconnect the N/G tube from suction and irrigate both lumens with a small amount of air (5 to 7 ml).

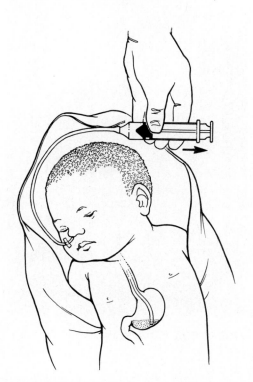

FIGURE 59.2 *Aspirating stomach contents to check placement.*

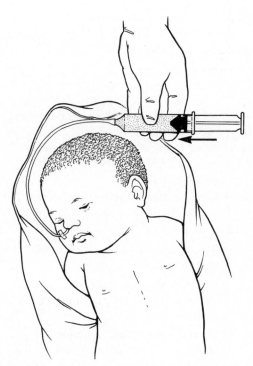

FIGURE 59.3 *Injecting air to check placement. Listen with stethoscope over gastric area.*

DOCUMENTATION

- Date and time of tube insertion, if applicable.
- Size and type of tube used, if applicable.
- Naris used and any resistance to passage of tube, if applicable.
- Type of drainage system used and type and amount of suction applied, if applicable.
- Amount, color, and consistency of returned gastric contents.
- Date, time, type, and amount of fluid when tube irrigated.

POTENTIAL RELATED NURSING DIAGNOSES

Fluid volume deficit: *high risk*

Swallowing, impaired

Pain, acute

POTENTIAL RELATED MEDICAL DIAGNOSES

Nausea and vomiting

Abdominal surgery

REFERENCES

Mott, S., James, S., and Sperhac, A. 1990. *Nursing care of children and families.* Redwood City, Calif.: Addison-Wesley.

Swearingen, P. 1991. *Photo-atlas of nursing procedures 2E.* Redwood City, Calif.: Addison-Wesley.

60 Gastric Lavage

PSYCHOSOCIAL CONSIDERATIONS: Explain the procedure in developmentally appropriate terms. Explain that the tube is soft and that the stomach will be washed with water. Do not tell a child, toddler, or preschooler that gagging is likely. Perform quickly. If lavage is for drug overdose, the child may be combative or resentful. Parents may be asked to leave the room. Allow therapeutic play, if possible.

TIME: 20 to 30 minutes

PURPOSE

To irrigate the stomach by the instillation and withdrawal of a rinsing fluid to prepare for surgery, relieve vomiting, clean the stomach, assess and treat upper gastrointestinal bleeding, and so on.

OBJECTIVES

- To irrigate the stomach.
- To prevent aspiration.
- To prevent injury.

EQUIPMENT

Nasogastric (N/G) tube, appropriate size

Syringe with adapter *or* irrigation tray

Two basins

Stethoscope

Water-soluble lubricant

Tape

Blanket for restraint

Gloves, nonsterile

Normal saline (0.9% sodium chloride) or other irrigating solution, per the physician's plan of care

Towels

SAFETY ISSUES

- **This procedure is contraindicated after ingestion of corrosive substances, such as lye, because of the danger of perforation.**
- **Iced lavage is controversial. Check with the specific physician. Iced solution may cause bradycardia and/or hypothermia.**

ESSENTIAL STEPS

1. Prepare the child and family.
2. Assemble the equipment.
3. Wash hands and put on gloves.
4. Position the child. Elevate the head of the bed or hold the child in an upright position. Restrain as necessary. Use a blanket for a mummy restraint, if necessary.
5. Insert the tube as specified in "Nasogastric Tube Insertion."
6. Aspirate stomach contents by gravity or with a syringe. (See Fig. 60.1)
7. Instill irrigating solution. (See Fig. 60.2) To determine the amount of solution to instill, consider the size of the child, the child's tolerance, and the total quantity ordered by the physician (usually 30 to 60 ml for an infant to 1-year-old, 60 to 90 ml for a 1- to 5-year-old, or 90 to 120 ml for a 6- to 12-year-old).
8. Repeat steps 6 and 7 until the gastric return is clear or the entire amount of irrigating solution is used, or according to the physician's plan of care. Place the discarded solution into the basins.
9. Evaluate the necessity to remove or leave the tube in place.
10. Measure gastric content before discarding and subtract the amount of solution instilled from the amount removed.

DOCUMENTATION

- Date and time of tube insertion.
- Size and type of tube used.
- Naris used.
- Color and consistency of gastric contents.
- Type and amount of solution instilled and amount returned.
- Any difference between amount of solution instilled and amount returned.
- Child's tolerance of the procedure.

POTENTIAL RELATED NURSING DIAGNOSES

Aspiration: *high risk*

Pain, acute

Fluid volume deficit: *high risk*

Injury: *high risk*

Nutrition, altered, less than body requirements

Swallowing, impaired

Skills Checklist

☐ Prepare the child and family.
☐ Assemble the equipment.
☐ Wash hands and put on gloves.
☐ Position the child.
☐ Insert the tube.
☐ Aspirate stomach contents.
☐ Instill irrigating solution. Aspirate.
☐ Measure stomach contents.
☐ Document.

POTENTIAL RELATED MEDICAL DIAGNOSES

Poisoning

Gastrointestinal bleeding

Preoperative preparation, especially following barium swallow

Pyloric stenosis

REFERENCES

Mott, S., James, S., and Sperhac, A. 1990. *Nursing care of children and families.* Redwood City, Calif.: Addison-Wesley.

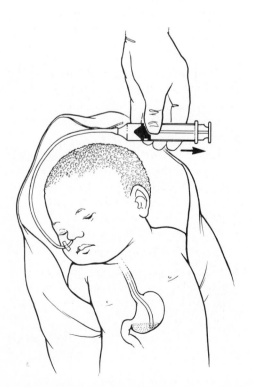

FIGURE 60.1 *Aspirating stomach contents.*

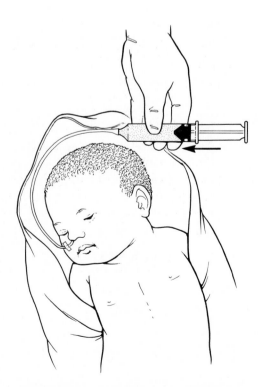

FIGURE 60.2 *Instilling irrigating solution.*

61 Gastroesophageal Reflux Care

PSYCHOSOCIAL CONSIDERATIONS: Explain the procedure to parents. Infants become frustrated at being tied down or restrained. Take the child out of the harness or the infant seat every 2 hours to provide stimulation and position change. Give parents support.

TIME: 5 minutes

PURPOSE

To reduce gastroesophageal reflux (GER) in the infant.

OBJECTIVES

- To prevent aspiration.
- To prevent vomiting and resulting nutritional depletion.

EQUIPMENT

Foam wedge

GER harness (newborn or infant) *or* infant seat *or* rolls or bolsters

S SAFETY ISSUES

- Check circulation to the perineal area and lower extremities with each diaper change when the child is in a GER harness.
- The child with GER is at risk for aspiration. Observe respirations and auscultate breath sounds with each set of vital signs.

ESSENTIAL STEPS

1. Prepare the family.
2. Assemble the equipment.

3. If using a GER harness:

   Cover the wedge with a sheet.

   Place the wedge at the head of the bed with the wide angle parallel to the end of the mattress.

   Using a slipknot, tie the bottom harness straps to the crib rungs at the head of the bed. (See Fig. 61.1)

   Place a protective cover (such as a cloth diaper) over the bottom straps.

   Place the infant in the harness following manufacturer's directions, ensuring that the infant is positioned entirely on the wedge. (See Figs. 61.2 and 61.3)

   The infant must remain in an upright position, prone, with straps parallel and over the back, unless otherwise indicated.

   Feed the infant in an upright position. Avoid rocking and excessive movement. Burp after every ½ oz.

   Place the infant in a GER harness immediately after feeding, or hold in an upright position (≥30° angle).

   The infant should remain on the wedge and in the harness for 2 hours after feeding, if possible.

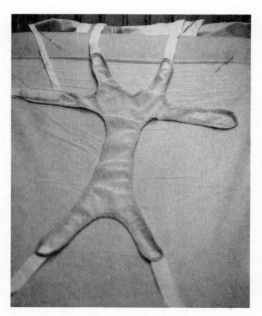

FIGURE 61.1 *GER harness positioned on the bed.*

Frequently check the infant while in the harness and change the head position, alternating sides.

4. If placing the child in an infant seat, follow steps 6 through 9 under number 3.

5. If using rolls or bolsters, place the child prone, with the head of the bed elevated 30°. Place rolls or bolsters around the infant to maintain position. Follow steps 6 through 9 under number 3.

DOCUMENTATION

- Time in harness, in infant seat, or positioned with rolls or bolsters.
- Circulation to perineal area and lower extremities when in GER harness.
- Any emesis. Amount, forcefulness, and relationship to feeding, positioning, and activity.
- Intake and output.

POTENTIAL RELATED NURSING DIAGNOSES

Parenting, altered

Aspiration: *high risk*

Fluid volume deficit: *high risk*

Injury: *high risk*

Nutrition, altered, less than body requirements

Skills Checklist

☐ Prepare the family.
☐ Assemble the equipment.
☐ Place the child in a GER harness, if appropriate.
  • Cover the wedge with a sheet.
  • Place the wedge at the head of the bed.
  • Lay the harness flat on the bed.
  • Tie the bottom harness straps to the crib rungs.
  • Place the infant prone in an upright position.
  • Place straps around the waist.
  • Fasten the top straps parallel and over the child's back.
☐ Place the child in an infant seat, if appropriate.
☐ Position the child prone, if appropriate.
  • Elevate the head of the bed 30°.
  • Support the child with rolls or bolsters.
☐ Document.

POTENTIAL RELATED MEDICAL DIAGNOSES

GER

Chronic vomiting

Colic

REFERENCES

Zahr, L., and Trentini, P. 1989. Gastroesophageal reflux, fundoplication, and dumping: Literature review and case study. *Issues in Comprehensive Pediatric Nursing* 12, no. 5: 385–93.

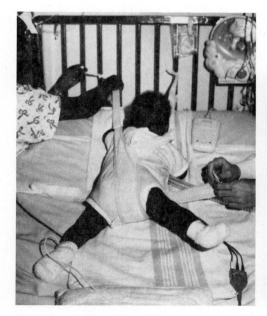

FIGURE 61.2 *Child positioned over the harness, with straps tied.*

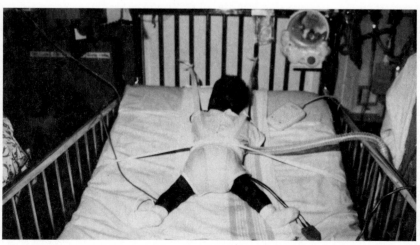

FIGURE 61.3 *Straps tied to the bed, not to side rails.*

62 Gastrostomy Button

- Use sterile water as an irrigant for infants less than 6 months of age; otherwise, use tap water or distilled water.
- Use a decompression tube prior to feeding if abdominal distention is noted. This should not be a routine practice, as button valve damage can result. (A valve in the gastrostomy button prevents backflow of feeding.)

PSYCHOSOCIAL CONSIDERATIONS: Explain the procedure in developmentally appropriate terms. Do not tell the child to make believe that food, such as steak, carrots, or potatoes, is being instilled; the child may fear the food substance is too large. Instead, explain that the substance is a food supplement.

TIME: 10 to 15 minutes

PURPOSE

To provide nutrition safely through a gastrostomy button.

OBJECTIVES

- To provide nutrition through a gastrostomy button.
- To prevent injury and trauma.

EQUIPMENT

Decompression tube of corresponding size, if appropriate

Adapter

Feeding bag and tubing *or* large (60 ml) syringe

Formula

Water, sterile, tap *or* distilled

ESSENTIAL STEPS

1. Prepare the child and family.
2. Assemble the equipment.
3. Wash hands.
4. Remove the plug from the button. (See Figs. 62.1 and 62.2)
5. Insert a hollow adapter for feeding. (See Fig. 62.3)
6. When using a feeding set:

   Add the appropriate amount of formula to the feeding set and prime the tubing.

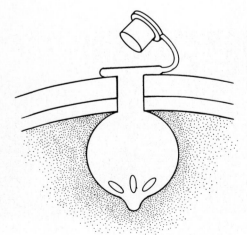

FIGURE 62.1 *Gastrostomy button with the plug open.*

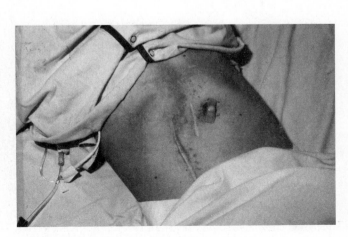

FIGURE 62.2 *Gastrostomy button.*

Connect the end of the feeding set to the adapter. (See Fig. 62.4)

7. When using a 60 ml syringe:

    Remove the plunger from the syringe.

    Attach the syringe to the adapter and pour in the appropriate amount of formula.

8. Flush with 5 ml of water, unless specifically ordered otherwise.

9. Disconnect the tubing or syringe.

10. Remove the adapter.

11. Reinsert the plug.

DOCUMENTATION

- Date and time.
- Type of formula.
- Amount of feeding.
- Amount and type of water used to flush.
- Child's response.

POTENTIAL RELATED NURSING DIAGNOSES

Swallowing, impaired

Nutrition, altered, less than body requirements

Self-care deficit, feeding

Sensory/perceptual alterations, gustatory

Skills Checklist

☐ Prepare the child and family.
☐ Assemble the equipment.
☐ Wash hands.
☐ Remove the plug.
☐ Insert the adapter.
☐ Instill feeding.
☐ Flush.
☐ Disconnect the tubing or syringe.
☐ Remove the adapter.
☐ Reinsert the plug.
☐ Document.

POTENTIAL RELATED MEDICAL DIAGNOSES

Musculoskeletal disorder

Tracheoesophageal fistula

Coma

REFERENCES

Huth, M., and O'Brien, M. 1987. The gastrostomy feeding button. *Pediatric Nursing* 13, no. 4: 241–45.

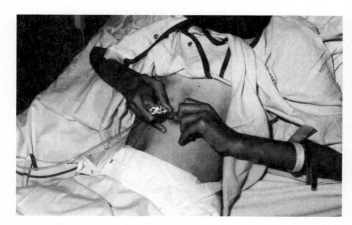

FIGURE 62.3 *Connecting the tubing to the button.*

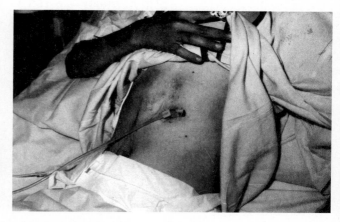

FIGURE 62.4 *Infusing formula.*

63 Gastrostomy Feedings: Bolus

PSYCHOSOCIAL CONSIDERATIONS: Explain the procedure in developmentally appropriate terms. Allow infants to suck a pacifier during feeding. Do not ask the child to make believe that food, such as steak, carrots, or potatoes, is being instilled. Explain that the substance is a food supplement.

TIME: 15 to 30 minutes; the time it would take to bottle-feed the same amount

PURPOSE

To deliver safe and accurate bolus gastrostomy tube feedings.

OBJECTIVES

- To administer feedings.
- To prevent injury and trauma.
- To minimize complications, such as diarrhea and vomiting.

EQUIPMENT

Syringe

Gavage set with bottle *or* 60 ml syringe

Formula, warmed to room temperature

Water, sterile, tap *or* distilled

Catheter adapter

Injection cap(s)

Stopcock

Gloves, nonsterile (if secretions from gastrostomy may soil hands)

SAFETY ISSUES

- The physician will specify if the gastrostomy tube is to be left unclamped after feedings.
- Check residuals before each feeding. Return residual volumes to the child to decrease the possibility of electrolyte imbalance and digestive enzyme deficits.
- Ready-to-feed formula may hang for up to 12 hours. Some institutions may allow only a 4-hour hang time for any formula.
- Use sterile water as an irrigant for infants less than 6 months of age. Otherwise, use tap water or distilled water.
- Rinse gavage sets with tap water after every use; reuse up to 24 hours. Change gavage sets, catheter adapters, injection caps, and stopcocks every 24 hours.

ESSENTIAL STEPS

1. Prepare the child and family.
2. Assemble the equipment.
3. Wash hands.
4. Position the child on the back with the upper body elevated, if possible. If not possible, place the child on the right side with the head slightly elevated or in a prone position with the head to one side.
5. Check the residual by unclamping the gastrostomy tube and aspirating with a syringe. Refer to the physician's plan of care concerning residual. If more than half of the ordered feeding amount is in residual, feeding is usually held and the physician notified.
6. Check the gastrostomy site for leakage and/or signs of infection. Notify the physician of either of these.
7. If using a gavage set:

    Attach the bottle with the appropriate amount of formula to the gavage set and prime the tubing.

Connect the end of the gavage set to the gastrostomy tube.

8. If using a 60 ml syringe:

   Remove the plunger from the syringe.

   Attach the syringe to the gastrostomy tube and pour in the appropriate amount of formula. (See Fig. 63.1)

9. Allow formula to flow by gravity for at least 15 to 30 minutes. The rate should not exceed 5 ml per 5 to 10 minutes for infants weighing less than 3.5 kg.

10. Encourage infants to suck on a pacifier during feedings.

11. When feeding is complete, disconnect the gavage set or syringe.

12. Flush the gastrostomy tube with 10 to 20 ml of water unless specifically directed otherwise by the physician's plan of care.

13. Close the end of the gastrostomy tube by covering the catheter adapter with an injection cap or stopcock.

14. Position the child with the head elevated and on the right side, if possible, for 1 hour after feeding.

DOCUMENTATION

- Amount and appearance of residual.
- Appearance of gastrostomy tube site.
- Type of formula.
- Patency and ease of flow.
- Volume of feeding and amount of time given over.
- Amount and type of water used to flush tube.

POTENTIAL RELATED NURSING DIAGNOSES

Nutrition, altered, less than body requirements

Fluid volume deficit: *high risk*

Swallowing, impaired

Self-care deficit, feeding

Skills Checklist

☐ Prepare the child and family.
☐ Assemble the equipment.
☐ Wash hands.
☐ Position the child.
☐ Check residual.
☐ Check the gastrostomy site for leakage and/or signs of infection.
☐ Infuse formula.
☐ Flush the tubing. Close end of gastrosomy tube.
☐ Document.

POTENTIAL RELATED MEDICAL DIAGNOSES

Bronchopulmonary dysplasia

Cerebral palsy

Trauma

Coma

REFERENCES

Mott, S., James, S., and Sperhac, A. 1990. *Nursing care of children and families.* Redwood City, Calif.: Addison-Wesley.

Swearingen, P. 1991. *Photo-atlas of nursing procedures 2E.* Redwood City, Calif.: Addison-Wesley.

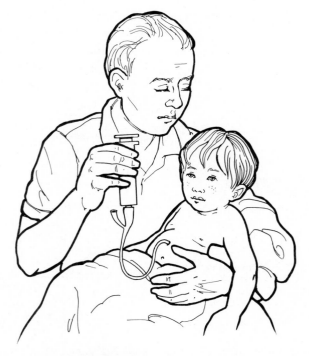

FIGURE 63.1 *Gastrostomy feeding.*

64 Gastrostomy Tube Change

PSYCHOSOCIAL CONSIDERATIONS: Explain the procedure in developmentally appropriate terms. The child may fear pain if this is the initial replacement. Allow the child to ventilate fears. Use a doll or puppet play to demonstrate the process.

TIME: 5 to 10 minutes

PURPOSE

To maintain enteral access via gastrostomy tube by keeping the tube intact.

OBJECTIVES

- To maintain access to the stomach.
- To prevent injury.

EQUIPMENT

Gastrostomy tube, same size and type as tube being replaced (see Figs. 64.1 and 64.2)

Gloves, nonsterile

Two 10 ml syringes, one needle

Water *or* normal saline (0.9% sodium chloride), to inflate balloon

Water-soluble lubricant

Catheter adapter

Stopcock *or* cap

Normal saline (0.9% sodium chloride), sterile water, *or* hydrogen peroxide (to clean site)

Gauze and tape for dressing (for Foley catheter only)

Nipple, sterile (for Foley catheter only)

Cotton-tip applicators

ESSENTIAL STEPS

1. Prepare the child and family. Have the parent restrain the child's hands, keeping them away from the clean tube.
2. Assemble the equipment. Verify the replacement tube is the correct size.
3. Remove the old tube.

   Wash hands and put on gloves.

   Remove the dressing and tape, if present.

   Attach the syringe to the balloon port of the Foley or MIC catheter and pull back the plunger to empty the balloon of water.

   Gently pull the tube out.

4. Insert the new tube.

   Test the balloon by filling it with water or normal saline and observing for leaks. Deflate balloon by aspirating water.

   Use 5 ml of liquid for Foley catheters.

   Use 7 ml of liquid for MIC catheters.

   Lubricate the catheter with water-soluble lubricant or water.

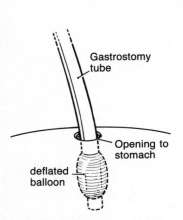

FIGURE 64.1 *Foley catheter gastrostomy tube.*

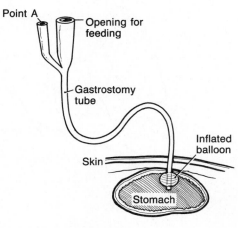

FIGURE 64.2 *Placement of the gastrostomy tube.*

Insert the tube into the stoma until the stomach contents drain out the open end of the tube.

Attach the water- or saline-filled syringe to the balloon port on the catheter. Inflate the balloon (should inflate easily) and remove the syringe.

Gently pull back on the tube until resistance is felt.

Insert the catheter adapter and stopcock or cap.

Clean the site with normal saline, sterile water, or hydrogen peroxide using cotton-tip applicators.

If using a Foley catheter,

>   Apply dressing and tape the tube securely.

>   Cut off the tip of a nipple and use around the base of the tube for support. (See Fig. 64.3)

If using an MIC tube, adjust the silicone disk to hold the tube securely. (See Fig. 64.4)

DOCUMENTATION

- Date and time of tube change.
- Assessment of child and gastrostomy site after the procedure.
- Any problems with removal and/or replacement of tube and name of the physician notified for problems.
- Condition of skin at site.
- Type and size of replacement tube.

Skills Checklist

- ☐ Prepare the child and family.
- ☐ Assemble the equipment.
- ☐ Wash hands and put on gloves.
- ☐ Deflate the balloon.
- ☐ Remove the old tube.
- ☐ Test the balloon.
- ☐ Insert the gastrostomy tube.
- ☐ Inflate the balloon.
- ☐ Clean the site.
- ☐ Document.

POTENTIAL RELATED NURSING DIAGNOSES

Anxiety

Infection: *high risk*

Nutrition, altered, less than body requirements

Swallowing, impaired

Activity intolerance

POTENTIAL RELATED MEDICAL DIAGNOSES

Tracheoesophageal reflux

Strictures

Near-drowning

Muscular dystrophy

Neurologic deficits

Head injuries

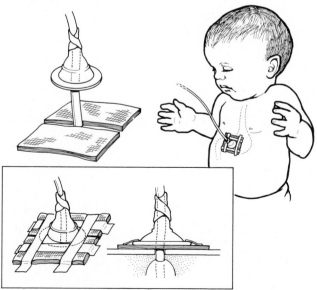

FIGURE 64.3 *Dressing application with a Foley catheter G-tube.*

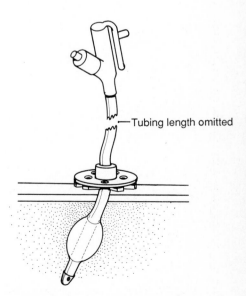

Tubing length omitted

FIGURE 64.4 *MIC gastrostomy tube.*

65 Heat Lamps

PSYCHOSOCIAL CONSIDERATIONS: Explain the procedure in developmentally appropriate terms. Provide privacy; keep the door to the room closed. Have a parent or significant person near to reassure the child that exposure of genitalia is all right at this time. Compare the heat lamp to the sun. Do not strap an infant in place. Provide distraction.

TIME: 10 to 15 minutes

PURPOSE

To promote healing of a wound, decrease wound exudation, improve circulation, and/or prevent heat loss during treatments.

OBJECTIVES

- To facilitate healing.
- To prevent heat loss.
- To prevent injury to the skin by heat.

EQUIPMENT

Heat lamp with timer and one 60-watt bulb.

Pillows or sand bags for positioning the child.

SAFETY ISSUES

- To prevent burning, do not place the lamp closer than 18 inches to the child.
- Do not place a sheet or a towel over the lamp, as doing so may cause a fire.
- Check the child's skin every 5 minutes to assess for redness.
- Avoid using lotion or baby oil on skin while the child is under the heat lamp, as this may contribute to tissue damage.
- Currently, heat lamps are not used as extensively as they have been in the past. Lately, the goal in wound healing is to keep the wound moist rather than dry. The use of heat lamps is controversial.

ESSENTIAL STEPS

1. Prepare the child and family. Position the child, using pillows or sand bags. Tell the family that the child will need to lie still. Make sure that the child's skin is clean.

2. Assemble the equipment.

3. Wash hands.

4. Assess skin and expose the area for application.

5. Place the lamp 18 to 24 inches from the area to be treated. (See Fig. 65.1)

6. Set the timer for 15 minutes. Assess the status of the child, including temperature, after initiating treatment.

7. Maintain proper positioning of the lamp and child during treatment.

DOCUMENTATION

• Date and time treatment performed.
• Assessment of child's temperature and skin condition.

POTENTIAL RELATED NURSING DIAGNOSES

Diarrhea

Infection: *high risk*

Skin integrity, impaired: *high risk*

Tissue integrity, impaired

POTENTIAL RELATED MEDICAL DIAGNOSES

Surgical procedures

Abcess

Decubitus

Infection

Diaper dermatitis, severe

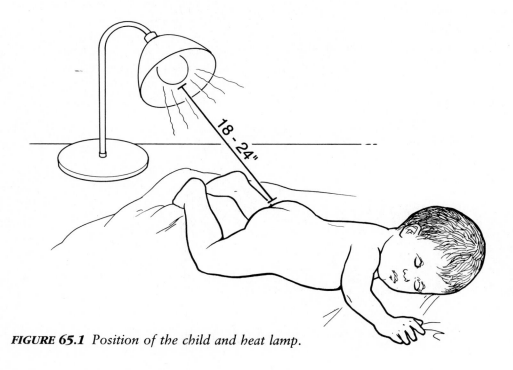

FIGURE 65.1 *Position of the child and heat lamp.*

66 Implantable Venous Access Device (IVAD): Blood Drawing

PSYCHOSOCIAL CONSIDERATIONS: Explain the procedure in developmentally appropriate terms. Avoid using terms with mixed meanings, such as *draw blood* and *stick*. Encourage the child to express feelings.

TIME: 10 to 15 minutes

PURPOSE

To obtain a blood sample from an implantable venous access device (IVAD) system.

OBJECTIVES

• To obtain a blood sample.
• To prevent injury or trauma.

EQUIPMENT

Two povidone-iodine swabs *or* alcohol swabs

Gloves, nonsterile

10 ml syringe

Vial of normal saline (0.9% sodium chloride), sterile

Three-way stopcock

5 ml syringe

Smooth-edge clamps

Lab tubes for blood

Syringe for drawing blood sample

Two sterile needles

ESSENTIAL STEPS

1. Prepare the child and family.
2. Assemble the equipment.
3. Wash hands and put on gloves.
4. Prepare and access the site according to procedure for "Implantable Venous Access Device: Site Preparation and Accessing."
5. Draw up 10 ml of normal saline.
6. Attach normal-saline–filled syringe to the side port of the stopcock and prime both ports to expel air.
7. Attach the empty 5 ml syringe to the other port of the stopcock. Keep the end and ports of the stopcock sterile.
8. Attach the primed stopcock and syringes to the clamped extension tubing. Some institutions may not use the stopcock.
9. Remove the clamp.
10. Turn the stopcock off to normal saline and withdraw 3 to 5 ml of blood for discard.
11. Turn the stopcock off to the child and remove the syringe with the discard blood.
12. Attach the syringe for the blood sample, turn the stopcock off to normal saline, and withdraw the appropriate amount of blood for sample(s). (See Fig. 66.1)

13. Turn the stopcock off to the blood-sample syringe and flush with normal saline.

14. Refer to "Implantable Venous Access Device: Heparin-Locking" or "Implantable Venous Access Device: Infusion of Fluids and Dressing Application."

DOCUMENTATION

- Amount of blood withdrawn.
- Time.
- Date.
- Ease of withdrawal.

POTENTIAL RELATED NURSING DIAGNOSES

Injury: *high risk*

Infection: *high risk*

Anxiety

Fear

Skin integrity, impaired: *high risk*

Fluid volume deficit: *high risk*

Skills Checklist

☐ Prepare the child and family.
☐ Assemble the equipment.
☐ Wash hands and put on gloves.
☐ Draw up saline.
☐ Prepare the stopcock; attach to extension tubing.
☐ Withdraw blood.
☐ Flush with normal saline.
☐ Attach the IV or heparin lock.
☐ Document.

POTENTIAL RELATED MEDICAL DIAGNOSES

Cancer

Chemotherapy

REFERENCES

Gullatte, M. 1989. Managing an implanted infusion device. *RN* 52, no. 1: 45–49.

McAfee, T., Garland, L., and McNabb, T. 1990. How to safely draw blood from a vascular device. *Nursing 90* 20, no. 11: 42–43.

Viall, C. 1990. Your complete guide to central venous catheters. *Nursing 90* 20: 34–41.

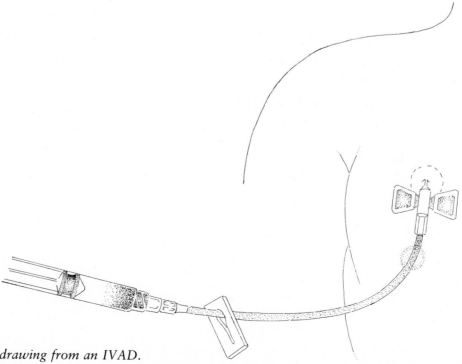

FIGURE 66.1 *Blood drawing from an IVAD.*

67 IVAD: Heparin-Locking

PSYCHOSOCIAL CONSIDERATIONS: Explain the procedure in developmentally appropriate terms. Be honest.

TIME: 10 to 15 minutes

PURPOSE

To heparin-lock the implantable venous access device (IVAD).

OBJECTIVES

- To keep the IVAD patent.
- To prevent injury or trauma.

EQUIPMENT

Gloves, nonsterile

10 ml syringe

Vial of normal saline (0.9% sodium chloride), sterile

5 ml syringe

3 to 5 ml of heparin solution (units/ml vary from 10 to 100, per institution policy)

Three-way stopcock

Smooth-edge clamps

Two povidone-iodine swabs *or* alcohol swabs

Needle, sterile

SAFETY ISSUES

- **Ensure placement and patency of the needle before injecting heparin.**
- **Heparinize an IVAD every 3 to 4 weeks when it is not being used. The amount of heparin used varies from 10 units to 100 units according to institution policy. Institutions may also prescribe heparin based on units/kg.**

ESSENTIAL STEPS

1. Prepare the child and family.
2. Assemble the equipment.
3. Wash hands.

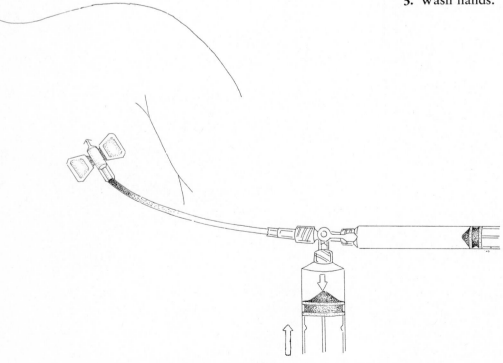

FIGURE 67.1 *Aspirating for blood return.*

4. Place supplies on a sterile field.

5. Put on gloves.

6. Draw up 10 ml of normal saline.

7. Draw up 3 to 5 ml of heparin solution.

8. Connect the normal-saline–filled syringe to the side port of the stopcock and prime the stopcock. Attach the heparin-filled syringe to the other port.

9. If heparin-locking the system after an infusion, omit step 10 and follow steps 11 through 16.

10. If heparin-locking the system following blood drawing, replace the blood-sample syringe with the syringe containing heparin solution. Refer to "Implantable Venous Access Device: Blood Drawing." Omit steps 11 through 14 and continue with step 15.

11. Clamp extension tubing.

12. Clean the IV tubing/extension connection site with a povidone-iodine or alcohol swab for 30 seconds. Remove the IV tubing and connect the stopcock with the attached normal-saline- and heparin-filled syringes.

13. Remove the clear occlusive dressing and tape that is anchoring the needle.

14. With the stopcock off to the heparin syringe, aspirate with the normal-saline–filled syringe to check for blood return; then flush the system with 10 ml of normal saline. (See Fig. 67.1) (Note: Decrease the amount of normal saline to no less than 4 ml, depending on the child's size and fluid requirements.)

15. Turn the stopcock off to the saline syringe and flush the system with 3 to 5 ml of heparin solution.

16. To avoid reflux, maintain positive injection pressure at the end of the heparin flush while simultaneously withdrawing the needle. (See Figs. 67.2 and 67.3)

Skills Checklist

☐ Prepare the child and family.
☐ Assemble the equipment.
☐ Wash hands.
☐ Set up sterile field.
☐ Put on gloves.
☐ Draw up heparin solution and normal saline. Connect syringes to the stopcock.
☐ Clean the IV tubing/extension connection. Remove IV tubing and connect the stopcock.
☐ Aspirate for blood return and flush with normal saline.
☐ Flush with heparin solution.
☐ Document.

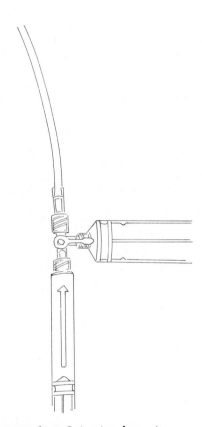

FIGURE 67.2 *Injecting heparin.*

17. To heparin-flush the system routinely, prepare and access the site following the procedure for "Implantable Venous Access Device: Site Preparation and Accessing." Then

Attach a heparin-filled syringe to the clamped extension tubing or needle.

Unclamp the tubing.

Flush the system with heparin solution.

Maintain positive injection pressure at the end of the heparin flush while simultaneously withdrawing the needle—to avoid reflux.

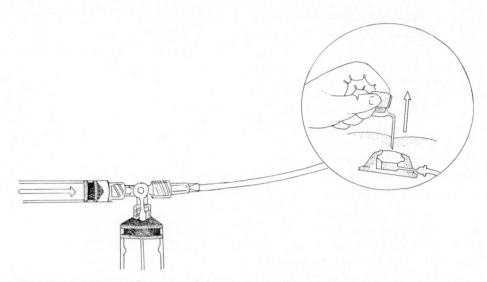

FIGURE 67.3 *Injecting heparin while removing the needle.*

DOCUMENTATION

- Amount and concentration of heparin.
- Ease of flushing.

POTENTIAL RELATED NURSING DIAGNOSES

Anxiety

Injury: *high risk*

Infection: *high risk*

Skin integrity, impaired: *high risk*

Fluid volume deficit: *high risk*

POTENTIAL RELATED MEDICAL DIAGNOSES

Cancer

Chemotherapy

REFERENCES

Gullatte, M. 1989. Managing an implanted infusion device. *RN* 52, no. 1: 45–49.

Viall, C. 1990. Your complete guide to central venous catheters. *Nursing 90* 20: 34–41.

68 IVAD: Infusion of IV Fluids and Dressing Application

PSYCHOSOCIAL CONSIDERATIONS: Explain the procedure in developmentally appropriate terms. Allow the child to ventilate feelings or concerns.

TIME: 10 to 15 minutes

PURPOSE

To administer infusion of IV fluids through the implantable venous access device (IVAD) system.

To apply a dressing to the access site, to stabilize the needle, and to maintain sterility of the system.

OBJECTIVES

- To administer IV fluids.
- To apply a new dressing.
- To prevent infection.
- To prevent injury and trauma.

EQUIPMENT

IV pump and tubing primed with appropriate IV solution

Smooth-edge clamps

Central venous catheter dressing change kit, including tape, gauze pads, split gauze pads *or* clear occlusive dressing, povidone-iodine ointment, gloves, and povidone-iodine swabs

Clear occlusive dressing (such as Tegaderm or Op-Site), sterile

ESSENTIAL STEPS

1. Prepare the child and family.
2. Assemble the equipment.
3. Prepare and access the site according to "Implantable Venous Access Device: Site Preparation and Accessing."
4. Turn the pump on and drip fluid into the clamped extension tubing to displace air. Connect IV tubing to the clamped extension tubing. Some institutions use a straight needle for intermittent administration of medications and a 90° bent needle for continuous infusions.
5. Remove the clamp from the extension tubing and begin infusion.
6. Secure the needle to the child as indicated by the type of device used.

   When the needle device has a cushion or when the child has poor skin integrity, place silk tape over the needle and in butterfly fashion over the extension tubing. (See Figs. 68.1 and 68.2)

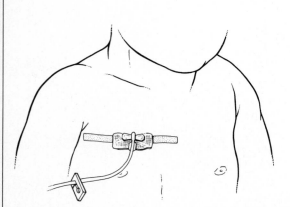

FIGURE 68.1 *Taped needle in an IVAD.*

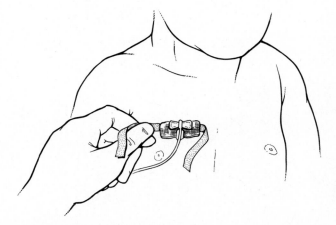

FIGURE 68.2 *Taping the needle.*

If the needle device has no cushion, place a sterile, double-folded, 2"×2" gauze underneath the hub of the Huber needle and secure it with tape. The Gripper needle has a foam pad already attached.

7. Add povidone-iodine ointment to the insertion site. This step is controversial; some studies have shown the ointment to provide a moist environment for bacteria. (Note: *Do not* place gauze over the needle insertion site as the needle needs to be checked every hour.)

8. Apply sterile clear occlusive dressing over the needle and portal area. (See Fig. 68.3)

9. Secure the IV connection site with tape. (See Fig. 68.4)

DOCUMENTATION

- Amount and type of infusion.
- Rate of infusion.
- Site of infusion.
- That dressing was changed.

POTENTIAL RELATED NURSING DIAGNOSES

Infection: *high risk*

Injury: *high risk*

Skin integrity, impaired: *high risk*

Anxiety

Fluid volume excess: *high risk*

Fluid volume deficit: *high risk*

Skills Checklist

☐ Prepare the child and family.
☐ Assemble the equipment.
☐ Prepare and access the site.
☐ Connect IV tubing to the extension tubing.
☐ Remove the clamp.
☐ Secure the needle.
☐ Apply occlusive dressing.
☐ Secure the IV connection.
☐ Document.

POTENTIAL RELATED MEDICAL DIAGNOSES

Chemotherapy

Cancer

REFERENCES

Gullatte, M. 1989. Managing an implanted infusion device. *RN 52*, no. 1: 45–49.

Viall, C. 1990. Your complete guide to central venous catheters. *Nursing 90 20:* 34–41.

Whitney, R. 1991. Comparing long term central venous catheters. *Nursing 91 21*, no. 4: 70–71.

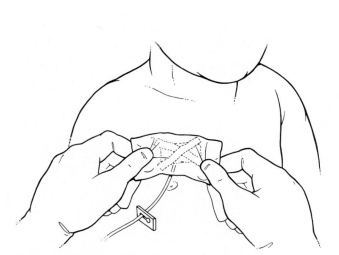

FIGURE 68.3 *Clear dressing over the needle and portal area.*

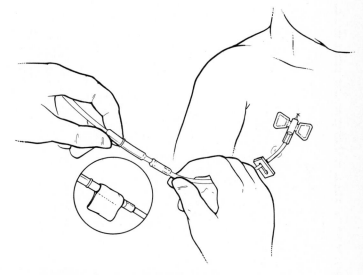

FIGURE 68.4 *Connecting IV tubing and securing connection.*

IVAD: Site Preparation and Accessing

PSYCHOSOCIAL CONSIDERATIONS: Explain the procedure in developmentally appropriate terms. Avoid using terms with mixed meanings, such as *stick*. Allow the child to ventilate feelings.

TIME: 10 to 15 minutes

PURPOSE

To provide an aseptic area for injections into the implantable venous access device (IVAD).

To obtain access to an IVAD.

OBJECTIVES

- To prepare the skin.
- To access the IVAD.
- To prevent injury or trauma.

EQUIPMENT

Gloves, sterile

10 ml syringe

Vial of normal saline (0.9% sodium chloride), sterile

90° bent Huber needle (22g or 20g) with attached extension set *or* 90° bent Huber needle (22g or 20g) with separate extension tubing (see Fig. 69.1) *or* Gripper needle with extension tubing (see Fig. 69.2)

Acetone alcohol swab sticks

Povidone-iodine swab sticks (or other antiseptic if child is allergic to iodine)

Needle, sterile

Smooth-edge clamps

ESSENTIAL STEPS

1. Prepare the child and family. (See Fig. 69.3)
2. Assemble the equipment.
3. Wash hands.
4. Palpate the site to locate the portal septum. (See Fig. 69.4)

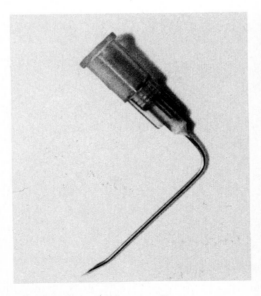

FIGURE 69.1 *Huber needle.*

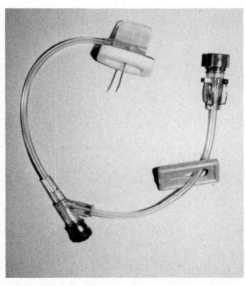

FIGURE 69.2 *Gripper needle.*

5. Put on sterile gloves. Use the interior lining of the sterile glove packet as a sterile field on which to arrange the equipment if desired.

6. Draw up 10 ml of normal saline and prime the extension tubing with the Huber or Gripper needle attached to displace air.

7. Open swab stick packets, maintaining sterility.

8. Clean the area with each acetone alcohol swab stick, starting over the portal and moving outward in a circular motion to cover an area 4" in diameter. Some institutions clean with povidone-iodine only because alcohol dries the skin.

Skills Checklist

- ☐ Prepare the child and family.
- ☐ Assemble the equipment.
- ☐ Wash hands.
- ☐ Palpate the site.
- ☐ Put on gloves.
- ☐ Draw up normal saline.
- ☐ Clean the site.
- ☐ Insert the needle.
- ☐ Aspirate.
- ☐ Flush.
- ☐ Attach IV fluids or heparin-lock.
- ☐ Document.

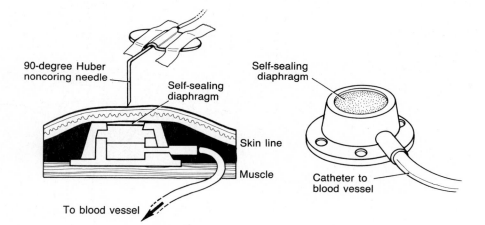

90-degree Huber noncoring needle

Self-sealing diaphragm

Self-sealing diaphragm

Skin line

Muscle

Catheter to blood vessel

To blood vessel

FIGURE 69.3 *Position of the IVAD.*

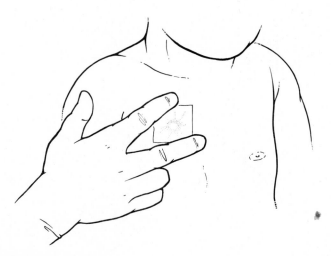

FIGURE 69.4 *Palpating the IVAD site.*

9. Clean the area with each povidone-iodine swab stick using the same technique described for acetone alcohol swab sticks in Step 8. (See Fig. 69.5)

10. Insert the Huber or Gripper needle perpendicular to the septum and push firmly through the skin and portal septum until it hits the bottom of the portal chamber. (See Fig. 69.6)

11. Aspirate with a normal-saline–filled syringe to check for blood return.

12. Flush the system with 3 to 5 ml of normal saline to confirm patency of the system. Clamp extension tubing.

13. Refer to "Implantable Venous Access Device: Infusion of IV Fluids and Dressing Application," or "Implantable Venous Access Device: Blood Drawing," or "Implantable Venous Access Device: Heparin-Locking."

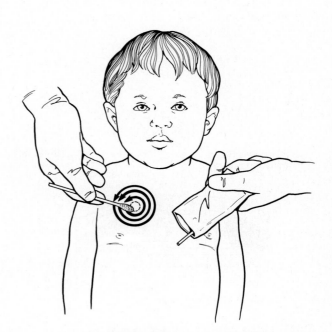

FIGURE 69.5 *Cleaning the IVAD site.*

DOCUMENTATION

- Skin preparation.
- Appearance of site around IVAD.
- Ease of entry.
- Ease of flushing.

POTENTIAL RELATED NURSING DIAGNOSES

Infection: *high risk*

Injury: *high risk*

Skin integrity, impaired: *high risk*

Anxiety

Fear

POTENTIAL RELATED MEDICAL DIAGNOSES

Cancer

Chemotherapy

REFERENCES

Gullatte, M. 1989. Managing an implanted infusion device. *RN 52*, no. 1: 45–49.

Viall, C. 1990. Your complete guide to central venous catheters. *Nursing 90* 20: 34–41.

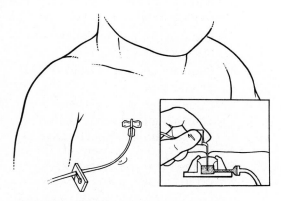

FIGURE 69.6 *Inserting the needle.*

IVAD: Urokinase for Occlusion

Three needles, sterile

Two 3 ml syringes

3 ml of heparin (units/ml vary from 10 to 100, per institution policy)

Straight Huber needle *or* Gripper needle

Three-way stopcock

ESSENTIAL STEPS

PSYCHOSOCIAL CONSIDERATIONS: Explain the procedure in developmentally appropriate terms. Avoid using terms with mixed meanings, such as *blocked catheter* and *clotted off*. Allow the child to express feelings.

TIME: 20 minutes

PURPOSE

To remove an occlusion from an implantable venous access device (IVAD) when the cause is suspected to be a blood clot or fibrin deposit.

OBJECTIVES

- To establish a patent IVAD.
- To prevent injury.

EQUIPMENT

Gloves, sterile

Two vials of normal saline (0.9% sodium chloride), sterile

Two 10 ml syringes

1 ml of urokinase 5,000 units/ml

1. Prepare the child and family.
2. Assemble the equipment.

   Wash hands and put on gloves.

   Draw up 2 ml of normal saline into one 10 ml syringe and 10 ml of normal saline into the other.

   Draw up 1 ml of urokinase into a 3 ml syringe.

   Draw up heparin into the other 3 ml syringe.

   Connect the 10 ml syringe containing 2 ml of normal saline and the straight Huber needle or Gripper needle to opposite sides of the three-way stopcock. Turn off to the side port.

3. Prepare and access the site according to "Implantable Venous Access Device: Site Preparation and Accessing."

4. Gently alternate between irrigation and aspiration with the 10 ml syringe.

5. If blood return is obtained, aspirate 4 to 5 ml of blood. Turn the stopcock off to the child. (If unable to obtain blood, notify the physician.)

6. Attach the 10 ml syringe of normal saline to sideport of stopcock and flush.

7. Remove 10 ml syringe and replace with 1 ml of urokinase in a 3 ml syringe. Flush with urokinase.

8. Wait 5 to 10 minutes and aspirate to remove small occlusions.

9. Repeat steps 4 through 8 as necessary.

10. When the occlusion is removed and the catheter is patent, flush with 3 ml of heparin before removing the needle and syringe assembly.

DOCUMENTATION

- Specific events leading to the occlusion.
- Amount and concentration of urokinase.
- Ease of flushing.
- Amount and concentration of heparin.

Skills Checklist

- ☐ Prepare the child and family.
- ☐ Assemble the equipment.
- ☐ Wash hands and put on gloves.
- ☐ Draw up normal saline.
- ☐ Draw up urokinase.
- ☐ Draw up heparin.
- ☐ Connect the normal-saline–filled syringe and the needle to the stopcock.
- ☐ Access the site.
- ☐ Alternate irrigation and aspiration.
- ☐ Aspirate blood.
- ☐ Flush with normal saline.
- ☐ Flush with urokinase.
- ☐ Flush with heparin.
- ☐ Document.

POTENTIAL RELATED NURSING DIAGNOSES

Injury: *high risk*

Infection: *high risk*

Anxiety

Fear

POTENTIAL RELATED MEDICAL DIAGNOSES

Universal application for IVADs

REFERENCES

Gullatte, M. 1989. Managing an implanted infusion device. *RN* 52, no. 1: 45–49.

Viall, C. 1990. Your complete guide to central venous catheters. *Nursing 90* 20: 34–41.

Intravenous: Catheter Securing and Dressing Change

PSYCHOSOCIAL CONSIDERATIONS: Explain the procedure in developmentally appropriate terms. Avoid using terms with mixed meanings, such as *stick*. Comfort the child after the procedure.

TIME: 5 to 10 minutes

PURPOSE

To standardize taping techniques in order to afford daily visualization of the insertion site and skin proximal to the site and to facilitate cleaning of the insertion site and changing of the dressing without jeopardizing the position of the IV device.

OBJECTIVES

- To secure the needle or catheter in place.
- To prevent trauma or injury.

EQUIPMENT

2″×2″ gauze, adhesive bandage, *or* clear occlusive dressing (such as Tegaderm or Op-Site), sterile

Povidone-iodine swab *or* alcohol swab

½″ adhesive tape

1″ adhesive tape

SAFETY ISSUES

- **Visualize peripheral IV sites daily.**
- **Prep IV sites with povidone-iodine and cover with a sterile dressing or adhesive bandage every 48 to 72 hours, per institution policy, unless manipulation might dislodge the IV. Clear occlusive dressings may remain in place for up to 7 days, unless they become wet or soiled.**

ESSENTIAL STEPS

1. Prepare the child and family.
2. Assemble the equipment.
3. Wash hands.

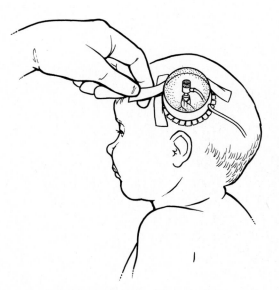

FIGURE 71.1 *Securing a scalp vein.*

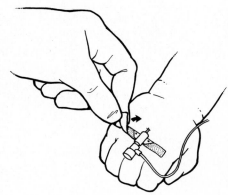

FIGURE 71.2 *Taping an IV.*

4. Inspect the site daily. Lift the 2″ by 2″ gauze or adhesive bandage or visualize through the transparent dressing. Check for erythema, drainage, swelling, and so on.

5. Using a povidone-iodine or alcohol swab, paint the insertion site in a circular fashion from the center to the periphery.

6. Place a folded 2″×2″ gauze over the clean site and secure with tape. Write the time, the date, and your initials on the adhesive tape anchoring the dressing. (See Figs. 71.1, 71.2, 71.3, 71.4, and 71.5)

DOCUMENTATION

- Appearance of IV site.
- Povidone-iodine or alcohol applied.
- Type of dressing applied.

POTENTIAL RELATED NURSING DIAGNOSES

Anxiety

Infection: *high risk*

Injury: *high risk*

Skin integrity, impaired

POTENTIAL RELATED MEDICAL DIAGNOSES

Universal application

REFERENCES

Tietjen, S. 1990. Starting an infant's IV. *American Journal of Nursing* 90, no. 5: 44–47.

Skills Checklist

☐ Prepare the child and family.
☐ Assemble the equipment.
☐ Wash hands.
☐ Inspect the site.
☐ Remove the old dressing, if applicable.
☐ Clean with povidone-iodine or alcohol swab.
☐ Apply a new dressing.
☐ Document.

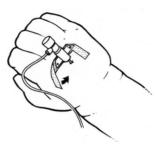

FIGURE 71.3 *Folding tape over phalanges.*

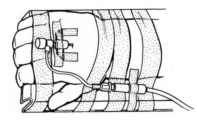

FIGURE 71.4 *Arm secured to an armboard.*

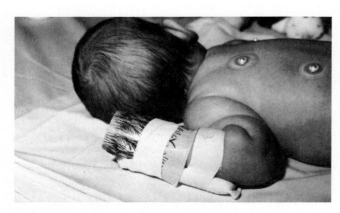

FIGURE 71.5 *Site protected by a paper cup.*

72 Intravenous: Cutdown

PSYCHOSOCIAL CONSIDERATIONS: Explain the procedure in developmentally appropriate terms. Avoid using terms with mixed meanings, such as *stick, cut,* and *cut into your vein*. Describe what the child will see, feel, and hear. Allow the child to scream or yell but not to move. Help the child to hold still; restrain as necessary. Use distraction. Ensure that the local anesthetic has had time to be effective. Provide comfort following the procedure.

TIME: 15 to 30 minutes

PURPOSE

To assist the physician in cannulating a blood vessel under direct visualization for placement and maintenance of an indwelling line.

OBJECTIVES

- To facilitate IV access.
- To prevent injury.

EQUIPMENT

Gloves, sterile

Cutdown tray, including a 5 ml syringe, 4″×4″ gauze, povidone-iodine solution and ointment, suture material

Longline catheter *or* angiocath

T connector (optional)

Mask (for the physician)

Gloves, nonsterile

Gown, sterile (optional)

Vial of normal saline (0.9% sodium chloride), sterile

Solution and administration set (refer to "Intravenous: Peripheral Infusion")

Adhesive tape

Local anesthetic, syringe, and small-gauge needle

 SAFETY ISSUES

- **Use sterile technique.**

ESSENTIAL STEPS

1. Prepare the child and family.
2. Assemble the equipment.
3. Wash hands and put on clean gloves.
4. Assist the physician as necessary. (See Fig. 72.1)
5. Apply povidone-iodine ointment to the cutdown site, at physician's discretion, after suturing.

6. Apply a sterile dressing. Mark the date and time on the dressing.

7. Observe the site hourly for patency/infiltration. Assess the insertion site daily for complications.

8. Refer to "Intravenous: Catheter Securing and Dressing Change" for care of a peripheral IV.

DOCUMENTATION

- Date, time, type, and gauge of catheter.
- Name of physician inserting the catheter.
- Number of incisions made.
- Number of sutures placed, if any.
- Child's tolerance of the procedure.
- When dressing changed; appearance of catheter exit site at that time.

POTENTIAL RELATED NURSING DIAGNOSES

Anxiety

Pain, acute

Injury: *high risk*

Tissue integrity, impaired

POTENTIAL RELATED MEDICAL DIAGNOSES

Any medical diagnosis requiring an IV access where usual peripheral accesses are not available.

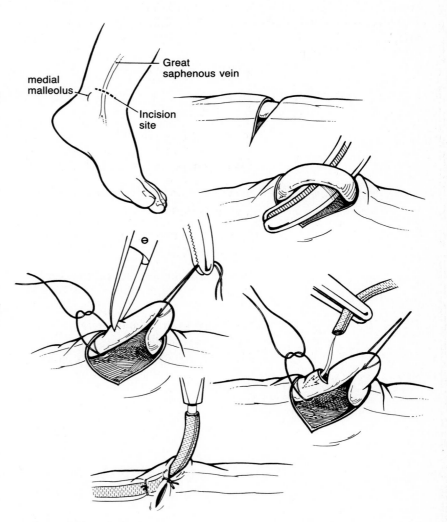

FIGURE 72.1 *IV cutdown.*

73 Intravenous: Heparin Flush

PSYCHOSOCIAL CONSIDERATIONS: Explain the procedure in developmentally appropriate terms. Tell the child that you are not going to remove or move the needle. The child may associate the IV needle with pain and fear the procedure. Children over the age of 4 may benefit from *supervised* needle play, such as drawing up saline or injecting a doll or puppet.

TIME: 5 minutes

PURPOSE

To maintain patency of a *peripheral* heparin lock.

OBJECTIVES

• To maintain a patent peripheral heparin lock.
• To prevent injury and trauma.

EQUIPMENT

Heparinized saline solution (units/ml vary per institution policy) (See Fig. 73.1)

Syringe with a needle (preferably a small-gauge needle)

Povidone-iodine swabs *or* alcohol swabs

 SAFETY ISSUES

• Currently some institutions are exploring the use of saline instead of heparin as a flush.
• Check vials of heparin carefully. Units/ml vary widely.

ESSENTIAL STEPS

1. Prepare the child and family.
2. Assemble the equipment.
3. Draw up 1 ml of heparinized saline, more if extension tubing is used. (See Fig. 73.2)

   Butterfly tubing holds approximately 0.3 ml of solution.

   T-connector tubing holds approximately 0.2 ml of solution.
4. Wash hands.
5. Clean the infusion plug with a povidone-iodine or alcohol swab.
6. Aspirate to check for blood return prior to injecting heparin, per institution procedure.
7. Inject all but the last 0.1 ml of heparinized saline.

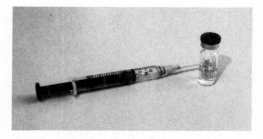

FIGURE 73.1 *Heparin and syringe.*

8. Inject the last 0.1 ml while removing the needle to prevent a backflow of blood or air accumulation in the cap. (See Figs. 73.3 and 73.4)

DOCUMENTATION

- Time.
- Presence of blood return.
- Amount and concentration of heparinized saline administered.
- Ease of flushing.
- Appearance of site.

POTENTIAL RELATED NURSING DIAGNOSES

Anxiety

Skin integrity, impaired

Tissue integrity, impaired

Infection: *high risk*

POTENTIAL RELATED MEDICAL DIAGNOSES

Universal application for IV accesses with a heparin lock

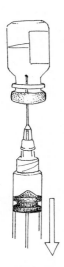

FIGURE 73.2 *Drawing up heparin.*

Skills Checklist

- ☐ Prepare the child and family.
- ☐ Assemble the equipment.
- ☐ Wash hands.
- ☐ Clean the infusion plug.
- ☐ Aspirate to check for blood return.
- ☐ Inject all but the last 0.1 ml of heparinized saline.
- ☐ Remove the needle while injecting the last 0.1 ml of heparinized saline.
- ☐ Document.

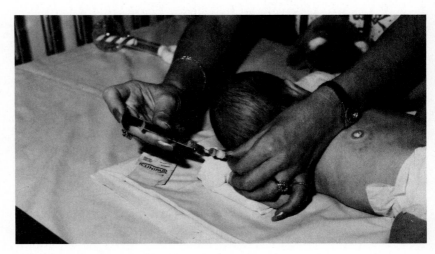

FIGURE 73.3 *Injecting heparin.*

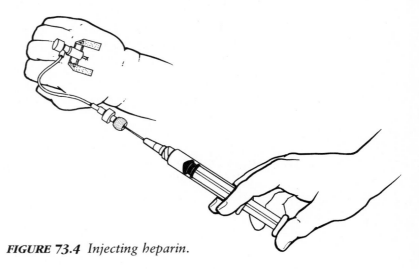

FIGURE 73.4 *Injecting heparin.*

Intravenous: Heparin Lock

PSYCHOSOCIAL CONSIDERATIONS: Explain the procedure in developmentally appropriate terms. Avoid using terms with mixed meanings, such as *stick* or *shot*. Explain to toddlers and preschoolers immediately prior to the procedure. Perform the procedure quickly without *excessive* explanation that may raise anxiety. *Do not* tell a child "it won't hurt." Be honest. Do not perform the procedure while the child is asleep. Encourage therapeutic play with a doll or puppet.

TIME: 5 to 10 minutes

PURPOSE

To allow for intermittent venous access without a continuous IV infusion or repetitive percutaneous IV punctures.

OBJECTIVES

- To allow IV access without continuous fluids.
- To prevent injury during the procedure.

EQUIPMENT

Gloves, nonsterile

Tourniquet

Tape

Normal saline (0.9% sodium chloride) sterile

One of the following heparin lock systems:

    Angiocath with injection cap

    Angiocath with T connector and injection cap

    Butterfly with injection cap

Povidone-iodine swabs or alcohol swabs

Heparinized saline solution (units/ml vary, per institution policy) *or* normal saline (0.9% sodium chloride) (see Fig. 74.1)

Syringe with 25g 5/8″ needle (not necessary when using the recently developed systems that do not require a needle for the heparin flush)

SAFETY ISSUES

- **Heparinized saline solution must be preservative free for children under 6 months of age.**
- **Check vials of heparin carefully. Units/ml vary widely.**

ESSENTIAL STEPS

1. Prepare the child and family.
2. Ensure that the IV device is stable and will not move.
3. Assemble the equipment.

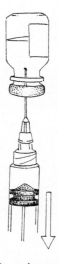

FIGURE 74.1 *Drawing up heparin.*

4. Wash hands and put on gloves.

5. Establish venous access using the angiocath or butterfly:

   Refer to "Intravenous: Peripheral Insertion."

   Fill the catheter tubing with normal saline in order to clear it. (See Fig. 74.2)

   After the vein has been successfully cannulated, connect the injection cap to the angiocath, the butterfly, or the T connector.

   Clean the injection cap with a povidone-iodine or alcohol swab.

   Inject 1 ml of heparinized saline solution or normal saline into the heparin lock system, injecting the last 0.1 ml while removing the needle to prevent a backflow of blood. (See Fig. 74.3)

   If using a T connector, ensure that the clamp on it is closed.

DOCUMENTATION

- Date and time.
- Type of heparin lock system.
- Site.
- Appearance of site at least every shift.
- Name of individual starting heparin lock.
- Child's tolerance of procedure.
- Heparinized saline flush, concentration, and amount.

POTENTIAL RELATED NURSING DIAGNOSES

Anxiety

Pain, acute

Infection: *high risk*

Injury: *high risk*

Skills Checklist

☐ Prepare the child and family.
☐ Assemble the equipment.
☐ Wash hands and put on gloves.
☐ Perform venipuncture, if applicable.
☐ Connect the injection cap.
☐ Flush with heparin.
☐ Document.

POTENTIAL RELATED MEDICAL DIAGNOSES

Infection

Postoperative pain management

Antibiotic therapy

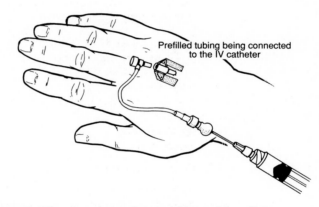

Prefilled tubing being connected to the IV catheter

FIGURE 74.2 *Clearing the catheter tubing with saline.*

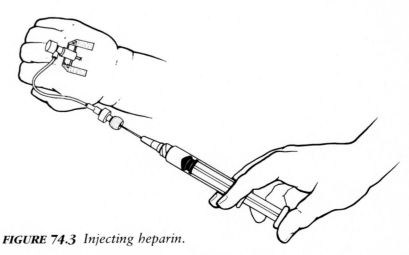

FIGURE 74.3 *Injecting heparin.*

75 Intravenous: Peripheral Infusion

PSYCHOSOCIAL CONSIDERATIONS: Explain the procedure in developmentally appropriate terms. Avoid using terms with mixed meaning, such as *stick* and *insert*. Allow the child to voice fears. Be honest with the child. If asked, tell the child that the procedure might hurt.

TIME: Varies

PURPOSE

To correctly administer IV solutions through a peripheral vein with minimal discomfort to the child and with maximum safety.

OBJECTIVES

- To administer IV solutions.
- To prevent injury and trauma.

EQUIPMENT

IV solution label
IV solution
IV pole
Administration set
Infusion pump, if appropriate
Extension tubing and stopcock, if appropriate
Injection cap, if a stopcock is used

SAFETY ISSUES

- Prior to hanging a new IV solution bag, check the manufacturer's label three times:

    When selecting the solution and checking it against the physician's plan of care.

    When making a label for the solution.

    When hanging the solution.

- Document intake and output for all patients receiving IV solutions.
- Inspect the site hourly.
- Do not turn off the audible pump alarm. Set the alarm to go off when the hourly or desired volume has been infused.

ESSENTIAL STEPS

1. Prepare the child and family.
2. Assemble the equipment.
3. Wash hands.
4. Check the physician's plan of care for IV fluid *replacement* or *maintenance*. The document should include:

    Date and time the order was written.

    Type of solution and concentration to be used.

    Rate in ml/hour.

5. Read the IV solution label three times and check it against the order. Some institutions require two RNs to double-check IV solutions.
6. Check the solution to make sure it is clear.
7. Assemble the appropriate administration set.
8. Use aseptic technique to open the IV solution and attach the administration set.

9. Prime the tubing with the IV solution, keeping the end of the tubing sterile with a cap or needle.

10. Complete and attach a label to the bag. *Do not* cover the manufacturer's label or expiration date. Record the following information on the label: name, room, type of solution, additives, medications, date and time bottle opened, nurse's name.

11. Label the administration set with the date and time opened.

12. Identify the child by checking the identification band.

13. Assess the status of the child and of the IV site prior to beginning the infusion.

14. Hang the solution.

15. If an IV site is *infiltrated* or inflamed, remove the IV cannula and restart the IV.

16. Irrigate a peripheral IV cannula with a small volume (1 to 2 ml) of IV solution when evaluating for patency.

17. Report to the physician any significant change in the child's fluid status. (See Table 75.1)

TABLE 75.1
Frequency of Change Schedule

Intravenous Equipment	Times for Change
IV solutions (stock and nonstock)	every 24°
Peripheral IV dressings	every 72°
IV administration sets and extension tubing	every 72°
IV administration sets used with heparin locks	every 72°
Peripheral percutaneous IV sites	every 72°
Stopcocks and infusion caps	every 72°

SOURCE: Centers for Disease Control Guidelines.

Skills Checklist

☐ Prepare the child and family.
☐ Assemble the equipment.
☐ Wash hands.
☐ Read the IV solution label three times.
☐ Open the IV solution and attach the administration set.
☐ Prime the tubing. Label the bag and the administration set.
☐ Identify the child by checking the identification band.
☐ Begin the infusion.
☐ Regulate the IV rate.
☐ Document.

DOCUMENTATION

• Type and concentration of solution.
• Time hung.
• Infusion rate.
• IV pump, if applicable.
• Assessment of signs and symptoms of infiltration and phlebitis.

POTENTIAL RELATED NURSING DIAGNOSES

Fear

Anxiety

Infection: *high risk*

Fluid volume deficit

Skin integrity: impaired

Injury: *high risk*

POTENTIAL RELATED MEDICAL DIAGNOSES

Universal application

76 Intravenous: Peripheral Insertion

PSYCHOSOCIAL CONSIDERATIONS: Explain the procedure in developmentally appropriate terms. Allow the child to cry or yell but not to move. Avoid using terms with mixed meanings, such as *stick*. Younger children may benefit from therapeutic play with a doll or puppet.

TIME: 10 to 15 minutes

PURPOSE

To provide an IV route via a superficial vein in an extremity or, for an infant, in the scalp; for obtaining blood samples or infusing products intravenously.

OBJECTIVES

- To establish a venous access.
- To prevent injury.

EQUIPMENT

Gloves, nonsterile (must fit well so as not to impede manual dexterity)

Povidone-iodine swabs *or* 70% isopropyl alcohol swabs

IV solution with administration set, if ordered

Topical anesthetic *or* normal saline (0.9% sodium chloride; with preservative), sterile

26g or 27g needle, if normal saline used

Tourniquet (rubber band may be used for scalp veins)

21g or 22g needle

One of the following IV cannulas:
  Winged-needle unit (butterfly)
  Over-the-needle catheter

Lab tubes, if blood samples are needed

Tape

2″ × 2″ gauze sponges *or* clear occlusive dressing (such as Tegaderm or Op-Site), sterile

Paper or plastic cup for cap

Restraints and an arm board

Razor or scissors, if needed

SAFETY ISSUES

- **Ensure that the child is properly restrained.**

ESSENTIAL STEPS

1. Prepare the child and family.
2. Assemble the equipment.
3. Wash hands and put on gloves.
4. Select a site.

   Carefully examine all extremities before choosing a site. Avoid the child's dominant hand, if possible.

   Start venipunctures distally and work proximally.

   Consider the following contraindications. Discuss a contraindicated site with a physician before using it. In cases where the child has

   Hydrocephalus or possible hydrocephalus: Do not use the scalp.

   Undergone Blalock-Taussig procedure: Do not use the arm on the side on which the procedure was done (usually the left side).

Infection, osteomyelitis, or cellulitis: Do not use the affected extremity.

Undergone cardiac catherization: Do not use the leg with the catherization site.

Vasospasm secondary to deep lines with discoloration of an extremity: Do not use the affected extremity.

5. Prepare the site.

For scalp veins, clip hair as close as possible to the skin or shave as needed. (Clipping is preferred because it is less likely to lead to ingrown hairs and infection.) (See Fig. 76.1)

Prep the skin by applying friction and cleaning from the center to the periphery using povidone-iodine swabs. *Allow to dry for 30 seconds.* Wipe the iodine off with alcohol if necessary to visualize the vein. If a child is iodine-sensitive, scrub for at least 1 minute with an alcohol swab and allow to dry for 30 seconds.

6. To insert the IV device:

Numb the site with a topical anesthetic or by injecting 0.1 to 0.2 ml of sterile normal saline (with preservative) intradermally with a 26g or 27g needle, if appropriate.

Apply a tourniquet.

Grasp the extremity firmly. Palpate the vein by pulling the skin over it taut with a finger above the point of entry.

Prestick with a 21g or 22g needle before inserting the IV device, if desired. This decreases the shearing effect of the IV device and increases comfort.

Point the needle with the bevel up in the direction of the course of the vein at a 20° angle.

Pierce the skin, lower the angle of the needle, and enter the vein. (See Fig. 76.2)

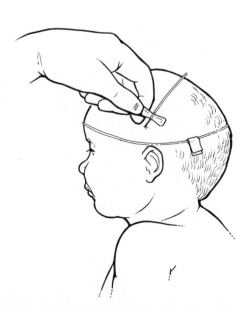

FIGURE 76.1 *Starting a scalp vein IV.*

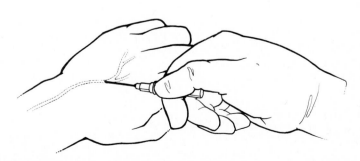

FIGURE 76.2 *Inserting the needle into the skin.*

Observe for a backflow of blood.

When using a winged infusion device, advance the needle gently until it is well within the lumen.

When using a catheter-over-needle device, stabilize the needle and advance the catheter until it is well within the lumen. Remove the needle once the catheter is advanced. Do not reinsert the needle. (See Fig. 76.3)

Collect blood samples, if needed.

Release the tourniquet, connect the IV tubing, and start the infusion.

Assess for patency and discontinue if infiltration occurs.

If the IV start is unsuccessful, apply pressure for 2 to 3 minutes.

After three unsuccessful attempts, request assistance from another individual.

7. To tape the IV,

Anchor the catheter/needle in place with tape. Do not tape directly over the insertion site. Use nonallergenic or sensitive-skin tape on neonates and infants. To prevent pressure under the hub, avoid applying tape too tightly. (See Figs. 76.4, 76.5, and 76.6)

Cover the IV site with a sterile dressing. Mark the date and time on the dressing. Cover the site with a clear occlusive dressing for better visualization if desired.

Protect the site with a paper or plastic cup cap if applicable. Pad the edges if necessary.

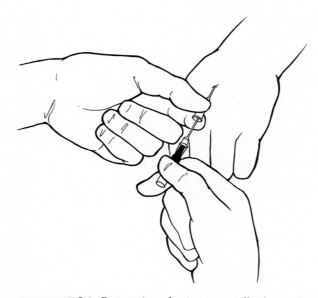

FIGURE 76.3 *Removing the inner needle from the catheter.*

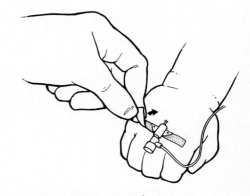

FIGURE 76.4 *Taping the IV.*

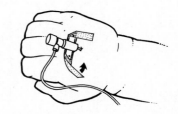

FIGURE 76.5 *Taping the IV.*

8. Secure the extremity to an arm board, being careful to protect pressure points with padding, if appropriate. (See Fig. 76.7)

9. Adjust the IV flow rate as ordered.

DOCUMENTATION

- Date and time.
- Name of individual starting the IV.
- Size and type of device used.
- Insertion site.
- Any blood samples sent to the lab.
- Appearance of site.
- Type of dressing applied.
- Number of attempts or difficulty starting IV.
- Child's tolerance of procedure.

POTENTIAL RELATED NURSING DIAGNOSES

Anxiety

Fear

Pain, acute

Skin integrity, impaired

Infection: *high risk*

POTENTIAL RELATED MEDICAL DIAGNOSES

Any diagnosis requiring IV fluids or IV medications

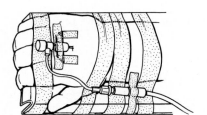

FIGURE 76.7 *IV secured with an arm board.*

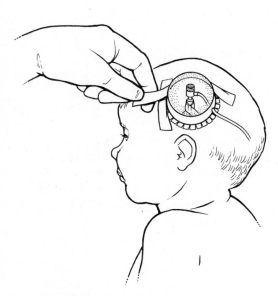

FIGURE 76.6 *Taping a scalp IV.*

77 Isolette, Closed

PSYCHOSOCIAL CONSIDERATIONS: Explain the procedure to the family. Allow the family to touch the infant and to remove the infant from the isolette as possible. Avoid bumping the isolette or closing portholes sharply or noisily as the noise is magnified inside the isolette.

TIME: Varies

PURPOSE

To provide a neutral thermal environment.

OBJECTIVES

• To maintain a neutral thermal environment.
• To prevent injury.

EQUIPMENT

Isolette

SAFETY ISSUES

• Record the infant's temperature every 30 to 60 minutes over the first 2 hours or until the temperature stabilizes at 36° to 36.5°C (axillary); 96.8° to 97.7° F. Then record the temperature every 4 hours or per the physician's plan of care.

• Check an infant's temperature every 30 minutes during the weaning process.

• Keep the on/off switch on while the infant is in the isolette.

• Keep port doors closed at all times except during care and transport.

ESSENTIAL STEPS

1. Prepare the infant and family.

2. Assemble the equipment.

3. Wash hands.

4. Obtain the isolette. (See Fig. 77.1)

5. Stabilize the isolette temperature before placing the infant inside.

   Ensure that the mode and meter switches are on air.

   Plug the isolette into an electrical supply and switch on. This causes the audible alarm to sound. After 5 seconds, reset the audible alarm by pressing the reset button and releasing it.

   Select the required air temperature. (See Table 77.1) If a high temperature is required, start with 34°C (93.2°F). After 40 minutes, select the final setting. Do not set the temperature above 35.9°C (96.6°F). Total stabilization time is approximately 45 to 60 minutes.

6. Place blankets, diapers, and other needed cloth items inside the isolette to get warm.

7. Place the baby inside the warm isolette. Ensure that the mattress and/ or the blanket do not cover thermometers at the rear of the isolette or block the air passages around the baby tray.

8. Notify the physician if the infant's temperature is unstable after the initial 2 hours.

9. To wean or discontinue,

   Obtain an order for discontinuing.

   Reset the digital switch to 0.5°C increments below the previous setting at 30-minute intervals, for as long as the infant's temperature remains at or above 36.4°C (axillary); 97.5°F.

   Transfer the infant from the isolette to an open crib when the isolette temperature setting is 30°C (86°F) and the baby's temperature is stable for 30 minutes at 36° to 36.5°C (axillary); 96.8° to 97.7°F.

   Monitor the infant's temperature after removal from the isolette per the physician's plan of care.

DOCUMENTATION

- Infant's temperature.
- Time infant placed in or removed from isolette.
- Temperature of isolette.
- Position of infant.
- Time weaning initiated and infant's response to weaning.

Skills Checklist

☐ Prepare the infant and family.
☐ Assemble the equipment.
☐ Wash hands.
☐ Stabilize isolette temperature.
☐ Place cloth items in the isolette to get warm.
☐ Place the infant in the isolette.
☐ Monitor the infant's temperature.
☐ Document.

POTENTIAL RELATED NURSING DIAGNOSES

Hypothermia

Skin integrity, impaired: *high risk*

Hyperthermia

POTENTIAL RELATED MEDICAL DIAGNOSES

Prematurity

Surgery

REFERENCES

Fanaroff MB, A. A., and Klaus MD, M. H. 1979. *Care of the high risk neonate.* Philadelphia, Pa.: W. B. Saunders Co.

Mott, S., James, S., and Sperhac, A. 1990. *Nursing care of children and families.* Redwood City, Calif.: Addison-Wesley.

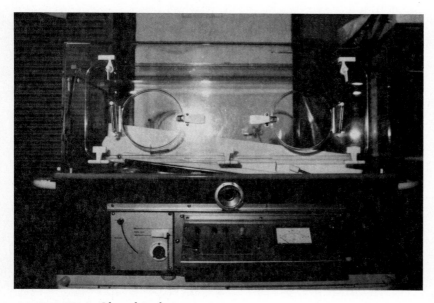

FIGURE 77.1 *Closed isolette.*

TABLE 77.1 *Neutral Environmental Temperatures*

Age and Weight	Starting Temperature (°C)	Range of Temperature (°C)
0–6 Hours		
<1,200 gm	35.0	34.0–35.4
1,200–1,500 gm	34.1	33.9–34.4
1,501–2,500 gm	33.4	32.8–33.8
>2,500 gm (& >36 wk gest time)	32.9	32.0–33.8
6–12 Hours		
<1,200 gm	35.0	34.0–35.4
1,200–1,500 gm	34.0	33.5–34.4
1,501–2,500 gm	33.1	32.2–33.8
>2,500 gm (& >36 wk gest time)	32.8	31.4–33.8
12–24 Hours		
<1,200 gm	34.0	34.0–35.4
1,200–1,500 gm	33.8	33.3–34.3
1,501–2,500 gm	32.8	31.8–33.8
>2,500 gm (& >36 wk gest time)	32.4	31.0–33.7
24–36 Hours		
<1,200 gm	34.0	34.0–35.0
1,200–1,500 gm	33.6	33.1–34.2
1,501–2,500 gm	32.6	31.6–33.6
>2,500 gm (& >36 wk gest time)	32.1	30.7–33.5
36–48 Hours		
<1,200 gm	34.0	34.0–35.0
1,200–1,500 gm	33.5	33.0–34.1
1,501–2,500 gm	32.5	31.4–33.5
>2,500 gm (& >36 wk gest time)	31.9	30.5–33.3
48–72 Hours		
<1,200 gm	34.0	34.0–35.0
1,200–1,500 gm	33.5	33.5–34.0
1,501–2,500 gm	32.3	31.2–33.4
>2,500 gm (& >36 wk gest time)	31.7	30.1–33.2

TABLE 77.1 *Neutral Environmental Temperatures (continued)*

Age and Weight	Starting Temperature (°C)	Range of Temperature (°C)
72–96 Hours		
<1,200 gm	34.0	34.0–35.0
1,200–1,500 gm	33.5	33.0–34.0
1,501–2,500 gm	32.2	31.1–33.2
>2,500 gm (& >36 wk gest time)	31.3	29.8–32.8
4–12 days		
<1,500 gm	33.5	33.0–34.0
1,501–2,500 gm	32.1	31.0–33.2
>2,500 gm (& >36 wk gest time)		
4–5 days	31.0	29.5–32.6
5–6 days	30.9	29.4–32.3
6–8 days	30.6	29.0–32.2
8–10 days	30.3	29.0–31.8
10–12 days	30.1	29.0–31.4
12–14 Days		
<1,500 gm	33.5	32.6–34.0
1,501–2,500 gm	32.1	31.0–33.2
>2,500 gm (& >36 wk gest time)	29.8	29.0–30.8
2–3 Weeks		
<1,500 gm	33.1	32.3–34.0
1,501–2,500 gm	31.7	30.5–33.0
3–4 Weeks		
<1,500 gm	32.6	31.6–33.6
1,501–2,500 gm	31.4	30.0–32.7
4–5 Weeks		
<1,500 gm	32.0	31.2–33.0
1,501–2,500 gm	30.9	29.5–32.2
5–6 Weeks		
<1,500 gm	31.4	30.6–32.3
1,501–2,500 gm	30.4	29.0–31.8

SOURCE: A. A. Fanaroff, MB, and M. H. Klaus, MD, 1979, *Care of the high risk neonate* (Philadelphia, Pa: W. B. Saunders Co.).

Biopsy needles (physician should specify size: short, medium, large)

For specimen:

    Carson formalin

    B5 fixative (or as specified)

    Single-edge razor blade

    Round petri dish

    Dental wax

    Fine-tip forceps

3″ foam tape

Eight 4″ × 3″ gauze sponges, sterile

PSYCHOSOCIAL CONSIDERATIONS: Explain the procedure in developmentally appropriate terms. Avoid using terms with mixed meanings, such as *stick into kidney*. Provide comfort to the child.

TIME: 15 to 20 minutes; also monitor for 4 hours postbiopsy

PURPOSE

To obtain a tissue sample of the kidney for diagnostic purposes.

OBJECTIVES

- To perform a biopsy of a kidney.
- To prevent injury, trauma, and hemorrhage.

EQUIPMENT

Premedication, as ordered

Drapes, sterile

Gown, sterile (optional, depending on physician's preference)

Gloves, sterile

Disposable basic biopsy tray (without needle), including 1% lidocaine, gauze, a syringe, a prep sponge, and barriers

Two 18g 3″ spinal needles

Povidone-iodine solution or, if child is iodine-sensitive, other cleaning solution

20 ml vial of normal saline (0.9% sodium chloride)

Two 18g 1½″ needles

Two 10 ml syringes

Gloves, nonsterile

Hypaque dye 50% (amount to be given according to child's weight; this dye is most commonly used unless the child is iodine-sensitive)

SAFETY ISSUES

- **Check for informed consent.**

ESSENTIAL STEPS

1. Prepare the child and family:

    Assure that all preprocedural requirements are met. Administer premedication per the physician's plan of care.

    Transport the child to X-ray via stretcher, if appropriate.

    Place the child on the X-ray table in the appropriate position:

        Prone, with radiotranslucent cushion under abdomen, during the procedure.

        Supine, if posttransplant.

2. Assemble the equipment:

    Using sterile technique, open the biopsy tray and needles.

    Pour povidone-iodine solution into the appropriate containers.

    Draw up normal saline into a 10 ml syringe.

3. Prior to the biopsy, the X-ray technician will take a scout film of the kidney.

4. Wash hands and put on clean gloves.

5. Position the child and help to hold still. (See Fig. 78.1)

6. The physician injects hypaque contrast medium intravenously.

7. During the procedure, observe for respiratory distress or any change in the child's status. Monitor vital signs.

8. Assist the physician in processing tissue into appropriate containers. Label all specimens. Send specimens to the lab.

9. For postbiopsy care,

Apply direct pressure to the needle site until local bleeding stops.

Apply a pressure dressing using folded 4″ × 3″ gauze and foam tape. Keep the dressing in place until the next morning.

Transport the child back to the room and check vital signs.

Have the child remain on bedrest until morning. Some institutions send the child to the intensive care unit for monitoring overnight.

Monitor vital signs and blood pressure every 15 minutes for the first hour, every 30 minutes for the next hour, and then every 4 hours.

Collect and label all urine specimens for 2 hours postbiopsy and then every 2 hours until clear. Report any gross hematuria to the physician.

DOCUMENTATION

- Date and time.
- Vital signs.
- Tolerance to procedure.
- Dressing applied.
- Intake and output; appearance of urine.

POTENTIAL RELATED NURSING DIAGNOSES

Infection: *high risk*

Tissue perfusion, altered, renal

Skin integrity, impaired: *high risk*

Skills Checklist

☐ Prepare the child and family. Check for informed consent.
☐ Administer premedication.
☐ Assemble the equipment.
☐ Wash hands and put on gloves.
☐ Position the child and help to hold still.
☐ Monitor for any respiratory distress. Monitor vital signs.
☐ Apply pressure to the needle site.
☐ Apply pressure dressing.
☐ Instruct on bedrest.
☐ Monitor vital signs.
☐ Collect and label urine specimens.
☐ Document.

POTENTIAL RELATED MEDICAL DIAGNOSES

Urinary tract infection, recurrent

Mass on the kidney

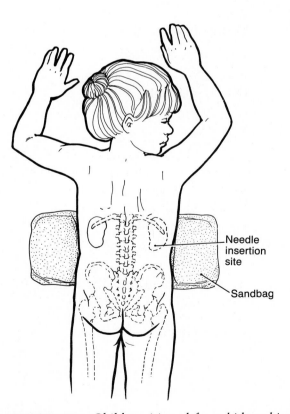

FIGURE 78.1 *Child positioned for a kidney biopsy.*

Needle insertion site

Sandbag

79 Liver Biopsy

PSYCHOSOCIAL CONSIDERATIONS: Explain the procedure in developmentally appropriate terms. Avoid using terms with mixed meanings, such as *remove part of the liver* and *stick*. Allow the child to cry or scream but not to move. Describe the feeling of cold solutions used for cleaning prior to skin preparation. The child may feel a burning sensation with the local anesthetic. The child may feel pressure when the biopsy needle is inserted. Comfort and hold the child after the procedure.

TIME: 5 to 10 minutes

PURPOSE

To assist the physician in obtaining liver tissue for microscopic examination and/or a culture to diagnose and/or confirm liver disease.

OBJECTIVES

- To obtain a liver specimen.
- To prevent injury.

EQUIPMENT

Medication, if ordered

Masks and/or gowns (optional)

Gloves, nonsterile

Gloves, sterile, for individual performing liver biopsy

Blanket for mummy restraint, if appropriate

1% xylocaine (with or without epinephrine) or other ordered anesthetic

Soft tissue biopsy tray, including a large-bore liver biopsy needle, a syringe, sterile drapes, and specimen containers

4″ × 4″ gauze, sterile

Tape

Fixative and/or media obtained from the lab

SAFETY ISSUES

- **Check for informed consent.**
- **Watch for decreased blood pressure and increased pulse, which can signify problems such as hemorrhage or shock.**

ESSENTIAL STEPS

1. Prepare the child and family. Check with the physician for desired preprocedural labs, NPO (nothing by mouth) period, and special assays of tissue.

   Obtain baseline vital signs.

   Premedicate, per the physician's plan of care.

   The physician may ask the family to leave the room during the procedure.

2. Assemble the equipment.

3. Wash hands and put on clean gloves.

4. Position the child supine. (See Fig. 79.1) Restrain the child, if necessary. Use a blanket for a mummy restraint or ask for additional assistance.

5. After the biopsy, place 4″ × 4″ gauze over the site and apply manual pressure directly to the site for 5 to 10 minutes.

6. Apply a sterile pressure dressing.

7. Place the child on the right side for a minimum of 3 hours. Place a sand bag between the child and the bed to increase pressure on the site, per the physician's plan of care, to prevent hemorrhage.

8. Take postprocedural vital signs per the physician's plan of care. Take vital signs every hour for 8 to 12 hours.

9. Observe the site for signs of hemorrhage. Check every 15 minutes for the first hour, every hour for the next 4 hours, every 2 hours twice, then every 4 hours for the next 24 hours.

10. Label specimen(s) and send to the lab.

11. Obtain postprocedure hemogram per the physician's plan of care.

DOCUMENTATION

- Date, time, and name of physician performing the procedure.
- Pre- and postprocedural assessments, including vital signs and site checks for hemorrhage.
- Child's response.
- Amount of biopsy specimen removed.

POTENTIAL RELATED NURSING DIAGNOSES

Anxiety

Fear

Pain, acute

Injury: *high risk*

Infection: *high risk*

Skills Checklist

☐ Prepare the child and family.
- Check for informed consent.
- Obtain baseline vital signs.
- Premedicate, if ordered.

☐ Assemble the equipment.

☐ Wash hands and put on gloves.

☐ Position the child.

☐ Postbiopsy, place 4″ × 4″ gauze over the site and apply pressure.

☐ Apply a sterile pressure dressing.

☐ Place the child on the right side.

☐ Monitor vital signs. Check for hemorrhage.

☐ Label specimen(s) and send to the lab.

☐ Document.

POTENTIAL RELATED MEDICAL DIAGNOSES

Liver disease

Bleeding disorders

REFERENCES

Mott, S., James, S., and Sperhac, A. 1990. *Nursing care of children and families.* Redwood City, Calif.: Addison-Wesley.

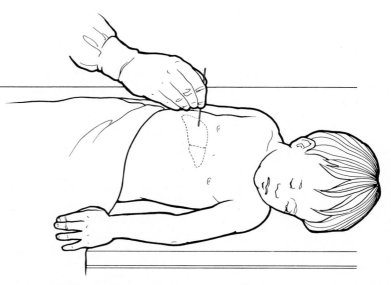

FIGURE 79.1 *Child positioned for a liver biopsy.*

80 Lumbar Puncture

PSYCHOSOCIAL CONSIDERATIONS: Explain each step in developmentally appropriate terms, just prior to performing the step. Avoid using terms with mixed meanings, such as *stick* and *puncture*. Avoid the word *spine*, as the child may be afraid of paralysis. Position the child. Explain that the child needs to hold still and that you will help. Speak soothingly and close to the child's face. Describe the feeling of cold solutions used for cleaning prior to skin preparation.

TIME: 20 to 30 minutes

PURPOSE

To obtain a specimen of spinal fluid for diagnostic purposes.

To measure cerebrospinal fluid pressure.

To inject intrathecal medications as indicated.

OBJECTIVES

- To assist in obtaining a specimen.
- To prevent injury.
- To reduce risks for nosocomial infection.

EQUIPMENT

Medication, if ordered

Gloves, nonsterile

Povidone-iodine solution

Gloves, sterile, for person performing lumbar puncture

Disposable lumbar puncture tray, including a 22g 1½″ spinal needle, a syringe, collection tubes, sterile drapes, a sponge for cleaning the skin, 2″ × 2″ gauze, and an adhesive bandage

Spinal fluid manometer, sterile, if requested by the physician

Spinal needle, per request, if other than supplied on the tray

ESSENTIAL STEPS

1. Prepare the child and family.

   Check for informed consent, if required.

   Administer premedication, if applicable.

2. Assemble the equipment.

3. Wash hands and put on clean gloves.

4. Position and restrain the child as necessary, per the physician's preference:

   Sitting with head bent forward. (See Fig. 80.1)

   Lateral recumbent, with knees and neck in flexed position. Small children will need help to maintain this position. (See Fig. 80.2)

5. Postprocedure, place 2″ × 2″ gauze over the site and apply pressure for 2 to 3 minutes. Apply a bandage.

6. Verify with the physician that tubes were collected in numerical sequence. Tubes are numbered 1, 2, and 3.

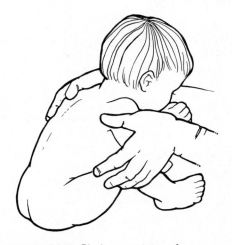

FIGURE 80.1 *Sitting position for a lumbar puncture.*

7. Label tubes and send to the lab. The first tube is usually for culture and gram stain, the second for glucose and protein, and the third for cell count.

8. Assess the puncture site for leakage and to determine the need to restrict activity every 4 hours for the next 24 hours.

9. Following intrathecal chemotherapy, the child should be positioned with hips elevated for 30 minutes postprocedure. Intrathecal meds must be preservative-free.

DOCUMENTATION

- Time and date.
- Medication administered, if appropriate.
- Person performing lumbar puncture.
- Child's tolerance of procedure.
- Appearance of spinal fluid.
- Pressure reading, if applicable.
- That specimen(s) were sent to lab.

POTENTIAL RELATED NURSING DIAGNOSES

Infection: *high risk*

Anxiety

Body temperature, altered: *high risk*

Pain, acute

Hyperthermia

Injury: *high risk*

Mobility, impaired physical

Tissue perfusion, altered, cerebral

POTENTIAL RELATED MEDICAL DIAGNOSES

Meningitis

Sepsis

Seizures

Cancer

REFERENCES

Mott, S., James, S., and Sperhac, A. 1990. *Nursing care of children and families.* Redwood City, Calif.: Addison-Wesley.

Skills Checklist

☐ Prepare the child and family.
  • Check for informed consent, if appropriate.
  • Administer premedication, if applicable.
☐ Assemble the equipment.
☐ Wash hands and put on gloves.
☐ Position the child and assist in maintaining the position.
☐ Apply pressure to the puncture site with 2″ × 2″ gauze.
☐ Apply a bandage.
☐ Label the specimen(s) and send to the lab.
☐ Assess the puncture site.
☐ Document.

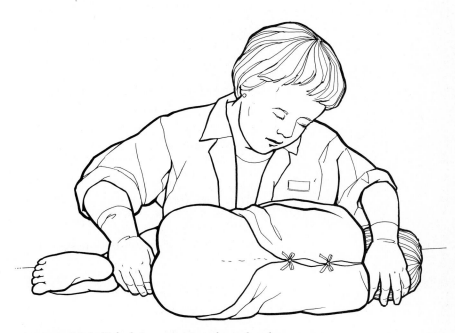

FIGURE 80.2 *Side-lying position for a lumbar puncture.*

Lab Values

Color: Clear
Cell Count
  Neonate: <15 leukocytes/mm^3
  Child: 0–5 leukocytes/mm^3
Protein
  Neonate: 60–120 mg/dL
  Child: 15–45 mg/dL
Glucose: 1/2–2/3 serum glucose level

81 Medication Administration: Oral Digoxin

PSYCHOSOCIAL CONSIDERATIONS: Explain the procedure in developmentally appropriate terms. Let the child play with the stethoscope before taking the apical pulse. Hold and comfort the child after the procedure.

TIME: 2 to 3 minutes

PURPOSE

To provide for the safe administration of digoxin (Lanoxin).

OBJECTIVES

- To administer the medication.
- To prevent injury during administration.
- To obtain the desired effect of the medication.

EQUIPMENT

Stethoscope
Medication and calibrated dropper *or* TB syringe

SAFETY ISSUES

- The physician should have written the order in milligrams with the dosage measured to the nearest 0.05 ml.
- Two RNs should check the order, calculations, container, and measured amount before administration.
- Auscultate the apical pulse (AP) for 1 full minute. Hold digoxin and notify the physician if the heart rate (HR) is irregular and/or if:

    The HR of a 0- to 2-year-old is less than 90.

    The HR of a 2- to 5-year-old is less than 80.

    The HR of a 5- to 12-year-old is less than 70.

    The HR of a 12-year-old or older is less than 60.

- Use the same type of measuring device for each dose, for example, a calibrated dropper provided with the medication or a tuberculin (TB) syringe. Varying the device can alter drug blood levels. (See Fig. 81.1)
- Notify the physician if the child vomits the dose within 30 minutes, but do not repeat the dose unless the physician specifies.
- To change the maintenance dosage schedule, ensure that at least 12 hours have elapsed between doses.
- Refer to "Medication Administration: General Procedure."

ESSENTIAL STEPS

1. Prepare the child and family.
2. Assemble the equipment. Refer to "Medication Administration: General Procedure."
3. Wash hands.
4. Identify the child by checking the identification band.
5. Auscultate the AP for 1 full minute.
6. Administer the dose. Refer to "Medication Administration: Oral."
7. For administration through a nasogastric (N/G) tube:

   Draw up the dosage with the calibrated dropper or TB syringe.

   Attach an open syringe to the N/G tube.

   Drop or squirt the medication into the open syringe.

   Flush as usual.

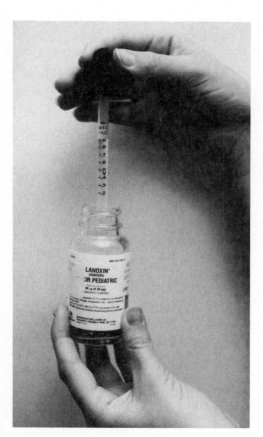

FIGURE 81.1 *Drawing up digoxin.*

DOCUMENTATION

- Medication.
- Dose.
- Route.
- Time.
- Apical pulse.
- Presence or absence of murmurs.

POTENTIAL RELATED NURSING DIAGNOSES

Activity intolerance

Aspiration: *high risk*

Cardiac output, decreased

Fluid volume excess

Injury: *high risk*

Tissue perfusion, altered, cardiopulmonary

POTENTIAL RELATED MEDICAL DIAGNOSES

Congenital cardiac defects

Congestive heart failure

REFERENCES

Pagliaro, L., and Pagliaro, A., eds. 1987. *Problems in pediatric drug therapy.* Hamilton: Drug Intelligence Publications.
Skidmore-Roth, L. 1991. *Mosby's 1991 nursing drug reference.* St. Louis, Mo.: C. V. Mosby.

Compatible IV fluid (0.9% sodium chloride or 0.45% sodium chloride); *not dextrose*
Infusion pump
.22 micron in-line filter
Appropriate tubing
Resuscitative equipment

PSYCHOSOCIAL CONSIDERATIONS: Explain the procedure in developmentally appropriate terms. Avoid using terms with mixed meanings, such as *shot* and *stick*. The child may fear medication going into the veins. Restrain the child appropriately, especially if child is in the clonic seizure stage.

TIME: 20 minutes to 1 hour

PURPOSE

To administer phenytoin by IV infusion, using safety precautions to prevent precipitation and side effects.

OBJECTIVES

- To prevent and/or treat seizures.
- To prevent precipitate.
- To administer medication.
- To prevent injury related to administration.

EQUIPMENT

Cardiac/respiratory monitor
Gloves, nonsterile
Medication

S SAFETY ISSUES

- **Mixing in solutions other than saline may cause precipitation.**
- **The infusion rate should not exceed 1 mg/kg/minute.**
- **Use an infusion pump.**
- **Place the child on a cardiac/respiratory monitor during the infusion.**
- **Observe the IV site frequently during administration. Stop the infusion immediately if any signs of extravasation, pain at the site of injection, hypotension, bradycardia, or respiratory depression occur. Notify the physician.**
- **Refer to "Medication Administration: General Procedure."**

ESSENTIAL STEPS

1. Prepare the child and family.
2. Assemble the equipment. Refer to "Medication Administration: General Procedure."
3. Wash hands.
4. Identify the child by checking the identification band.

5. Perform baseline assessment, including vital signs.

6. Put on gloves.

7. For a peripheral line, dilute the solution between 1 mg/ml and 10 mg/ml. A central line may have a concentration of up to 20 mg/ml.

8. Flush before and after Dilantin infusion with saline.

9. Start the infusion immediately after preparation. Infusion time should not exceed 1 hour.

10. Observe for particulate matter. Stop the infusion if precipitate is noted and notify the physician.

11. Monitor vital signs during and after the administration of medication.

DOCUMENTATION

- Medication.
- Dose.
- Route.
- Time.
- Vital signs before, during, and after administration.
- Child's response.

POTENTIAL RELATED NURSING DIAGNOSES

Anxiety

Fear

Urinary incontinence, stress

Powerlessness

Cardiac output, decreased

Tissue integrity, impaired

Skills Checklist

☐ Prepare the child and family.
☐ Assemble the equipment.
☐ Wash hands.
☐ Identify the child by checking the identification band.
☐ Perform baseline assessment, including vital signs.
☐ Put on gloves.
☐ Flush the line with saline.
☐ Infuse the medication.
☐ Observe for particulate matter.
☐ Flush the line with saline.
☐ Monitor vital signs during and after the administration of medication.
☐ Document.

POTENTIAL RELATED MEDICAL DIAGNOSES

Epilepsy

Status epilepticus

Meningitis

Encephalitis

REFERENCES

Pagliaro, L., and Pagliaro, A., eds. 1987. *Problems in pediatric drug therapy.* Hamilton: Drug Intelligence Publications.

Skidmore-Roth, L. 1991. *Mosby's 1991 nursing drug reference.* St. Louis, Mo.: C. V. Mosby.

Lab Values

Therapeutic Dilantin Blood Level: 10–20 mcg/ml.

83 Medication Administration: Ear

- Refer to "Medication Administration: General Procedure."

PSYCHOSOCIAL CONSIDERATIONS: Explain the procedure in developmentally appropriate terms. Avoid the use of terms with mixed meanings. Do not attempt such humor with the child as describing fictitious things in the ears, such as tomatoes, a garden, or worms. Prepare the child for the sensation of coldness prior to administration of the medication.

TIME: 2 to 3 minutes

PURPOSE

To administer medication in a safe, effective manner.

To follow practices in accordance with state and federal regulations.

OBJECTIVES

- To administer the medication.
- To prevent trauma to the ear.
- To obtain the desired effect of medication.

EQUIPMENT

Medication with a dropper
Cotton ball

ESSENTIAL STEPS

1. Prepare the child and family.
2. Assemble the equipment. Refer to "Medication Administration: General Procedure."
3. Wash hands.
4. Ensure that the medication is nearly body temperature. Hold the medication in a hand to warm it.
5. Identify the child by checking the identification band.
6. Place the child with the affected ear turned upward.
7. Straighten the external auditory canal by gently pulling the pinna
   Down and back in children 3 years and under. (See Fig. 83.1)
   Up and back in children older than 3 years.
8. Instill the ear medication. (The tip of the dropper should not touch the child.) Have the child remain with the affected ear upward for 5 minutes.
9. Place a cotton ball loosely in the ear, unless the child has excessive otic drainage.

DOCUMENTATION

- Medication.
- Dose.
- Route.
- Time.
- Child's response to medication.

POTENTIAL RELATED NURSING DIAGNOSES

Sensory-perceptual alterations, auditory

Anxiety

Injury: *high risk*

POTENTIAL RELATED MEDICAL DIAGNOSES

Otitis media

Cerumen

REFERENCES

Mott, S., James, S., and Sperhac, A. 1990. *Nursing care of children and families*. Redwood City, Calif.: Addison-Wesley.

Skills Checklist

☐ Prepare the child and family.
☐ Assemble the equipment.
☐ Wash hands.
☐ Hold medication to warm to body temperature.
☐ Identify the child by checking the identification band.
☐ Position the child.
☐ Instill medication.
☐ Place a cotton ball in the ear.
☐ Document.

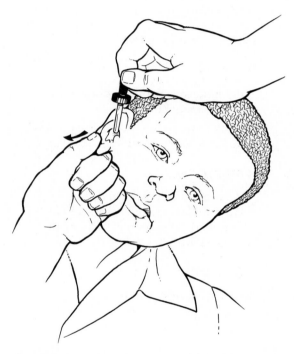

FIGURE 83.1 *Administering ear medication.*

84 Medication Administration: Eye

PSYCHOSOCIAL CONSIDERATIONS: Explain the procedure in developmentally appropriate terms. Avoid the use of terms with mixed meanings. Show the child the small amount of medication that will be used. Perform the procedure quickly and comfort the child after completion. Distract the child to prevent rubbing of the eyes after administration of the drops or application of the ointment.

TIME: 2 to 3 minutes

PURPOSE

To administer medication in a safe, effective manner.

To follow practices in accordance with state and federal drug regulations.

OBJECTIVES

- To administer the medication.
- To prevent trauma to the eye(s).
- To obtain the desired effect of the medication.

EQUIPMENT

Blanket for restraint, if appropriate

Cotton ball

Medication

Facial tissue

SAFETY ISSUES

- Refer to "Medication Administration: General Procedure."
- Store ophthalmic drops and ophthalmic ointment at room temperature.

ESSENTIAL STEPS

1. Prepare the child and family. Avoid administration when the child is crying, if possible. Restrain the child if necessary, using a blanket for a mummy restraint to prevent the child's hands from interfering.

2. Assemble the equipment. Refer to "Medication Administration: General Procedure."

3. Wash hands.

4. Identify the child by checking the identification band.

5. Wipe the child's eyes gently with a warm, moist cotton ball to remove any crusted drainage.

6. If using ophthalmic drops:

   Expose the lower conjunctival sac and drop the medication into the sac's center. Ask a child who is old enough to follow instructions to lie back and look up. Retract the lower lid and place drops in the saclike area formed by doing this. Ask an older child to close the eyes and blink. (See Fig. 84.1)

Wipe off excess solution by blotting with a cotton ball or tissue from the inner to the outer canthus. If medicating both eyes, use a new cotton ball or tissue for the second eye.

7. If using ophthalmic ointment:

Warm the ointment by holding the tube in a hand.

Apply the ointment to the lower conjunctival sac from the inner canthus laterally. Close the child's eye and gently massage to distribute the medication. Ask an older child to close and blink or roll the eyes. (See Fig. 84.2)

DOCUMENTATION

- Medication.
- Dose.
- Route.
- Time.
- Child's response to medication.

POTENTIAL RELATED NURSING DIAGNOSES

Sensory-perceptual alterations, visual

POTENTIAL RELATED MEDICAL DIAGNOSES

Eye infection

Excessive tearing

REFERENCES

Hahn, K. 1989. Administering eye medications. *Nursing 89* 19, no. 9: 80.

Mott, S., James, S., and Sperhac, A. 1990. *Nursing care of children and families.* Redwood City, Calif.: Addison-Wesley.

Skills Checklist

- ☐ Prepare the child and family.
- ☐ Assemble the equipment.
- ☐ Wash hands.
- ☐ Identify the child by checking the identification band.
- ☐ Remove crusted drainage.
- ☐ Instill eyedrops or apply ointment.
- ☐ Document.

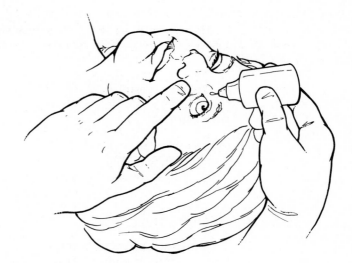

FIGURE 84.1 *Administering eyedrops.*

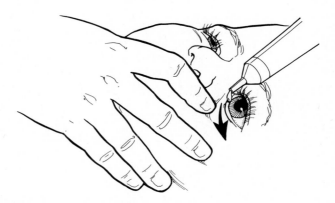

FIGURE 84.2 *Administering eye ointment.*

Medication Administration: General Procedure

PSYCHOSOCIAL CONSIDERATIONS: Explain the procedure in developmentally appropriate terms. Avoid using terms with mixed meanings, such as *stick, shot,* and *candy.* Be honest when describing how a medication will taste or feel. Children often fear that medications may cause pain or discomfort or make them sick. Do not conceal medications in bottles of formula or in meals. Fully awaken the child prior to giving an injection.

TIME: Varies

PURPOSE

To administer medication in a safe, effective manner.

To follow practices in accordance with state and federal drug regulations.

OBJECTIVES

- To administer medication safely.
- To prevent injury.
- To obtain the desired effect of medication.

EQUIPMENT

Medication

Appropriate equipment for administering medication (such as a syringe, dropper, or nipple)

References

- The physician's orders for medication should be legible and should include the following. If any of these items is missing, call the physician to get the needed information.

  Name of the child.

  Name of the medication.

  Dosage required.

  Frequency of administration required.

  Route of administration.

  Date and time the order is written.

  Signature of physician or countersignature.

- Medication dosages should be written in

  Units.

  Metric weights *or* metric volumes.

  Number of capsules, drops, suppositories, and so on, if applicable.

- Discontinue Schedule II narcotic and sedative orders after 72 hours unless the order indicates an exact number of doses to be administered *or* stipulates an exact period of time for administration.

- Some institutions may require double-checking certain drugs, such as digitalis, cyclosporin, and neuromuscular blocking agents. This includes verifying information on the physician's plan of care, the medication label or container, calculations, and the amount of the drug measured for administration.

- Document rationale for any medication not given within 30 minutes of the scheduled time.

- Adhere to the Five Rights of medication administration: right patient, right drug, right dose, right route, and right time.

ESSENTIAL STEPS

1. Prepare the child and family.
2. Assemble the equipment.

    Check the physician's plan of care.

    Check for drug allergies. Ask parents about past responses to particular medications, which may be significant even if they are not listed as allergies.

    Compare the dosage ordered to the recommended dosage for that child's size or age to verify that it is appropriate.

    Compare the information on the medication label with the medication administration record or medication card when obtaining the medication and again before administering it to the child.

    Check the expiration date of the medication.

3. Wash hands.
4. Identify the child by checking the identification band.
5. Assess the status of the child.
6. Administer the medication. If for any reason the medication is not given, or if the child does not retain it, notify the physician as soon as possible.

DOCUMENTATION

- Medication.
- Dose.
- Route.
- Time.
- Child's response.
- Rationale for altered routine of medication administration, as when the medication is withheld or when the child does not retain it.

Skills Checklist

- ☐ Prepare the child and family.
- ☐ Assemble the equipment.
- ☐ Check the physician's plan of care.
- ☐ Check for drug allergies.
- ☐ Verify the dosage.
- ☐ Check medication, including the expiration date.
- ☐ Wash hands.
- ☐ Identify the child by checking the identification band.
- ☐ Assess the status of the child.
- ☐ Administer the medication.
- ☐ Document.

POTENTIAL RELATED NURSING DIAGNOSES

Airway clearance, ineffective

Anxiety

Fear

Swallowing, impaired

POTENTIAL RELATED MEDICAL DIAGNOSES

Universal application

REFERENCES

Byington, K. 1991. Your guide to pediatric drug administration. *Nursing 91* 21, no. 8: 82–92.

Carr, D. 1989. New strategies for avoiding medication errors. *Nursing 89* 19, no. 10: 39–45.

Litwack, Kim. 1991. Administering preoperative medications. *Nursing 91* 21, no. 8: 44–47.

McGovern, K. 1988. Ten golden rules for administering drugs safely. *Nursing 88* 18, no. 8: 34–41.

Mott, S., James, S., and Sperhac, A. 1990. *Nursing care of children and families.* Redwood City, Calif.: Addison-Wesley.

PSYCHOSOCIAL CONSIDERATIONS: Explain the procedure in developmentally appropriate terms. Avoid the use of terms with mixed meanings, such as *stick* and *kill bugs*. Be honest.

> **TIME:** Varies with medication

> ### PURPOSE
>
> To administer IV medications correctly with minimal discomfort to the child and with maximum safety.

> ### OBJECTIVES
>
> • To administer IV medications safely.
> • To prevent injury and trauma.
> • To obtain the desired effect of the medication.

 SAFETY ISSUES

• Refer to "Medication Administration: General Procedure."

• Determine if the medication is compatible with the IV solution. If it is not, inform the physician of the need for a new order.

• Follow the manufacturer's instructions for drugs requiring reconstitution.

• Decide which method of medication administration is the most appropriate (for example, via metriset or retrograde method). Base a decision on the child's fluid status, on the properties of the medication (including the amount of dilution required), and on the type of IV administration set to be used.

• Refer to the following procedures for Equipment, Essential Steps, and Documentation:

> Continuous Infusion.
>
> Retrograde, With and Without Fluid Removal.
>
> Volumetric Chamber.
>
> Heparin Lock.
>
> Piggyback.
>
> IV Push.

Continuous Infusion

EQUIPMENT

Medication administration record *or* medication card

IV solution

Medication

Label

Administration set and extension tubing

Povidone-iodine swabs *or* alcohol swabs

Infusion pump

Stopcock and infusion plug, if needed

ESSENTIAL STEPS

1. Prepare the child and family.
2. Assemble the equipment. Refer to "Medication Administration: General Procedure."
3. Wash hands.
4. Aseptically open the IV solution.
5. Withdraw and discard any IV solution greater than the ordered amount, per agency policy. (Note: Manufacturers overfill containers with more IV solution than is stated on the bottle. To obtain the correct dilution, discard the overfill or account for it in the total amount.)

6. Clean outlet port with povidone-iodine or alcohol swabs. Add the medication to the IV solution through the outlet port.

7. Mix the IV solution and medication thoroughly, observing for cloudiness. Inform the pharmacy and/or the physician of any cloudiness. Do not administer a cloudy IV solution.

8. Label the IV bottle with the child's name, the type of IV fluid, the volume, the medication, the dose, the time, and the date.

9. Attach a sterile IV administration set and prime the set, per the manufacturer's instructions.

10. Identify the child by checking the identification band.

11. Assess the status of the child (including the IV site) before infusing the medication.

12. Set the infusion pump at the ordered rate. Set the pump to alarm when the hourly volume has infused. Leave the audible alarm on. (See Fig. 86.1)

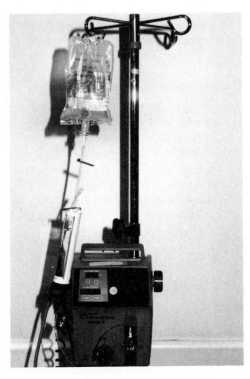

FIGURE 86.1 *IV pump and tubing.*

Skills Checklist

Continuous Infusion
☐ Prepare the child and family.
☐ Assemble the equipment.
☐ Wash hands.
☐ Open the IV solution.
☐ Withdraw and discard overfill.
☐ Add medication. Mix solution and medication thoroughly.
☐ Label the IV bottle.
☐ Prime the administration set.
☐ Identify the child by checking the identification band.
☐ Assess the status of the child.
☐ Set the infusion pump.
☐ Administer solution.
☐ Document.

Retrograde
☐ Prepare the child and family.
☐ Assemble the equipment.
☐ Wash hands.
☐ Dilute the medication in a syringe.
☐ Label the syringe.
☐ Determine the infusion rate.
☐ Identify the child by checking the identification band.
☐ Assess the status of the child.
☐ Retrograde with or without fluid removal:
  • Turn the IV flow off to the child.
  • Clean the injection port(s).
  • Inject the medication.
  • Turn the IV flow on to child.
  • Label the IV tubing.
  • Infuse medication.
  • When the medication has infused, adjust the IV to the hourly rate.
☐ Document.

Volumetric Chamber
☐ Prepare the child and family.
☐ Assemble the equipment.
☐ Wash hands.
☐ Draw up the medication.
☐ Label the syringe.
☐ Determine the appropriate volume of IV solution needed to dilute medication in the metriset.
☐ Determine the rate of infusion.
☐ Identify the child by checking the identification band. Assess the status of the child.
☐ Fill the metriset to the predetermined diluent volume.
☐ Clean the metriset injection site.
☐ Add the drug. Label the metriset.
☐ Infuse the medication.
☐ Document.

Heparin Lock

- ☐ Prepare the child and family.
- ☐ Assemble equipment.
- ☐ Wash hands.
- ☐ Draw up medication. Label the syringe.
- ☐ Determine appropriate volume of IV solution.
- ☐ Determine rate of infusion.
- ☐ Prime administration set.
- ☐ Identify the child by checking the identification band.
- ☐ Assess the status of the child.
- ☐ Clean metriset injection site, fill metriset, add medication.
- ☐ Label the metriset.
- ☐ Clean heparin lock infusion plug.
- ☐ Attach needle to end of IV tubing and insert this needle into heparin lock infusion plug.
- ☐ Secure tubing, infuse medication.
- ☐ Withdraw IV set needle and tubing from heparin lock.
- ☐ Document.

Piggyback

- ☐ Prepare the child and family.
- ☐ Assemble the equipment.
- ☐ Wash hands.
- ☐ Spike the medication bag and prime the tubing.
- ☐ Attach a small-gauge needle to the end of the administration set.
- ☐ Determine the rate of infusion.
- ☐ Identify the child by checking the identification band.
- ☐ Assess the status of the child.
- ☐ Clean the injection port of the primary IV.
- ☐ Insert the needle from the secondary tubing into the injection port and secure.
- ☐ Hang the medication higher than the primary IV.
- ☐ Regulate the IV with a roller clamp on the primary tubing. Infuse the medication.
- ☐ Document.

IV Push

- ☐ Prepare the child and family.
- ☐ Assemble the equipment.
- ☐ Wash hands.
- ☐ Determine the rate of infusion.
- ☐ Draw up the medication.
- ☐ Clean the injection port closest to the child.
- ☐ Insert the needle of the medication syringe into the port.
- ☐ Pinch or clamp the IV tubing distal to the port.
- ☐ Administer the medication.
- ☐ Remove the syringe. Unclamp the tubing and adjust the IV rate.
- ☐ Document.

13. Assess the child while the medication is infusing. Record observations.

14. If an infiltration occurs, discontinue the IV and restart the IV infusion as quickly as possible.

DOCUMENTATION

- Type and concentration of IV solution.
- Volume of IV solution.
- Medication.
- Dose.
- Time.
- Rate of infusion.
- Child's response.

Retrograde, With and Without Fluid Removal

EQUIPMENT

Medication administration record (MAR) *or* medication card

Medication in a syringe with a 25g needle

Syringe with a 25g needle, if displacing fluid

Povidone-iodine swabs *or* alcohol swabs

Label

ESSENTIAL STEPS

1. Prepare the child and family.

2. Assemble the equipment. Check the manufacturer's instructions on the administration set to determine if retrograde is feasible and if fluid removal will be required. (See Table 86.1) Refer to "Medication Administration: General Procedure."

3. Wash hands.

4. Dilute the medication in the syringe according to the manufacturer's instructions, as appropriate.

5. Label the syringe containing the medication.

6. Determine the infusion rate; refer to the manufacturer's instructions. To determine the rate, consider the volume of medication to be retrograded, a 10 ml flush, and the volume of tubing between the child and the site where the medication is to be added. (See Table 86.2) For example, the total volume to be infused might be

10 ml flush + 2 ml diluted med + 2.5 ml extension tubing
= 14.5 ml (rounded up to 15 ml)

Set the pump to infuse the volume over 30 minutes:

$$\frac{60 \text{ gtt/ml}}{30 \text{ minutes}} \times 15 \text{ ml} = 30 \text{ ml/hr}$$

7. Keep the syringe containing the medication with the MAR or medication card.

8. Identify the child by checking the identification band.

9. Assess the status of the child (including the IV site).

10. To retrograde without fluid removal:

Invert the metriset. Clamp off the air vent.

Empty the drip chamber by squeezing.

Return the metriset to its hanging position. Unclamp the air vent.

Turn the stopcock to the off position or pinch the tubing so that the IV flow is off to the child. (The flow *must* be off to the child to prevent an IV bolus push of medication.)

Ensure that the roller clamp is completely open.

TABLE 86.1 *Administration Set Table*
(Examples of Different Brands of Tubing)

Administration Set	Vol. Retrograded without Fluid Removal	Vol. Retrograded with Fluid Removal
McGaw Metriset	≤2.7 ml	Not Used
I-Med Accuset (and Micro)	Not Used	≤2.5 ml
Abbott Soluset	≤1 ml	≤7 ml*
McGaw Metriset with stopcock and extension tube(s)	Not Used	>2.7 ml

*If 7 ml or more is retrograded, some medication may be displaced in the discarded syringe.

TABLE 86.2 *IV Tubing Volumes*
(Examples of Different Volumes)

Tubing Type	Volume in Tubing
Medlon Extension	1.1 ml
20″ Extension (Abbott)	2.5 ml
Medlon Y-set extension	1.7 ml
Soluset (Abbott)	12.0 ml
Soluset (Abbott Pump Tubing)	
● From drip chamber to end	18.0 ml
● Between 2 Y-injection ports	7.0 ml
● From upper Y-injection to end of tubing	8.0 ml
Micro Imed	
● From metriset to end of tubing	14.0 ml
● Between 2 Y-injection ports (below the cassette)	2.5 ml
● From upper Y-injection port (below cassette) to end of tubing	3.0 ml
Micro Abbott (Pump Tubing)	
● From metriset to end of tubing	9.8 ml
● Between 2 Y-injection ports (below the cassette)	2.4 ml
● From upper Y-injection port (below cassette) to end of tubing	2.8 ml

Clean the infusion plug or injection port closest to the child with a povidone-iodine or alcohol swab and insert the medication syringe into the plug using a 25g needle.

Inject the *diluted* medication. Check the drip chamber to ensure that the microdrip is visible.

Open the stopcock to the child or unpinch the tubing.

Remove the syringe.

Label the IV tubing to indicate that a medication is infusing.

Fill the metriset with an appropriate volume of IV fluid.

Set the flow rate to deliver the drug as determined in Step 6.

When the medication has infused, remove the label on the IV tubing and adjust the infusion to the ordered rate.

11. To retrograde with fluid removal (see Fig. 86.2):

Clean the upper injection site/infusion plug with a povidone-iodine or alcohol swab and insert the empty syringe using a 25g needle.

Clean the infusion plug on the stopcock or injection port closest to the child with a povidone-iodine or alcohol swab and insert the medication syringe.

Turn the stopcock to the off position or pinch the tubing so that the IV flow is off to the child.

Inject the medication slowly. (Fluid from the tubing will displace into the empty syringe.)

Open the stopcock to the child or unpinch the tubing.

Remove the syringes.

Label the IV tubing to indicate that a medication is infusing.

Adjust the rate to deliver the drug as determined in Step 6.

When the medication has infused, remove the label on the IV tubing and adjust the infusion to the ordered rate.

DOCUMENTATION

- Medication.
- Dose.
- Route.
- Time.
- Volume of IV fluid infused.
- Child's response.

Volumetric Chamber

EQUIPMENT

MAR or medication card

Povidone-iodine swabs *or* alcohol swabs

Medication in a syringe with a 25g needle

Label

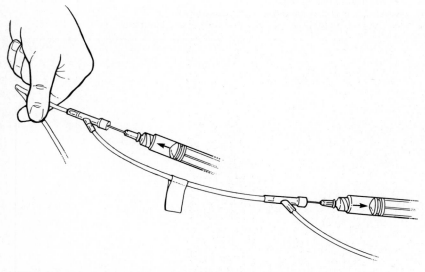

FIGURE 86.2 *Giving IV medication by retrograde.*

ESSENTIAL STEPS

1. Prepare the child and family.

2. Assemble the equipment. Refer to "Medication Administration: General Procedure."

3. Wash hands.

4. Draw up the volume of medication required for the dose.

5. Label the syringe containing the medication.

6. Determine the appropriate volume of the IV solution needed to dilute the medication in the metriset using the manufacturer's information.

7. Determine the rate of the infusion using the manufacturer's information. Include the volume required to flush the tubing (see Table 86.2) in determining this rate. To be most effective, infuse the medication (including the flush) within the recommended infusion time.

8. Identify the child by checking the identification band.

9. Assess the status of the child (including the IV site).

10. Confirm that the correct IV solution is hanging.

11. Check the metriset for the presence of any medication labels.

12. Check the IV bottle label(s) to see if the solution contains an additive and/or medication. Note that

    Some meds may be incompatible with certain additives.

    Certain meds may be ordered and given together (such as some oncology drugs).

13. Fill the metriset to the predetermined diluent volume. (See Fig. 86.3)

14. Clean the metriset injection site with a povidone-iodine or alcohol swab. Use a small-gauge needle on the medication syringe to pierce the injection site. Add the IV drug. (See Fig. 86.4)

15. Thoroughly mix the drug and the IV solution.

16. Label the metriset to indicate that a medication is infusing.

17. Adjust the rate to deliver the medication and flush in the recommended time. Infuse the medication.

18. Allow the metriset to empty, and add the appropriate volume of flush, which is the same as the volume of the IV tubing listed on the tubing box. If a second IV medication is to be given immediately following the first, use a 10 ml fluid barrier to prevent mixing of the medications. (See Table 86.2)

19. Following infusion of the medication and the flush, adjust the rate of infusion to the ordered rate and remove the label on the metriset.

DOCUMENTATION

- Medication.
- Dose.
- Route.
- Time.
- Volume of IV fluid infused.
- Child's response.

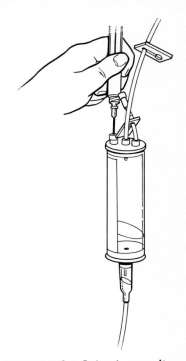

FIGURE 86.4 *Injecting medication into the buretrol.*

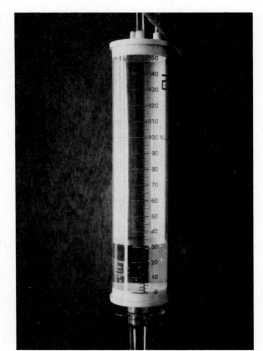

FIGURE 86.3 *IV buretrol/metriset.*

Heparin Lock

EQUIPMENT

MAR *or* medication card

Medication in a syringe with a 25g needle

Label

IV administration set and IV solution

Povidone-iodine swabs *or* alcohol swabs

25g 5/8″ needle

Gloves, nonsterile, if appropriate

Tape

Heparin or normal saline in a syringe with a 25g needle

ESSENTIAL STEPS

1. Prepare the child and family.

2. Assemble the equipment. Refer to "Medication Administration: General Procedure."

3. Wash hands.

4. Withdraw the appropriate volume (dose) of the medication into a sterile syringe. Label the syringe.

5. Determine the appropriate volume of the IV solution needed to dilute the medication in the metriset using the manufacturer's information.

6. Determine the rate of infusion using the manufacturer's information. Include the volume required to flush the tubing. (See Table 86.2) Infuse all medication (including the flush) within the recommended time in order to be most effective.

7. Prime the administration set with the IV solution.

8. Identify the child by checking the identification band.

9. Assess the status of the child (including the IV site).

10. Fill the metriset to the predetermined volume.

11. Clean the metriset injection site with a povidone-iodine or alcohol swab. Use a small-gauge needle on the medication syringe to pierce the injection site. Add the IV drug.

12. Gently mix the drug and the IV solution.

13. Label the metriset to indicate that a medication is infusing.

14. Clean the heparin lock infusion plug with a povidone-iodine or alcohol swab.

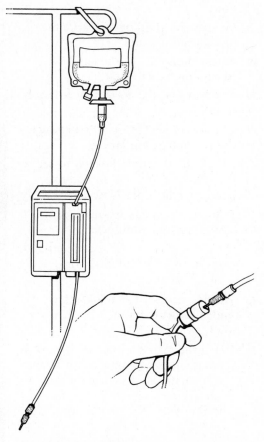

FIGURE 86.5 *Administering medication via a heparin lock.*

15. Attach a sterile, 25g 5/8″ needle to the end of the IV administration set tubing and insert this needle into the center of the heparin lock. A longer needle may puncture the heparin lock tubing. Use a new needle each time the heparin lock is entered. (See Fig. 86.5) *Or* put on gloves and connect the IV tubing directly to the uncapped end of the heparin lock. (Note: Connecting a needle to a heparin lock may be a safety hazard. When children move around, the needle can become disconnected and cause injury.)

16. Secure the IV tubing to the child's hand or arm board with tape.

17. Adjust the rate to deliver the medication and flush in the appropriate time.

18. Allow the metriset to empty, and add the appropriate volume of flush, which is the same as the volume of the IV tubing listed on the tubing box. If a second IV med is to be given, use a 10 ml flush between the two medications.

19. Withdraw the IV set needle and tubing from the heparin lock. Cover the end of the tubing with a sterile needle cap.

20. Irrigate the heparin lock with heparin or normal saline. Refer to "Intravenous: Heparin Flush."

DOCUMENTATION

- Medication.
- Dose.
- Route.
- Time.
- Volume of IV fluid infused.
- Child's response.

Piggyback

EQUIPMENT

MAR *or* medication card
Medication in a small IV bag
Secondary administration set
Small-gauge needle
Povidone-iodine swab *or* alcohol swab
Tape, if appropriate

ESSENTIAL STEPS

1. Prepare the child and family.

2. Assemble the equipment. Refer to "Medication Administration: General Procedure."

3. Wash hands.

4. Spike the medication bag and prime the tubing.

5. Attach a small-gauge needle to the end of the administration set.

6. Determine the rate of infusion according to the manufacturer's information.

7. Identify the child by checking the identification band.

8. Assess the status of the child (including the IV site).

9. Clean the injection port of the primary IV tubing with povidone-iodine or alcohol swabs. Use the port above the roller clamp.

10. Insert the needle from the secondary tubing into the injection port of the primary tubing, or attach tubing directly to the stopcock. If using the injection port, secure the connection with tape.

11. Hang the IV container with the medication higher than the primary IV.

12. Adjust the rate of flow with the roller clamp on the primary tubing.

13. When the medication has infused, remove the needle and secondary tubing from the primary port.

14. Adjust the rate of the primary IV.

DOCUMENTATION

- Medication.
- Dose.
- Route.
- Time.
- Amount of fluid infused.
- Child's response.

IV Push

EQUIPMENT

MAR *or* medication card

Medication

Syringe with a small-gauge needle

Povidone-iodine swab *or* alcohol swab

Syringe pump (optional)

ESSENTIAL STEPS

1. Prepare the child and family.
2. Assemble the equipment. Refer to "Medication Administration: General Procedure."
3. Wash hands.
4. Ensure that the medication can be safely given by IV push.
5. Determine the rate that the medication can be given by IV push.
6. Draw up the medication.

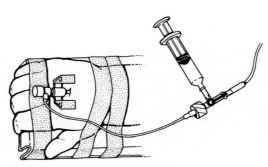

FIGURE 86.6 *IV push medication.*

7. Clean the injection port closest to the child with a povidone-iodine swab *or* alcohol swab.
8. Insert the needle of the medication syringe into the port. Pinch or clamp the IV tubing distal to the port.
9. Give medication. Observe the child carefully. (See Fig. 86.6)
10. Remove the syringe; unclamp the tubing and adjust the IV rate. *Or* insert the syringe into the syringe pump and set parameters. (See Figs. 86.7 and 86.8)

DOCUMENTATION

- Medication.
- Dose.
- Route.
- Time.
- Child's response.

POTENTIAL RELATED NURSING DIAGNOSES

Injury: *high risk*

Infection: *high risk*

POTENTIAL RELATED MEDICAL DIAGNOSES

Universal application

REFERENCES

Mott, S., James, S., and Sperhac, A. 1990. *Nursing care of children and families.* Redwood City, Calif.: Addison-Wesley.

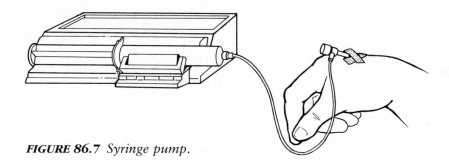

FIGURE 86.7 *Syringe pump.*

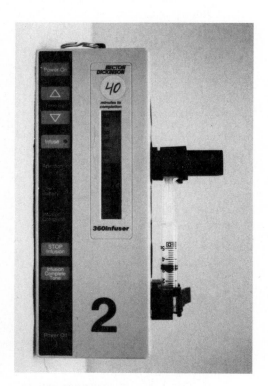

FIGURE 86.8 *Syringe pump.*

87 Medication Administration: Narcotics

PSYCHOSOCIAL CONSIDERATIONS: Explain the procedure in developmentally appropriate terms. Narcotics can affect thinking and may increase fear. Use simple, clear terms.

TIME: 3 to 5 minutes

PURPOSE

To administer medication in a safe, effective manner.

To comply with the regulations of controlled substances set forth by the hospital administration and the federal narcotics bureau.

To monitor the storing and issuing of drugs for floor stock and specific patient usage.

OBJECTIVES

- To administer narcotics safely.
- To prevent injury.
- To obtain the desired effect of medication.

EQUIPMENT

Refer to the appropriate medication administration procedure.

- Keep all controlled substances in a locked cabinet.
- Stop administration of Schedule II drugs (see Table 87.1) after 48 to 72 hours unless

    The physician has indicated the exact number of doses.

    The physician has stated an exact length of time for administration.

- Two RNs should double-check Schedule II drugs for correct drug and dosage.
- Refer to "Medication Administration: General Procedure."

ESSENTIAL STEPS

1. Prepare the child and family.

    Assess the child's pain level. Use a pain assessment tool, as appropriate.

    Assess vital signs.

2. Assemble the equipment.

    Verify that the narcotic order is current.

    Refer to "Medication Administration: General Procedure."

3. Wash hands.

4. Prepare medication. Refer to "Medication Administration: General Procedure" and the appropriate medication administration procedure.

    If wasting any narcotic, have another RN witness and sign.

    Sign out for the narcotic.

5. Identify the child by checking the identification band.

6. Administer the medication and ensure that appropriate safety measures are taken. Side rails should be up, the child and family should be instructed to call for help if the child needs to get out of bed, and so on.

7. Monitor vital signs. Utilize a pain management flow sheet to monitor pain level and response to interventions.

DOCUMENTATION

- Medication.
- Dose.
- Route.
- Time.
- Vital signs.
- Child's response.

POTENTIAL RELATED NURSING DIAGNOSES

Pain, acute

Pain, chronic

Anxiety

Fear

Gas exchange, impaired

Injury: *high risk*

Breathing pattern, ineffective

POTENTIAL RELATED MEDICAL DIAGNOSES

Pain

Preoperative medication

Postoperative medication

Sickle cell crisis

Cancer

Fracture

REFERENCES

Litwack, Kim. 1991. Administering Preoperative medications. *Nursing 91* 21, no. 8: 44–47.

Mott, S., James, S., and Sperhac, A. 1990. *Nursing care of children and families.* Redwood City, Calif.: Addison-Wesley.

Skills Checklist

☐ Prepare the child and family. Assess the child's pain level and vital signs.

☐ Assemble the equipment.

☐ Wash hands.

☐ Prepare the medication.

☐ Sign out for the narcotic.

☐ Identify the child by checking the identification band.

☐ Administer the medication. Institute safety measures.

☐ Monitor vital signs.

☐ Document.

TABLE 87.1
Examples of Controlled Drugs

Schedule II
B & O Suppositories
Cocaine Solution 4%
Codeine Sulfate
Dexamphetamine (Dexedrine)
Hydromorphone (Dilaudid)
Methadone (Dolophine)
Levorphanol (Levo Dromoran)
Dronabinol (Marinol)
Meperidine (Demerol)
Methylphenidate (Ritalin)
Morphine
Pentobarbital (Nembutal)
Sufentanyl (Sufenta)
Sublimaze (Fentanyl)

Schedule III
Tylenol with Codeine
ASA with Codeine
Methyprylon (Noludar)
Pentobarbital Supp. (Nembutal)
Paregoric

Schedule IV
Chloral Hydrate (Noctec)
Paraldehyde
Phenobarbital
Diazepam (Valium)
Lorazepam (Ativan)
Flurazepam (Dalmane)
Alprazolam (Xanax)
Midazolam (Versed)
Clorazepate Dipotassium (Tranxene)
Temazepam (Restoril)
Triazolam (Halcion)
Mephobarbital (Mebaral)
Clonazepam (Clonopin)
Propoxyphene Napsylate and APAP (Darvocet N-50) (Darvocet N-100)
Meprobamate with ASA (Equagesic)

Schedule V
Diphenoxylate HCl and Atropine SO_4 (Lomotil)
APAP with Codeine Elixir (Tylenol with Codeine Elixir)
Donnagel PG
Robitussin AC
Phenergan VC with Codeine
Terpin Hydrate with Codeine

88 Medication Administration: Nasal

PSYCHOSOCIAL CONSIDERATIONS: Explain the procedure in developmentally appropriate terms. Avoid using terms with mixed meanings. Comfort and console the child after administration.

TIME: 1 to 2 minutes

PURPOSE

To administer medication in a safe, effective manner.

To follow practices in accordance with state and federal drug regulations.

OBJECTIVES

- To administer the medication.
- To prevent injury and maintain comfort.
- To obtain the desired effect of the medication.

EQUIPMENT

Medication
Bulb syringe, if appropriate
Tissues

SAFETY ISSUES

- Refer to "Medication Administration: General Procedure."

ESSENTIAL STEPS

1. Prepare the child and family.
2. Assemble the equipment. Refer to "Medication Administration: General Procedure."
3. Wash hands.
4. Identify the child by checking the identification band.
5. Clean nares, if necessary. Ask a child old enough to follow instructions to blow his or her nose, if needed.
6. Place the child in a supine position with the head hyperextended. (See Fig. 88.1)
7. Instruct the child to breathe through the mouth.

8. Instill the medication. Avoid touching the dropper to the nose. Keep the child on his or her back for 2 to 3 minutes. Instruct a child old enough to follow instructions to sniff. Offer tissue for a runny nose, but caution against blowing the nose for 2 to 3 minutes.

DOCUMENTATION

- Medication.
- Dose.
- Route.
- Site(s).
- Time.
- Child's response.

POTENTIAL RELATED NURSING DIAGNOSES

Airway clearance, ineffective
Breathing pattern, ineffective
Fluid volume deficit: *high risk*
Aspiration: *high risk*

Skills Checklist

☐ Prepare the child and family.
☐ Assemble the equipment.
☐ Wash hands.
☐ Identify the child by checking the identification band.
☐ Clean nares.
☐ Position the child.
☐ Instill drops.
☐ Document.

POTENTIAL RELATED MEDICAL DIAGNOSES

Nasal congestion

Allergies

Diabetes insipidus (with vasopressin administration)

REFERENCES

Mott, S., James, S., and Sperhac, A. 1990. *Nursing care of children and families.* Redwood City, Calif.: Addison-Wesley.

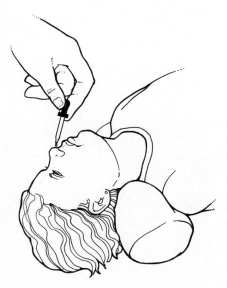

FIGURE 88.1 *Administering nasal medications.*

Medication Administration: Oral

Plastic dropper, nipple, or syringe, if appropriate (see Fig. 89.1)

Medication

Medicine cup, if appropriate

PSYCHOSOCIAL CONSIDERATIONS: A parent or a significant other may be able to administer the medicine more easily than a nurse. Avoid mixing the medication with favorite foods, as doing so may cause the child to dislike these food items. Comfort and console the child after administration.

TIME: 2 to 3 minutes per medication

PURPOSE

To administer medication in a safe, effective manner.

To follow practices in accordance with state and federal drug regulations.

OBJECTIVES

- To administer the medication.
- To prevent aspiration.
- To obtain the desired effect of the medication.

SAFETY ISSUES

- Keep the child's head elevated while administering the medication.
- After drawing up medication, give in small increments to prevent choking and aspiration.
- If the medicine is particularly strong or foul tasting, it may be mixed with a small amount of formula or food. Neonates can become bradycardic with strong-tasting medicine.
- Refer to "Medication Administration: General Procedure."

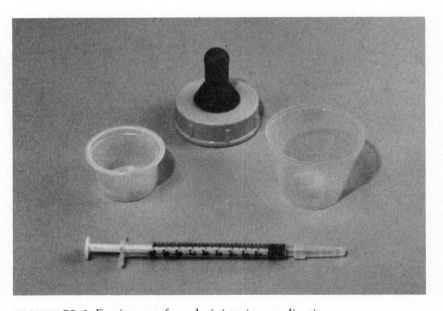

FIGURE 89.1 *Equipment for administering medications.*

ESSENTIAL STEPS

1. Prepare the child and family.
2. Assemble the equipment. Refer to "Medication Administration: General Procedure."
3. Wash hands.
4. Identify the child by checking the identification band.
5. For an infant:

    To administer tablets:

    > Crush the tablet and mix it into a small amount of formula, juice, or flavored syrup.

    > Administer in a syringe or dropper, if appropriate.

    To administer liquid medications:

    > Measure the volume to be administered in a medicine cup or syringe.

    > If a calibrated dropper comes with the medication, use that dropper to measure the dose volume.

    Position the child with the head elevated to prevent aspiration.

    If using a dropper or syringe, aim the tip toward the back of the buccal pouch. (See Fig. 89.2)

    If using a nipple, place the measured dose into the nipple and allow the infant to suck. (See Fig. 89.3)

    Administer the medicine slowly, allowing the child time to swallow.

Skills Checklist

☐ Prepare the child and family.
☐ Assemble the equipment.
☐ Wash hands.
☐ Identify the child by checking the identification band.
☐ Administer medication.
☐ Document.

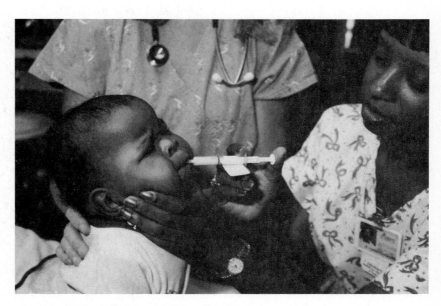

FIGURE 89.2 *Administering medication via syringe.*

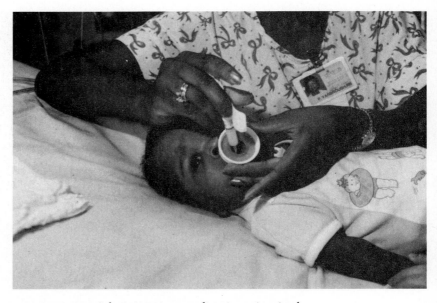

FIGURE 89.3 *Administering medication via nipple.*

251

6. For a toddler:

   To administer tablets:

   Crush the tablet and mix with a small amount of food or drink.

   Administer in a syringe or dropper, if appropriate.

   For liquid medications:

   Measure the volume to be administered in a medicine cup or syringe.

   If a calibrated dropper comes with the medication, use that dropper to measure the dose volume. (Note: Strong-tasting medicine may be given in liquids or food if necessary, such as chocolate syrup, applesauce, or jello. It may help to vary the substance in which the medication is mixed.)

   Position the child with the head elevated to prevent aspiration.

   If using a dropper or syringe, aim the tip toward the back of the buccal pouch.

   Administer the medicine slowly, allowing the child time to swallow.

7. For a child old enough to follow instructions:

   To administer tablets:

   If the child is unable to swallow tablets, crush non-enteric-coated tablets and mix with a flavored syrup, food, or drink.

To administer liquid medications:

Measure the volume to be administered in a medicine cup or syringe.

If a calibrated dropper comes with the medication, use that dropper to measure the dose volume.

If the medicine is foul or strong tasting, allow the child to choose what to mix with the medication. Strong-tasting medication can cause dyspnea if taken too rapidly.

DOCUMENTATION

- Medication.
- Dose.
- Route.
- Time.
- Child's response.

POTENTIAL RELATED NURSING DIAGNOSES

Airway clearance, ineffective

Aspiration: *high risk*

Injury: *high risk*

POTENTIAL RELATED MEDICAL DIAGNOSES

Universal application

REFERENCES

Mott, S., James, S., and Sperhac, A. 1990. *Nursing care of children and families.* Redwood City, Calif.: Addison-Wesley.

90 Medication Administration: Rectal

PSYCHOSOCIAL CONSIDERATIONS: Explain the procedure in developmentally appropriate terms. It is helpful if the parents or a significant other are near or holding the child to provide reassurance. Avoid using terms with mixed meanings, such as *stick into the bottom*. Talk soothingly to the child during the process. Provide distraction during the procedure. Awaken the child prior to administering the medication.

TIME: 3 to 4 minutes

PURPOSE

To administer medication in a safe, effective manner.

To follow practices in accordance with state and federal drug regulations.

OBJECTIVES

- To administer the medication.
- To prevent injury.
- To obtain the desired effect of the medication.

EQUIPMENT

Gloves, nonsterile, *or* finger cot

Lubricant

Medication

Bedpan and underpad, if needed

Syringe and red rubber or Foley catheter *or* enema bag, if needed

SAFETY ISSUES

- **Refer to "Medication Administration: General Procedure."**

1. Prepare the child and family.
2. Assemble the equipment. Refer to "Medication Administration: General Procedure."
3. Wash hands.
4. Identify the child by checking the identification band.
5. To insert a suppository:

    Cut lengthwise if suppository needs division.

    Position the child on a side with the knees flexed.

    Put on gloves or finger cot.

    Lubricate the suppository and insert gently. (See Fig. 90.1)

    Hold the buttocks together to prevent expulsion for a least 2 to 3 minutes.

6. To administer liquid rectal medication:

    Position the child on the left side.

    Put on gloves.

    Place a protective pad under the child.

    If using a syringe with a red rubber catheter:

    Attach the syringe to the rubber catheter.

    Lubricate the tip of the rubber catheter and gently insert it about 1″ to 2″ into the rectum.

    Instill the medication slowly. Do not use force against resistance.

    Hold the buttocks together to prevent immediate expulsion. (Have a bedpan available.)

    If using a syringe with a Foley catheter:

    Attach the syringe to the Foley catheter.

    Lubricate the tip of the Foley catheter and gently insert it about 1″ to 2″ into the rectum.

    Inflate the balloon 3 to 5 ml.

    Instill the medication slowly. Do not use force against resistance.

Clamp the Foley.

Apply slight tension to the Foley to prevent expulsion of the liquid.

If using a prepared enema (such as Fleets), follow the manufacturer's directions for steps to administer.

If using an enema bag:

Fill the tubing with the liquid, per the physician's plan of care.

Lubricate the tip of the tubing and gently insert it about 1″ to 2″ into the rectum.

Instill the medication slowly. Do not use force against resistance.

Hold the buttocks together to prevent immediate expulsion for at least 2 to 3 minutes. (Have a bedpan available.)

DOCUMENTATION

- Medication.
- Dose.
- Route.
- Time.
- Child's response.

POTENTIAL RELATED NURSING DIAGNOSES

Constipation

Swallowing, impaired

Anxiety

Hyperthermia

Injury: *high risk*

POTENTIAL RELATED MEDICAL DIAGNOSES

Hyperthermia

Infection

Constipation

Pain

NPO (nothing by mouth)

Unconsciousness

REFERENCES

Mott, S., James, S., and Sperhac, A. 1990. *Nursing care of children and families.* Redwood City, Calif.: Addison-Wesley.

Skills Checklist

Suppository

☐ Prepare the child and family.

☐ Assemble the equipment.

☐ Wash hands.

☐ Identify the child by checking the identification band.

☐ Position the child.

☐ Put on gloves or finger cot.

☐ Lubricate the suppository.

☐ Insert the suppository.

☐ Hold buttocks.

☐ Document.

Liquid Rectal Medication

☐ Prepare the child and family.

☐ Assemble the equipment.

☐ Wash hands.

☐ Identify the child by checking the identification band.

☐ Position the child.

☐ Put on gloves.

☐ Place a protective pad under the child.

☐ Attach the syringe to a catheter, or use an enema bag.

☐ Lubricate the end of the catheter or the tip of the enema bag tubing.

☐ Administer medication.

☐ Hold buttocks.

☐ Document.

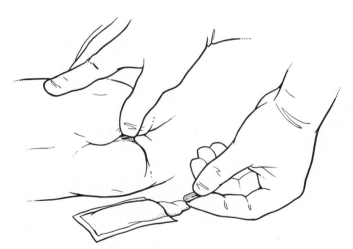

FIGURE 90.1 *Administering rectal medication.*

Medication Administration: Sub Q and IM Injection

PSYCHOSOCIAL CONSIDERATIONS: Explain the procedure in developmentally appropriate terms. Avoid the use of terms with mixed meanings, such as *stick* and *pinch*. To avoid prolonged worrying, do not tell toddlers or preschoolers of the procedure in advance. Tell the child it is okay to cry, just not to move. Do not tell the child ahead of time that it will hurt, as doing so may give preconceived ideas about the procedure. If the child asks, answer honestly and state that it may hurt; this answer allows for the child's own interpretation. Comfort and console the child after administration.

TIME: 3 to 5 minutes

PURPOSE

To administer the medication in a safe, effective manner.

To follow practices in accordance with state and federal drug regulations.

OBJECTIVES

- To administer the medication.
- To prevent injury to the tissue or muscle.
- To obtain the desired effect of the medication.

EQUIPMENT

Gloves, nonsterile

Povidone-iodine swab *or* alcohol swab

Medication

Syringe and needle, of length and gauge based on the size of the child and the characteristics of the medicine

Cotton ball *or* 2″ × 2″ gauze, if appropriate

Adhesive bandage

S SAFETY ISSUES

- Avoid using a needle longer than 1″ for infants and young children.
- In any one site, do not inject more than 1 ml of medication for an infant or more than 2 ml for a toddler or older child.
- Avoid using the dorsogluteal site for children under the age of 4. Complications from the use of this site in infants and small children are well documented.
- Avoid using the deltoid muscle for frequent intramuscular injections.
- Refer to "Medication Administration: General Procedure."

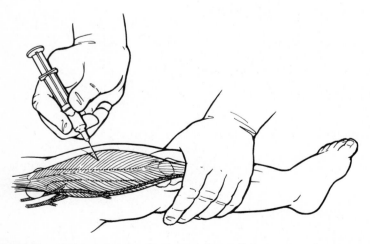

FIGURE 91.1 *Injecting into the vastus lateralis.*

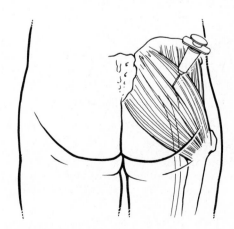

FIGURE 91.2 *Injecting into the dorsogluteal.*

1. Prepare the child and family.

2. Assemble the equipment. Refer to "Medication Administration: General Procedure."

3. Wash hands.

4. Identify the child by checking the identification band.

5. Select the appropriate site.

   Rotate subcutaneous (SQ) sites.

   For an intramuscular (IM) site, select from the following:

   Vastus lateralis, preferred for infants and small children. (See Fig. 91.1)

   Dorsogluteal, only to be used for children who have been walking for 1 or more years. (See Fig. 91.2) Give with the child prone, toes turned inward to relax the muscle.

   Ventrogluteal, second most preferred for infants and small children. (See Fig. 91.3) This should be the primary site in children over the age of 12.

   Deltoid, used only when giving a small amount of medication since its muscle mass is small. Do not inject thick, viscous medications into this muscle, and avoid repeated deltoid injections. (See Fig. 91.4)

6. Position the child and request assistance as necessary to restrain the child.

7. Put on gloves.

8. Clean the site with a povidone-iodine or alcohol swab.

9. Insert the needle using aseptic technique.

   When administering SQ medication, pinch up the skin and insert the needle at a 90° angle into the skin fold.

Skills Checklist

☐ Prepare the child and family.

☐ Assemble the equipment.

☐ Wash hands.

☐ Identify the child by checking the identification band.

☐ Select the appropriate site.

☐ Position the child.

☐ Put on gloves.

☐ Clean the skin.

☐ Administer the medication.

☐ Bandage.

☐ Discard the needle and syringe in the sharps disposal container.

☐ Document.

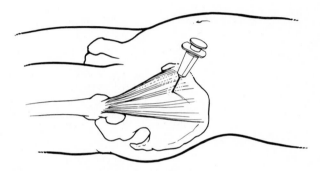

FIGURE 91.3 *Injecting into the ventrogluteal.*

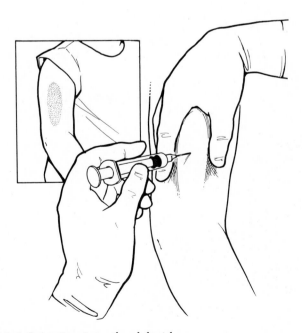

FIGURE 91.4 *Injecting into the deltoid.*

When administering IM injection:

In the vastus lateralis, insert the needle at a 90° angle.

In the dorsogluteal, insert the needle into the upper outer quadrant at a 90° angle to the skin.

In the ventrogluteal, stretch the skin taut and insert the needle at a 90° angle in the V formed by the two fingers. Inject into the middle third of the lateral muscle.

In the deltoid, grasp the muscle mass and angle the needle slightly upward toward the shoulder.

Using the Z-track technique, draw up a small amount of air (.2 ml) after drawing up medication. Pull the skin laterally about ½″. Keeping the skin taut, insert the needle at a 90° angle. After injecting the medication, withdraw the needle and release the skin. (See Fig. 91.5)

(Note: use this method only with large muscle masses such as the dorsogluteal or vastus lateralis. Injecting the .2 ml of air can prevent tracking of medication through subcutaneous tissue when the needle is withdrawn. This is especially important with irritating medications.)

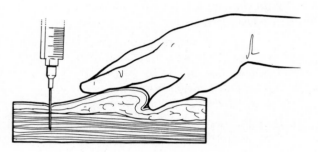

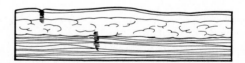

FIGURE 91.5 *Injection using the Z-track technique.*

10. Aspirate, observing for blood return. If blood is aspirated, remove the needle, discard the medication, and repeat Step 9.

11. Inject the medication and withdraw the needle.

12. Rub the area to increase the circulation and absorption for IM injections. For SQ injections, use a dry cotton ball or a 2″ × 2″ gauze and provide gentle pressure or rub lightly.

13. Apply a bandage, as needed.

14. Do not recap the needle.

15. Discard the needle and syringe in the sharps disposal container.

DOCUMENTATION

- Medication.
- Dose.
- Route.
- Time.
- Child's response.

POTENTIAL RELATED NURSING DIAGNOSES

Pain, acute

Fear

Skin integrity, impaired

POTENTIAL RELATED MEDICAL DIAGNOSES

Universal application

REFERENCES

Beecroft, P., and Redick, S. 1990. Intramuscular injection practices of pediatric nurses and site selection. *Nurse educator* 15, no. 4: 23–28.

Beecroft, P., and Redick, S. 1989. Possible complications of intramuscular injections on the pediatric unit. *Pediatric nursing* 15, no. 4: 333–36.

Hahn, K. 1990. Brush up on your injection technique. *Nursing 90* 20, no. 9: 54–58.

Litwack, Kim. 1991. Administering preoperative medications. *Nursing 91* 21, no. 8: 44–47.

Mott, S., James, S., and Sperhac, A. 1990. *Nursing care of children and families.* Redwood City, Calif.: Addison-Wesley.

92 Medication Administration: Topical

PSYCHOSOCIAL CONSIDERATIONS: The child may be afraid of gloves because the gloves feel unnatural. Apply medications quickly but gently. A parent or significant other may be able to perform this procedure more easily than a nurse. Children old enough to follow instructions may apply their own medication. Describe to the child any stinging, burning, or cold feeling that the medication might cause.

TIME: 2 to 3 minutes

PURPOSE

To administer medication in a safe, effective manner.

To follow practices in accordance with state and federal drug regulations.

OBJECTIVES

- To administer the medication.
- To obtain the desired effect of the medication.

EQUIPMENT

One of the following applicators:
   Gloves, sterile
   Applicators
   4″ × 4″ gauze, sterile

Medication

SAFETY ISSUES

- **Apply mittens, socks, or long sleeves as necessary to prevent the child from sucking the affected area(s).**
- **Refer to "Medication Administration: General Procedure."**

ESSENTIAL STEPS

1. Prepare the child and family.
2. Assemble the equipment. Refer to "Medication Administration: General Procedure."
3. Wash hands.
4. Identify the child by checking the identification band.

5. Assess the affected area.

6. Clean the affected area of dried medication or drainage when indicated.

8. Apply the medication using gloves, applicators, or gauze.

DOCUMENTATION

- Appearance of the area.
- Medication.
- Route.
- Time.
- Site(s) to which medication has been applied.
- Child's response.

POTENTIAL RELATED NURSING DIAGNOSES

Infection: *high risk*

Pain, acute

Skin integrity, impaired: *high risk*

POTENTIAL RELATED MEDICAL DIAGNOSES

Rash

Urticaria

Dryness

REFERENCES

Mott, S., James, S., and Sperhac, A. 1990. *Nursing care of children and families.* Redwood City, Calif.: Addison-Wesley.

Skills Checklist

☐ Prepare the child and family.
☐ Assemble the equipment.
☐ Wash hands.
☐ Identify the child by checking the identification band.
☐ Assess the skin.
☐ Clean the area, if indicated.
☐ Apply medication.
☐ Document.

93 Medication Administration: IV Phytonadione

- Do not infuse at a rate greater than 1 mg/minute.
- Use an infusion pump.
- Place the child on a cardiac/respiratory monitor during and for 1 hour after the infusion.
- Because IV administration of phytonadione can cause severe reactions, the IV route is indicated only in severe hypoprothrombinemia or when other routes of administration are not feasible.
- Refer to "Medication Administration: General Procedure."

PSYCHOSOCIAL CONSIDERATIONS: Explain the procedure in developmentally appropriate terms. Avoid using terms that may have mixed meanings, such as *stick* and *inject*. Tell the child that you will not disrupt or remove the IV needle.

TIME: Varies with dosage of medication

PURPOSE

To safely administer phytonadione by IV infusion. Phytonadione increases the clotting ability of the blood in conditions of hypoprothrombinemia caused by vitamin K deficiency.

OBJECTIVES

- To administer the medication.
- To prevent injury related to administration.
- To raise prothrombin levels and stop bleeding.
- To prevent precipitate.

EQUIPMENT

Cardiac/respiratory monitor

Gloves, nonsterile

Infusion pump and tubing

Phytonadione

Compatible IV fluid (preservative-free 5% dextrose in water, normal saline, or 5% dextrose and normal saline)

ESSENTIAL STEPS

1. Prepare the child and family. Check for known sensitivity to vitamin K.
2. Assemble the equipment. Refer to "Medication Administration: General Procedure."
3. Wash hands.
4. Identify the child by checking the identification band.
5. Establish a baseline assessment, including vital signs.
6. Put on gloves.

7. Administer medication immediately after dilution. Dilution is not necessary as long as the rate of administration does not exceed 1 mg/minute.

8. Monitor vital signs during and after administration of the medication.

9. Report any adverse reactions, such as anaphylaxis, shock, or cardiac or respiratory arrest.

DOCUMENTATION

- Medication.
- Dose.
- Route.
- Time.
- Vital signs before, during, and after administration.
- Child's response.

POTENTIAL RELATED NURSING DIAGNOSES

Anxiety

Fear

Injury: *high risk*

Tissue perfusion, altered, cardiopulmonary

POTENTIAL RELATED MEDICAL DIAGNOSES

Decreased clotting time

Newborn

Hemorrhage

Hypoprothrombinemia

Skills Checklist

- ☐ Prepare the child and family.
- ☐ Assemble the equipment.
- ☐ Wash hands.
- ☐ Identify the child by checking the identification band.
- ☐ Establish a baseline assessment, including vital signs.
- ☐ Put on gloves.
- ☐ Administer the medication.
- ☐ Monitor vital signs during and after administration of the medication.
- ☐ Document.

REFERENCES

Howry, L. B., Bendler, R. M., and Tso, Y. 1981. *Pediatric medications*. Philadelphia, Pa.: J. B. Lippincott Co.

McEvoy, G., and McQuarrie, G., eds. 1989. *American hospital formulary services drug information 89*. Bethesda, Md.: American Society of Hospital Pharmacists.

Trissel, L. A. 1988. *Handbook of injectable drugs,* 4th ed. Bethesda, Md.: American Society of Hospital Pharmacists.

Lab Values

PROTHROMBIN TIME TEST
Newborn: <17 seconds
All Other: 11–15 seconds

PARTIAL THROMBOPLASTIN TIME
Newborn: <90 seconds
All Other: Nonactivated—60–85 seconds
Activated—25–35 seconds

Monitor: Cardiac/Apnea

- Children with cardiac dysrhythmias or pacemakers should be on a monitor system capable of producing an ECG printout.
- Alarms should always be on while the child is unattended.
- Rate limits should not be set at 0.

PSYCHOSOCIAL CONSIDERATIONS: Explain the procedure in developmentally appropriate terms. The child may express feeling like a robot with all the wires and/or may fear electrocution. Explain the alarms and numbers to the child and parents.

TIME: Varies

PURPOSE

To monitor the cardiac and/or respiratory activity of the child.

OBJECTIVES

- To monitor cardiac and respiratory activity.
- To prevent injury.

EQUIPMENT

Alcohol swabs

Skin electrodes

Monitor with lead cable and wires

ESSENTIAL STEPS

1. Prepare the child and family.
2. Assemble the equipment.
3. Wash hands.
4. Wipe the appropriate skin electrode sites on the child with alcohol and allow to dry.
5. Apply appropriate-sized electrode. (See Table 94.1 and Fig. 94.1)
6. Turn on the monitor. Follow the manufacturer's instructions. (See Fig. 94.2)
7. Connect the appropriate leads to the electrodes. (See Fig. 94.3)
8. Adjust the sensitivity knobs until the cardiac and respiratory rates on the monitor correlate with the auscultated rates on the child.
9. Set high and low alarm limits.
10. Set apnea delay for the desired time frame.
11. Activate the alarms.

DOCUMENTATION

- Date and time monitor initiated.
- That alarm limits are set and on, each shift.
- ECG rate/rhythm and respiratory rate/rhythm, each shift.
- ECG strip printout labeled with the child's name, date, and time recorded, each shift, taped to documentation record.

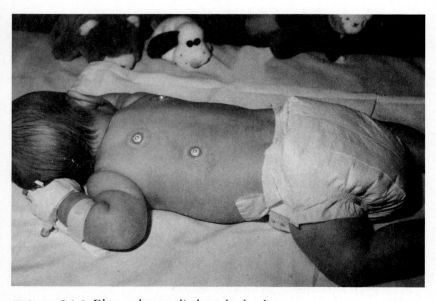

FIGURE 94.1 *Electrodes applied to the back.*

TABLE 94.1 *Recommended Sites for Electrode Placement*

**Chest Breathers
(Usually Older Children)**
RL: At the 6th or 7th ICS on the right MCL
LA: At the 6th or 7th ICS on the left MCL
RA: Near the atrium or below the right clavicle

**Abdominal Breathers
(Including Infants)**
RA: Directly under the right clavicle
LA + RL: Directly opposite each other at the
point of maximal respiration

Infants Less than 2,500 Grams

ON THE CHEST
RA: Directly under the right clavicle
RL: Beneath the RA electrode
LA: At the 6th or 7th ICS on the left MCL

ON THE BACK
RA: Right scapula
RL: Right lower back
LA: Left scapula

KEY: RA = right arm; electrode wire or lead is white. LL
= left leg; electrode wire or lead is green. LA = left arm;
electrode wire or lead is black. RL = right leg; electrode
wire or lead is green. ICS = intercostal space. MCL =
midclavicular line.

- Any changes in the monitoring system or cardiac/respiratory irregularities. Be specific as to whether the child's alarm sounded for apnea, tachypnea, bradycardia, or tachycardia. Document what the child was doing, the child's color, and vital signs.

POTENTIAL RELATED NURSING DIAGNOSES

Anxiety

Tissue perfusion, altered, cardiopulmonary

Cardiac output, decreased

Breathing pattern, ineffective

POTENTIAL RELATED MEDICAL DIAGNOSES

Congenital cardiac defects

Pneumonia

Apnea

Cardiac arrhythmias

Respiratory infections

Unconsciousness

Head injuries

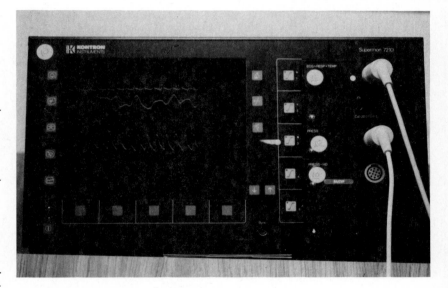

Skills Checklist

☐ Prepare the child and family.
☐ Assemble the equipment.
☐ Wash hands.
☐ Place electrodes.
☐ Turn on the monitor.
☐ Connect leads to the electrodes.
☐ Set alarms and limits.
☐ Set apnea delay.
☐ Activate alarms.
☐ Document.

FIGURE 94.2 *Cardiac/apnea monitor.*

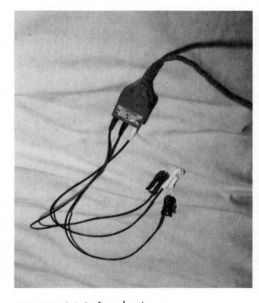

FIGURE 94.3 *Lead wires.*

265

95 Nasogastric Tube Insertion

Tape

Water-soluble lubricant

Gloves, nonsterile

Blanket for restraint, if appropriate

Pacifier, if appropriate

Pin and rubber band to secure tube to clothing

Emesis basin

Stethoscope

Syringe with an adapter

PSYCHOSOCIAL CONSIDERATIONS: Explain the procedure in developmentally appropriate terms. Explain that the tube is soft. Allow the child to touch the tube. Talk to the child in soothing tones while inserting the tube. Allow the child to swallow sips of water to facilitate tube insertion. Encourage therapeutic play, if possible.

TIME: 10 to 15 minutes

PURPOSE

To provide access to the gastrointestinal system to decompress the stomach, sample gastric contents, gavage or lavage, assess and treat gastrointestinal bleeding, or administer medications, electrolyte solutions, or nutrition.

OBJECTIVES

- To insert a nasogastric (N/G) tube safely and accurately.
- To prevent injury.

EQUIPMENT

Appropriate-sized N/G tube:

    A single-lumen N/G tube for gavage or lavage

    A double-lumen N/G tube (Argyle, Salem Sump, or Anderson Sump) for intermittent gastric decompression (one-time use only)

    A silicone N/G tube for long-term, continuous N/G feedings

 SAFETY ISSUES

- **Vagal nerve stimulation during insertion may cause bradycardia. Assess the apical pulse prior to and after insertion.**

- **A nasogastric tube in a child having had esophageal or gastric surgery should not be removed or moved except by the physician, unless otherwise indicated. If the tube comes out, do not reinsert it; notify the physician.**

- **Single-lumen N/G tubes (such as Argyle) may be used for infants and for children needing short-term therapy. Change these tubes every 3 days, inserting in alternate naris each time. Use a No. 5 or a No. 8 for infants less than 5 kg.**

- **Use prelubricated silicone indwelling N/G tubes (such as Corpak) for children receiving long-term therapy. Remove and clean the indwelling tube monthly (or sooner if it malfunctions or complications occur). Replace it in the opposite naris.**

ESSENTIAL STEPS

1. Prepare the child and family.

2. Assemble the equipment. See package insert for prelubricated silicone indwelling tubes.

   Assess patency of the nares.

   Use the tube to measure the distance from the child's nose to the earlobe and then to the point halfway between the xiphoid and the umbilicus. Mark the tube with tape at this measured distance. (See Fig. 95.1)

   Lubricate the tip of the tube (approximately 1″ to 3″).

3. Wash hands and put on gloves.

4. Restrain the child, as necessary. Use a blanket for a mummy restraint, if appropriate. Position the child on the right side or with the chest elevated 30° to 45°.

5. Encourage a child old enough to follow instructions to swallow during insertion. Offer a pacifier to babies older than 3 months who do not need to mouth-breathe.

6. Insert the N/G gently into the naris. If resistance is met, use the other naris. On an infant, it may be helpful to flex the neck to facilitate insertion into the esophagus. Insert the tube to the measured point. (See Fig. 95.2)

7. Check the back of the mouth for kinking of the tube.

8. Remove the tube quickly if the child coughs excessively, chokes, becomes cyanotic, or cannot speak or cry; these responses indicate that the tube is in the trachea. Reinsert the tube if necessary following steps 5 through 7.

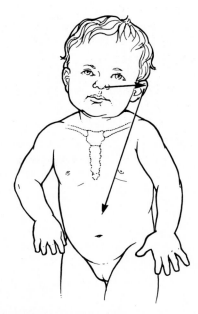

FIGURE 95.1 *Measuring the N/G tube length.*

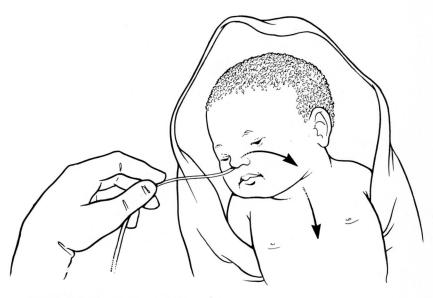

FIGURE 95.2 *Inserting an N/G tube.*

9. Check for proper placement in the stomach by aspirating the gastric contents and/or auscultating over the epigastric region while injecting a small amount (3 to 5 ml) of air through the N/G tube. Aspirate should be light green in color with a pH below 6. (See Figs. 95.3 and 95.4)

10. Secure the tube to the upper lip with tape, avoiding pressure on the nasal cartilage and occlusion of the opposite naris. Secure the tube to the cheek with a transparent occlusive dressing. Tape all connections.

11. Use a pin and a rubber band to secure the tube to clothing.

DOCUMENTATION

- Date and time of tube insertion.
- Purpose of the procedure (such as for gastric gavage, lavage, and so on).
- Size and type of tube used. If tube has numbering, the number seen as the tube exits the naris.
- Naris used.
- Amount, color, and consistency of returned contents.
- Lab tests done on gastric contents, if applicable.
- Child's tolerance of procedure.

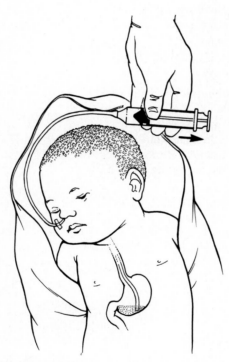

FIGURE 95.3 *Aspirating the stomach contents for placement.*

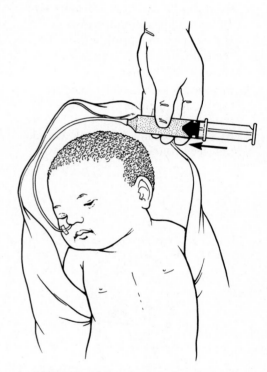

FIGURE 95.4 *Injecting air for a placement check. Listen with stethoscope over gastric area.*

POTENTIAL RELATED NURSING DIAGNOSES

Aspiration: *high risk*

Fluid volume deficit: *high risk*

Injury: *high risk*

Nutrition, altered, less than body requirements

Swallowing, impaired

Skin integrity, impaired: *high risk*

Pain, acute

POTENTIAL RELATED MEDICAL DIAGNOSES

Failure to thrive

Ingestion of substances

Hemorrhage

Nausea and vomiting

Poor sucking and swallowing reflexes

Prematurity

Congestive heart disease

REFERENCES

Camp, D., and Otten, N. 1990. How to insert and remove nasogastric tubes quickly and easily. *Nursing 90* 20: 59–64.

Mott, S., James, S., and Sperhac, A. 1990. *Nursing care of children and families.* Redwood City, Calif.: Addison-Wesley.

N/G Tube Size Chart

Premature	5 or 6 french
Newborn	
less than 8 pounds	6 french
greater than 8 pounds	8 french
Infant	8 french
Toddler and Preschooler	8 french
School-Age Child and Adolescent	10 french

These sizes serve only as guides; they can vary greatly, depending on the size of the child and the size of the naris. The nurse must make an independent judgment based on an assessment of the child.

96 Nasopharyngeal Swab

EQUIPMENT

Gloves, nonsterile, if contamination from secretions is likely

Bulb syringe, if appropriate

Penlight

Nasopharyngeal applicator (Calgi), sterile

Viral medium from lab, if needed

Culture container (such as a culturette), sterile, if needed

PSYCHOSOCIAL CONSIDERATIONS: Explain the procedure in developmentally appropriate terms. Avoid terms with mixed meanings. Perform the procedure quickly. Do not perform when the child is asleep. Teach the child and the family that they should not insert anything into the nose.

TIME: 2 to 3 minutes

PURPOSE

To obtain a specimen from the nasopharynx for diagnosis of a pathological condition or for an eosinophil count.

OBJECTIVES

- To obtain a specimen.
- To prevent injury during the procedure.

ESSENTIAL STEPS

1. Prepare the child and family.
2. Assemble the equipment.
3. Wash hands and put on gloves.
4. Have the child blow the nose. Use a bulb syringe for an infant. Check nostrils for patency with a penlight.
5. Bend the nasopharyngeal applicator into a curve; remove from package.
6. Insert applicator gently into the nostril as far as possible. Rotate quickly and remove. (See Fig. 96.1)
7. *For viral cultures,* carefully place the applicator into the sterile culture (viral) medium and close tightly. *For routine cultures,* place the applicator

into a sterile culture container (culturette with the swab stick removed). *For eosinophil count,* smear onto a glass slide and allow to air-dry before sending to the lab. *Pertussis* requires a culture tube and a smear and may be repeated with a second applicator, depending on the test.

8. Label the specimen and send to the lab immediately, keeping the viral culture specimen upright.

DOCUMENTATION

• Date and time specimen obtained.
• Naris(es) used.

POTENTIAL RELATED NURSING DIAGNOSES

Airway clearance, ineffective

Breathing pattern, ineffective

Infection: *high risk*

POTENTIAL RELATED MEDICAL DIAGNOSES

Infection

Rhinorrhea

Sinus infection

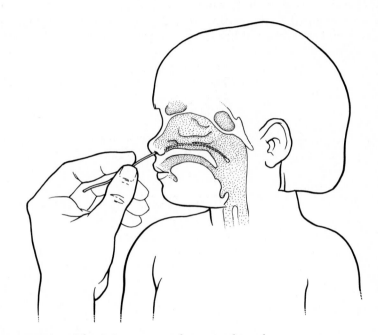

FIGURE 96.1 *Obtaining a nasopharyngeal swab.*

97 Neurological Assessment

Penlight
Tongue blade
Reflex hammer
Tape measure, for an infant
Tuning fork

PSYCHOSOCIAL CONSIDERATIONS: Explain the procedure in developmentally appropriate terms. Avoid using terms with mixed meanings. Neonates do not suffer psychological distress with this exam. Hold and comfort after the examination. Older children may fear strangers or fear being injured. If the child has a neurological impairment, the level of understanding may be altered.

TIME: 10 to 15 minutes

PURPOSE

To assess the neurological status of an infant or child.

OBJECTIVES

- To provide an ongoing assessment of neurological status.
- To prevent injury or trauma.

S | SAFETY ISSUES

- Signs and symptoms of increased intracranial pressure are

  Tachycardia.

  Bradycardia.

  Systolic hypertension.

  Widened pulse pressure.

  Respiratory depression.

  Apnea.

  Decreasing level of consciousness.

  Bulging fontanel.

  Vomiting, usually projectile.

  Shrill, high-pitched cry.

ESSENTIAL STEPS

1. Prepare the child and family.
2. Assemble the equipment.
3. Wash hands.
4. Assess vital signs.
5. To assess a child:

    Assess alertness, speech patterns, and behavior.

    Assess pupils for reactiveness, size, and equality. May turn off the lights and hand the child a penlight or a flashlight. When the child shines the light into his or her face, assess pupil reaction. (See Figs. 97.1, 97.2, and 97.3)

Skills Checklist

- ☐ Prepare the child and family.
- ☐ Assemble the equipment.
- ☐ Wash hands.
- ☐ Assess vital signs.
- ☐ Assess alertness.
- ☐ Assess infant's fontanels and head circumference.
- ☐ Assess pupils.
- ☐ Assess child's grips and strength or infant's movement of extremities.
- ☐ Assess child's gait.
- ☐ Assess child's orientation to time, place, and self.
- ☐ Assess child's recall of a series of numbers.
- ☐ Assess child's cranial nerves.
- ☐ Assess child's sensation.
- ☐ Assess reflexes.
- ☐ Assess infant's cry.
- ☐ Assess for presence of seizure activity in an infant.
- ☐ Document.

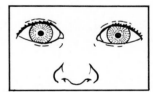

FIGURE 97.2 *Constricted pupils.*

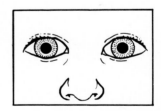

FIGURE 97.3 *Dilated pupils.*

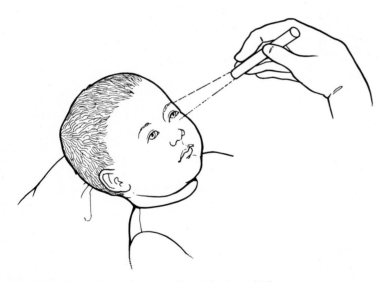

FIGURE 97.1 *Assessing pupils with a penlight.*

Assess grips and strength and compare bilaterally. (See Fig. 97.4)

Assess gait.

Assess orientation to time, place, and self (for older children).

Assess recall of a series of numbers. Give a series of no more than three numbers to a 4-year-old, four numbers to a 5-year-old, or five numbers to a 6-year-old.

Assess cranial nerves, including pupils.

Assess sensation. Use a broken tongue blade to test sharp and dull sensation. (See Fig. 97.5)

Assess deep tendon reflexes: biceps, triceps, branchioradialis, patellar, and Achilles tendon. Reflexes are graded in the following manner:
4+: hyperactive
3+: brisker than normal
2+: normal
1+: slightly diminished
0: absent

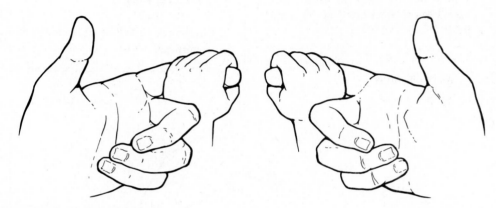

FIGURE 97.4 *Assessing grips.*

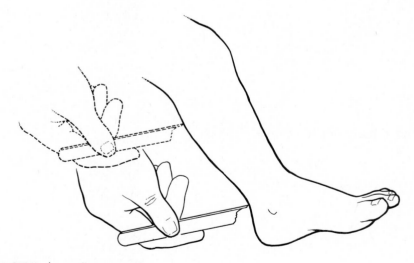

FIGURE 97.5 *Assessing sensation.*

6. To assess an infant:

Assess alertness.

Assess fontanels for fullness. (Posterior fontanel closes at approximately 5 months, anterior at approximately 12 to 18 months.)

Measure head circumference.

Assess pupils for reactiveness, size, and equality.

Assess movement of extremities.

Assess reflexes.

Assess cry (pitch and volume).

Assess for presence of seizure activity, such as rolling eyes, smacking noises, rigidity, and nonresponsiveness.

DOCUMENTATION

- Assessment findings.
- Any change in response.

POTENTIAL RELATED NURSING DIAGNOSES

Injury: *high risk*

Thought processes, altered

Tissue perfusion, altered, cerebral

Protection, altered

POTENTIAL RELATED MEDICAL DIAGNOSES

Head injury

Brain tumor

Hydrocephalus

Seizure disorder

Diabetes insipidus

Neurosurgical conditions

Syndrome of inappropriate secretion of antidiuretic hormone

REFERENCES

Reeves, K. 1989. Assessment of pediatric head injury: The basics. *Journal of Emergency Nursing:* 329–32.

Ostomy Care

PSYCHOSOCIAL CONSIDERATIONS: Explain the procedure in developmentally appropriate terms. Allow the child to assist as able.

TIME: 5 to 10 minutes for a bag change and stoma care; 15 to 20 minutes for irrigation

PURPOSE

To clean the stoma and the surrounding skin.

To irrigate and facilitate evacuation of feces.

OBJECTIVES

- To clean the stoma and the surrounding skin.
- To change the ostomy bag(s).
- To irrigate the ostomy.
- To prevent trauma and injury.

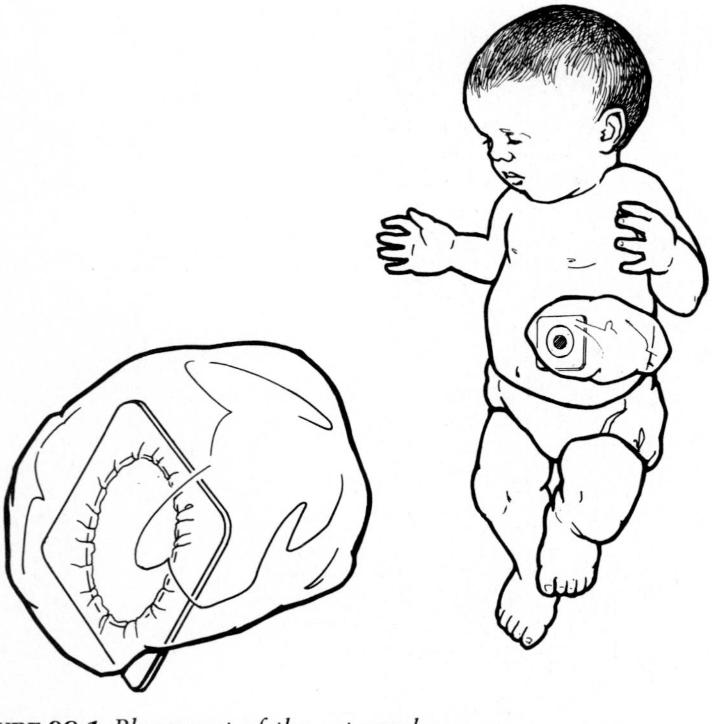

FIGURE 98.1 *Placement of the ostomy bag.*

EQUIPMENT

For a bag change and stoma care:

    Gloves, nonsterile

    Soap and water

    Washcloth

    Tissue paper

    Skin preparation

    Skin barrier, if not attached to ostomy bag

    Ostomy bag

In addition, for an ostomy irrigation:

    Irrigation bag and tubing

    Irrigating solution

    Drainage bag or sleeve

    Water-soluble lubricant

    Cone

S SAFETY ISSUES

- **Do not irrigate an ileostomy.**
- **Do not force the irrigating tube into the stoma. Insert the tip of the irrigating tube only up to 2″.**

ESSENTIAL STEPS

Stoma Care and Bag Change

1. Prepare the child and family.
2. Assemble the equipment.
3. Wash hands and put on gloves.
4. Remove the old bag.
5. Assess the stoma and the skin around the stoma.
6. Clean the skin and the stoma with soap and water.
7. Apply tissue over the stoma to prevent leakage.
8. Dry the skin around the stoma.
9. Apply skin preparation.
10. Remove tissue.
11. Apply skin barrier. Barrier should be ⅙″ to ⅛″ larger than the stoma.
12. Attach the bag, if the barrier is separate from the bag. (See Fig. 98.1)

13. Empty the ostomy bag when approximately two-thirds full.

Ostomy Irrigation

1. Prepare the child and family.
2. Assemble the equipment.
3. Wash hands and put on gloves.
4. Remove the old bag.
5. Fill the irrigation bag with irrigating solution and expel air from the tubing. Clamp the tubing.
6. Apply drainage bag over the stoma.
7. Lubricate the end of the irrigation tube.
8. Insert the tube through the cone.
9. Insert the tube into the stoma and fit the cone securely against the stoma. (See Fig. 98.2)
10. Hang the bag 12″ to 18″ above the stoma site.
11. Instill solution slowly. If cramping occurs, slow the rate or stop irrigation.
12. Remove the irrigant tube.
13. Secure the drainage bag.
14. Allow approximately 45 minutes for complete drainage.
15. Care for the stoma and apply a new bag, if applicable.
16. Assess the child's response.

DOCUMENTATION

- Appearance of skin and stoma.
- Amount and characteristics of bag contents.
- Care given.
- Amount and type of irrigating solution.
- Child's response.

POTENTIAL RELATED NURSING DIAGNOSES

Body image disturbance

Bowel incontinence

Diarrhea

Injury: *high risk*

Skills Checklist

Stoma Care and Bag Change
- ☐ Prepare the child and family.
- ☐ Assemble the equipment.
- ☐ Wash hands and put on gloves.
- ☐ Remove the old bag.
- ☐ Assess the stoma and skin.
- ☐ Clean the site.
- ☐ Apply skin preparation.
- ☐ Apply skin barrier.
- ☐ Apply the bag.
- ☐ Document.

Ostomy Irrigation
- ☐ Prepare the child and family.
- ☐ Assemble the equipment.
- ☐ Wash hands and put on gloves.
- ☐ Remove the old bag.
- ☐ Apply the drainage bag/sleeve.
- ☐ Instill irrigant.
- ☐ Allow 45 minutes for drainage.
- ☐ Care for the stoma and apply a new bag, if applicable.
- ☐ Document.

POTENTIAL RELATED MEDICAL DIAGNOSES

Short bowel syndrome

Hirschsprung's disease

Diverticulitis

REFERENCES

Mott, S., James, S., and Sperhac, A. 1990. *Nursing care of children and families.* Redwood City, Calif.: Addison-Wesley.

Swearingen, P. 1991. *Photo atlas of nursing procedures 2E.* Redwood City, Calif.: Addison-Wesley.

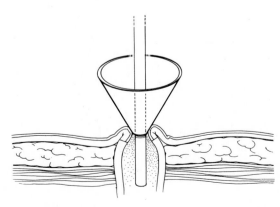

FIGURE 98.2 *Position of the irrigation cone in the stoma.*

99 Pacemakers: External Cardiac

PSYCHOSOCIAL CONSIDERATIONS: Explain the procedure in developmentally appropriate terms. The child may fear the monitor alarms or electrocution. Explain alarms to the child and parents.

TIME: Varies

PURPOSE

To provide safe operation of external cardiac pacemakers. To protect the child with external pacing wires from electric shock.

OBJECTIVES

- To monitor the operation of pacemakers.
- To prevent shock or injury.

EQUIPMENT

External pacemaker

External pacemaker wire(s), transvenous or transthoracic

Cardiac monitor programmed for pacemakers

Latex gloves

SAFETY ISSUES

- When handling external wires, wear latex gloves. Bare wires should not touch the child's or the care giver's skin. Avoid contact with electrically operated devices.
- Coil uninsulated pacemaker wires extending from the child and place them in a small (2 ml) blood tube with the rubber stopper in place (see Fig. 99.1), or coil them inside a finger cot. Securely tape the blood tube or finger cot to the child's chest.
- Ensure that pacer rate, sensitivity, and output are per the physician's plan of care.
- Ensure that the child is continuously attached to a cardiac monitor programmed for pacemakers.
- Place a new battery in the pacemaker before each patient use. Label the pacemaker with the date and time of battery placement.
- Protect temporary pacemaker dials with a plastic cover.
- Do not allow the child to operate electrical devices, such as electric toys, an electric razor, a blow dryer, or a curling iron.
- Avoid the use of electrocautery or diathermy equipment.

ESSENTIAL STEPS

1. Prepare the child and family.
2. Assemble the equipment.
3. Wash hands.
4. Check that pacemaker dials are set per the physician's plan of care (demand, A–V sequential pacing, or fixed rate).
5. Check that the electrode wires are securely attached to the pacemaker:

    The positive electrode (skin) connects to the positive terminal.

    The negative electrode (heart) connects to the negative terminal.
6. Connect the child to the cardiac monitor. Refer to "Monitor: Cardiac/Apnea."
7. Run a 6-second ECG strip. Label with the child's name, the date, and the time.
8. Secure the pacemaker or the connecting cable to the child's bed. *Do not secure to side rails.*
9. Repeat Steps 3 through 7 at the beginning of each shift and if any changes or problems are noted.

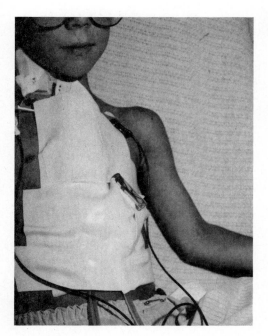

FIGURE 99.1 *Pacemaker wires in a tube.*

Skills Checklist

☐ Prepare the child and family.
☐ Assemble the equipment.
☐ Wash hands.
☐ Check the pacemaker dials and electrode wires.
☐ Connect the child to the cardiac monitor.
☐ Run a 6-second ECG strip.
☐ Secure the pacemaker.
☐ Document.

DOCUMENTATION

- Pacemaker settings and vital signs.
- 6-second ECG strip, attached.
- Name of the physician notified concerning any changes or problems.
- Mode (demand or fixed) and rate.
- Whether pacemaker is on or off.
- How frequently the child is paced and the child's underlying rhythm.

POTENTIAL RELATED NURSING DIAGNOSES

Cardiac output, decreased

Skin integrity, impaired: *high risk*

Injury: *high risk*

Tissue perfusion, altered, cardiopulmonary

Infection: *high risk*

POTENTIAL RELATED MEDICAL DIAGNOSES

Cardiothoracic surgery

Heart block

Congestive heart failure

REFERENCES

Mott, S., James, S., and Sperhac, A. 1990. *Nursing care of children and families.* Redwood City, Calif.: Addison-Wesley.

PSYCHOSOCIAL CONSIDERATIONS: Explain the procedure in developmentally appropriate terms. Avoid using terms with mixed meanings, such as *remove or drain fluid from your stomach*. Explain that it is okay to cry or yell, just not to move.

TIME: 15 to 20 minutes

PURPOSE

To remove fluid from the peritoneal cavity for diagnostic or therapeutic reasons.

OBJECTIVES

- To remove fluid from the peritoneal cavity.
- To decrease pressure on the peritoneal organs.
- To prevent injury and trauma.

EQUIPMENT

Gloves, sterile, for physician

Gloves, nonsterile

Povidone-iodine solution

Thoracentesis tray, which may include sterile drapes, 1% or 2% lidocaine, a syringe with a 25g needle, a thoracentesis needle, a large syringe, a three-way stopcock and tubing, sterile specimen containers, and 4″ × 4″ gauze sponges

Pressure dressing

Adhesive bandage, appropriate size

ESSENTIAL STEPS

1. Prepare the child and family.
   Ensure that the child's bladder is empty prior to the procedure.
   Obtain weight.
2. Assemble the equipment.
3. Wash hands and put on nonsterile gloves.
4. Position the child as indicated by the physician. Help the child to hold still by providing gentle restraint. (See Fig. 100.1)
5. Clean the skin with povidone-iodine solution.
6. Observe the child for signs of shock during and after the procedure.
7. After the procedure, apply pressure to the puncture site with a sterile gauze for 5 minutes. Apply a pressure dressing or, when oozing has stopped, a small bandage.

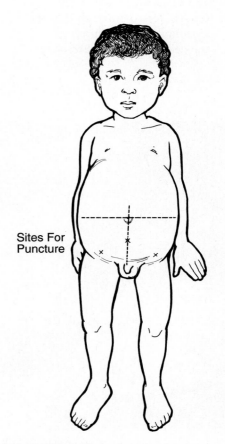

Sites For Puncture

***FIGURE 100.1** Paracentesis sites.*

8. Measure the quantity of fluid removed. Obtain the volume of fluid needed for lab test(s).

9. Comfort the child.

10. Send labeled specimen(s) to the lab immediately.

11. Take vital signs every 15 minutes for 1 hour, then every 4 hours. Obtain weight.

DOCUMENTATION

- Name of the physician performing the procedure.
- Time and date performed.
- Amount, color, and consistency of the fluid.
- That specimen has been sent to the lab.
- Any adverse effects of the procedure.
- Child's response.
- Vital signs, weights, and site checks.

POTENTIAL RELATED NURSING DIAGNOSES

Infection: *high risk*

Injury: *high risk*

Fluid volume excess

Breathing pattern, ineffective

Skin integrity, impaired

Tissue perfusion, altered, gastrointestinal

Skills Checklist

☐ Prepare the child and family. Ensure that the bladder is empty. Obtain weight.

☐ Assemble the equipment.

☐ Wash hands and put on gloves.

☐ Position the child.

☐ Clean the skin.

☐ Observe the child during and after the procedure.

☐ Apply pressure to the site after the procedure.

☐ Apply bandage.

☐ Measure the fluid and send specimen(s) to the lab.

☐ Take vital signs. Obtain weight.

☐ Document.

POTENTIAL RELATED MEDICAL DIAGNOSES

Cancer

Bowel obstruction

Perforation

Liver disease

Ascites

Renal failure

101 Phenylketonuria Screening

PSYCHOSOCIAL CONSIDERATIONS: Explain the procedure to the parents. Phenylketonuria (PKU) screening is performed on neonates, and the primary consideration is the neonate's response to pain. After the procedure, give the neonate to the parent for comforting, or hold and cuddle the neonate if the parent is not available.

TIME: 3 to 4 minutes

PURPOSE

To detect increasing phenylalanine levels in the blood.

OBJECTIVES

- To obtain a blood sample.
- To prevent injury.

EQUIPMENT

Gloves, nonsterile

Povidone-iodine swabs *or* alcohol swabs

Lancet

Guthrie test blotter

2″ × 2″ gauze, sterile, *or* cotton ball

Adhesive bandage

SAFETY ISSUES

- Do not squeeze the skin area for a prolonged time. This may alter the results of the screening by expressing a large amount of serum with a minimal number of red blood cells.
- Saturate the test blotter with blood for an accurate test.
- Perform the test 24 to 72 hours after feeding has been initiated. Delay this time period in a breast-feeding infant until breast milk, not colostrum, has been ingested for at least 24 hours.
- Some states repeat the test in 10 to 14 days.

ESSENTIAL STEPS

1. Prepare the child and family.
2. Assemble the equipment.
3. Wash hands and put on gloves.
4. Select the site, preferably the heel. Refer to "Blood Drawing: Heel and Finger Stick."
5. Prepare the skin with a povidone-iodine or alcohol swab.
6. Puncture the skin with a lancet. (See Figs. 101.1 and 101.2)

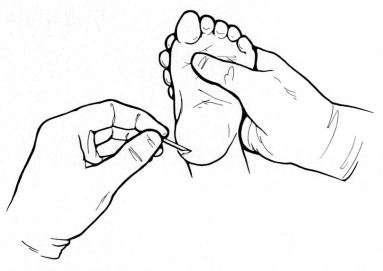

FIGURE 101.1 Puncturing the heel.

7. Completely saturate circles on the blotter with blood. (See Fig. 101.3)

8. Apply pressure with a sterile gauze or cotton ball until bleeding has stopped.

9. Apply a bandage to the site.

10. Label the specimen and send it to the lab.

11. Observe the site for adverse signs and symptoms, such as infection.

12. Instruct a parent on care of the site and removal of the bandage.

DOCUMENTATION

- Time blood obtained.
- Site used.
- That test has been sent to the lab.

POTENTIAL RELATED NURSING DIAGNOSES

Skin integrity, impaired

Infection: *high risk*

POTENTIAL RELATED MEDICAL DIAGNOSES

Phenylketonuria

Mental retardation

Newborn

REFERENCES

Mott, S., James, S., and Sperhac, A. 1990. *Nursing care of children and families.* Redwood City, Calif.: Addison-Wesley.

Skills Checklist

☐ Prepare the child and family.
☐ Assemble the equipment.
☐ Wash hands and put on gloves.
☐ Prepare the skin.
☐ Obtain a blood sample.
☐ Apply pressure to the site with a sterile gauze or cotton ball.
☐ Apply bandage.
☐ Send test kit to the lab.
☐ Document.

Lab Values

PHENYLALANINE LEVELS—NORMAL RANGES

Premature: 0.12–0.45 mmol/L
Newborn: 0.07–0.21 mmol/L

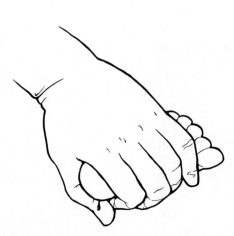

FIGURE 101.2 *Obtaining a droplet of blood for the PKU.*

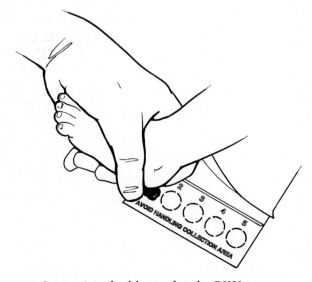

FIGURE 101.3 *Saturating the blotter for the PKU.*

102

Phototherapy and Photoradiometer

- Keep the infant's eyes covered at all times when under the lights.
- Cover genitalia in males and the lower abdomen in females when the infant is under the lights.
- Use an isolette unless the physician orders an open warmer.
- If the infant has a pulse oximeter, cover the probe site with a diaper while under the lights. Phototherapy can interfere with pulse oximeter readings.
- Change the infant's position every 2 hours to maximize exposure.

PSYCHOSOCIAL CONSIDERATIONS: Explain the procedure to the parents. The procedure can interrupt holding and touching and the bonding process for parents or significant others. Encourage parents to touch the infant and allow parents to hold the infant several times per day. Take care not to bump the isolette or make loud noises, as the noise level increases inside the isolette. Discuss the use of the protective coverings with parents and reassure them as needed.

TIME: 10 to 15 minutes for setup

PURPOSE

To increase the decomposition and excretion of bilirubin.

OBJECTIVES

- To decrease bilirubin levels.
- To prevent injury.
- To prevent dehydration.
- To maintain skin integrity.

EQUIPMENT

Phototherapy lights with plastic safety screen

Photoradiometer, if applicable

Cover for genitalia or abdomen, such as a flat isolation face mask with the nose piece removed

Eye patches

Isolette or open warmer

ESSENTIAL STEPS

1. Prepare the child and family.
2. Assemble the equipment. (See Figs. 102.1 and 102.2)
3. Wash hands.
4. Obtain phototherapy lights:

    Check the intensity of the light at the center of focus, where it is the greatest.

    The recommended *minimal intensity* for blue lights is 4.0 uw/cm2/nm.

The *maximal distance* of the light from the body is that distance which will allow no less than 4.0 uw/cm2/nm. If an intensity of at least 4.0 uw/cm2/nm cannot be obtained, insert new blue fluorescent bulbs. (The bulbs continue to light even when they have lost therapeutic effectiveness.)

The *minimal distance* for the light from the top of the isolette is 4″. If using an open warmer, position the light source 42 to 45 cm from the top surface of the infant.

5. Ensure that the plastic safety screen is in place on the lights.

6. Place the lights to provide maximum exposure to the child's body.

7. Check the intensity of light every shift, using a photoradiometer, if applicable. Press to read the intensity in uw/cm2/nm.

   If the reading is less than 4.0 uw/cm2/nm, move the light bank closer to the isolette, but no closer than 18″ above the child.

If the reading remains less than 4.0 uw/cm2/nm, try:

Raising the mattress.

Installing new bulbs.

Using a double bank of lights.

Returning the phototherapy lights and obtaining a new bank of lights.

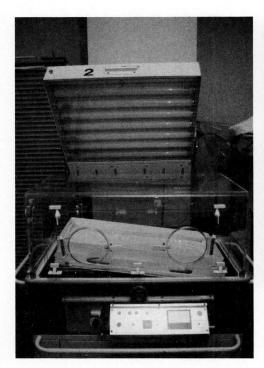

FIGURE 102.1 *Phototherapy lights with a safety cover.*

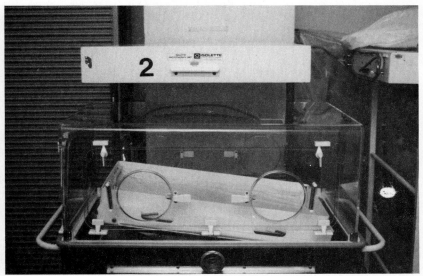

FIGURE 102.2 *Phototherapy lights.*

If the digital display shows a rhythmic blinking, then the intensity is greater than 19.9 uw/cm2/nm:

Move the lights further away from the isolette. The readings should be at least 4.0. Recheck the readings after making an adjustment in distance.

8. Remove the infant's clothing. Cover the genitalia of males or the lower abdomen of females with an isolation face mask.

9. To use eye patches:

Ensure that the baby's eyes are closed before covering.

Turn the lights off before removing the eye patches.

Remove the eye patches to assess eyes and perform eye care every 4 to 8 hours. Clean the eyes and assess.

10. Place the infant in an isolette or warmer.

11. Reposition the infant every 1 to 2 hours during phototherapy.

12. Check the infant's temperature every 4 hours.

13. Turn off phototherapy lights during bilirubin blood draws. Bilirubin levels are usually drawn by heel stick every 4 to 8 hours.

14. Check the infant every hour to ensure that all coverings are secure and in proper position.

15. Monitor intake and output, electrolytes, and stool frequency. Green, watery, projectile stools are characteristic of infants receiving phototherapy. Fluid requirements may increase during the procedure.

DOCUMENTATION

- Time phototherapy began and any interruption in therapy.
- Any problems arising from phototherapy; the name of the physician contacted.

- Light density in uw/cm2/nm each shift.
- That eye patches were in place. Eye assessment.
- That genitalia or lower abdomen covering was in place.
- Frequency of infant's position change.
- Infant's temperature.
- Intake and output, including stool consistency.
- Appearance of infant's jaundice. Increase or decrease.
- Time phototherapy ended.

POTENTIAL RELATED NURSING DIAGNOSES

Body temperature, altered: *high risk*

Fluid volume deficit: *high risk*

Hyperthermia

Social interaction, impaired

Parenting, altered: *high risk*

Injury: *high risk*

Hypothermia

Skin integrity, impaired: *high risk*

Infection: *high risk*

Tissue perfusion, altered, peripheral

POTENTIAL RELATED MEDICAL DIAGNOSES

Hyperbilirubinemia

Prematurity

ABO incompatibility

Rh disease

REFERENCES

Fanaroff, A. A., and Martin, J. R., eds. 1987. *Neonatal-perinatal medicine. Diseases of fetus and infant.* St. Louis, Mo.: C. V. Mosby.

Fetus and Newborn Committee. 1986. Use of phototherapy for neonatal hyperbilirubinemia. *Canadian Medical Association Journal* 134: 1,237–45.

Harper, R. G., and Yoon, J. J. 1987. *Handbook of neonatology.* Chicago: Yearbook Medical Publishers.

Korones, S. B. 1986. *High-risk newborn infants: The basis for intensive nursing care.* St. Louis, Mo.: C. V. Mosby.

Mott, S., James, S., and Sperhac, A. 1990. *Nursing care of children and families.* Redwood City, Calif.: Addison-Wesley.

Olds, S., London, M., and Ladewig, P. 1988. *Maternal-newborn nursing.* Menlo Park, Calif.: Addison-Wesley.

pH Probe Study (Esophageal pH Monitoring)

PSYCHOSOCIAL CONSIDERATIONS: Explain the procedure in developmentally appropriate terms. Avoid using terms with mixed meanings. Perform the probe placement quickly. Hold and comfort the child after the procedure.

TIME: 5 minutes for placement
20 to 30 minutes for a chest X-ray
12 hours for the actual procedure

PURPOSE

To determine the amount of reflux present, the duration of reflux, the frequency of reflux, and the effects of eating, sleeping, and positioning on reflux.

OBJECTIVES

- To confirm the diagnosis of gastroesophageal reflux (chalasia).
- To maintain functioning of the pH probe.
- To prevent injury.

EQUIPMENT

Gloves, nonsterile
Tape measure
pH probe
Water-soluble lubricant
Clear and adhesive tape
Transparent dressing
Electrode gel
Lead wire with electrode
Digitrapper
Flow sheet

ESSENTIAL STEPS

1. Prepare the child and family. *The child must be NPO for 2 hours prior to the procedure* to lessen the chance of aspiration during tube insertion. A physician's order to discontinue antacids and gastrointestinal drugs (such as cimetidine or ranitidine) is necessary during the study.
2. Assemble the equipment.
3. Wash hands and put on gloves.
4. Pass the probe through the child's naris or oral cavity, following measurements used by the institution. Tape in place.

5. Accompany the child to radiology for a chest X-ray.

6. Have placement verified by the radiologist and make any necessary adjustments. (Placement will be at T-7.)

7. Return the child to his or her room and start the test.

8. Place a well-gelled electrode with a sticker to the bony area of the back (the spine).

9. Plug the electrode and the probe into the Digitrapper. (See Fig. 103.1)

10. Place the Digitrapper on run and begin the pH probe flow sheet.

11. Resume diet, per the physician's plan of care.

12. Check the child at least once every 30 minutes and record on the flow sheet.

13. Check that the probe remains inserted at all times.

14. Check that the electrode grounding wire remains intact and attached to the child.

15. Feed the child the designated type and amount of fluid at the specified time.

16. Record pertinent information. Refer to step 3 Documentation.

17. Do not alter any of the dials on the Digitrapper.

Skills Checklist

☐ Prepare the child and family.
☐ Assemble the equipment.
☐ Wash hands and put on gloves.
☐ Insert the probe.
☐ Verify placement.
☐ Attach the electrode.
☐ Plug the electrode and probe into the Digitrapper.
☐ Turn the Digitrapper on.
☐ Monitor the child.
☐ Document.

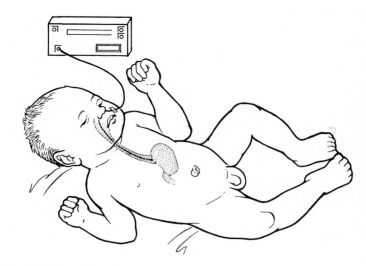

FIGURE 103.1 *pH probe.*

Lab Values

NORMAL RANGE
4–9 pH

18. To discontinue the study, perform the following steps:

    Turn off the Digitrapper.

    Remove the pH probe from the nose.

    Remove the ground wire from the back.

    Document the time that the study was stopped.

19. The child may resume a normal routine following the study, including fluids by mouth.

20. To troubleshoot:

    If a problem occurs with the probe, electrode, or Digitrapper, place the Digitrapper switch on standby. After the problem is resolved, turn the switch back to run. Note the time and document on the flow sheet.

    If the lead disconnects, reattach it to the Digitrapper.

    If the child's pH fluctuates wildly or if negative pH values occur, check all the connections and the electrode.

If the digital readout is no longer visible, notify the appropriate person.

If the pH probe falls out or is pulled out, turn the Digitrapper to standby and record the time. A repeat chest X-ray may be indicated to verify placement.

21. Tests are best run from 1800 to 0600. Infants sleep more during this time period.

DOCUMENTATION

- Time of probe insertion.
- Time study initiated.
- Every 30 minutes:

  Time and pH reading.

  Any change in position and level of consciousness.

  Activity (such as gagging, coughing, sneezing, fussing, vomiting); apnea, bradycardia, or seizures.

  Times feeding started and stopped.
- One time per shift:

  That the probe is in place. Any deviations.

  That ground wires are intact.

  That wires have been properly connected.
- Time study completed.

POTENTIAL RELATED NURSING DIAGNOSES

Anxiety

Nutrition, altered, less than body requirements

POTENTIAL RELATED MEDICAL DIAGNOSES

Gastroesophageal reflux (chalasia)

Vomiting

REFERENCES

Mott, S., James, S., and Sperhac, A. 1990. *Nursing care of children and families.* Redwood City, Calif.: Addison-Wesley.

Peterson, M. 1986. Esophageal pH monitoring. *Journal of Pediatric Nursing* 1, no. 5: 354–57.

104 Positioning

PSYCHOSOCIAL CONSIDERATIONS: Explain the procedure in developmentally appropriate terms. Children may be afraid of positioning because it sometimes causes them pain. Do not rush into the room and immediately reposition the child. Speak to the child in soothing terms. Encourage the child to assist with turning and in the selection of a position; this allows the child a sense of control.

TIME: 2 to 5 minutes

PURPOSE

To reposition the child to relieve pressure and increase circulation to skin areas and to prevent skin breakdown.

OBJECTIVES

- To reposition the child.
- To prevent injury or trauma.
- To prevent skin breakdown.

EQUIPMENT

Lotion for skin care

Pillow(s), if appropriate

Rolled blankets, if appropriate

Infant seat

Covered sandbags, if appropriate

SAFETY ISSUES

- Do not place a pillow under the head of an infant as doing so may cause the airway to become obstructed.
- Ensure that all extremities are in proper alignment. Check that arms and legs are not directly under the body or under another extremity, which could impede blood flow.
- For immobility, consider using passive range of motion; sheepskin/alternating pressure mattress; a footboard, boots, or high-top tennis shoes to prevent foot drop; and/or a rolled washcloth in the palm to maintain hand position.

ESSENTIAL STEPS

1. Prepare the child and family.
2. Assemble the equipment.
3. Wash hands.
4. Change the child's position slowly while supporting the head and body.
5. Assess the skin condition and use lotion for skin care. Massage areas over bony prominences. Remove any excess lotion from the skin.
6. If the child is to be on the side in a lying position:

   Place a small pillow under the child's head and a pillow or sandbag behind the child's back. (See Fig. 104.1)

   Support the upper extremities with a pillow or a blanket.

   Place a small pillow or blanket between the legs.

7. If the child is to be in a ventral recumbent position (on the abdomen):

   Place a small pillow under the head.

8. Use an infant seat to vary the position for the infant, if desirable. Ensure that the infant seat is stable and secure where it is placed. Use the safety straps to secure the infant in the seat. (See Fig. 104.2)

DOCUMENTATION

- Time of positioning.
- Position.
- Skin assessment and skin care.

POTENTIAL RELATED NURSING DIAGNOSES

Skin integrity, impaired: *high risk*

Activity intolerance

Tissue perfusion, altered, peripheral

Skills Checklist

☐ Prepare the child and family.
☐ Assemble the equipment.
☐ Wash hands.
☐ Assess and care for the skin.
☐ Reposition the child.
☐ Support the head and extremities.
☐ Document.

POTENTIAL RELATED MEDICAL DIAGNOSES

Fractures

Coma

Musculoskeletal disorders

REFERENCES

Mott, S., James, S., and Sperhac, A. 1990. *Nursing care of children and families.* Redwood City, Calif.: Addison-Wesley.

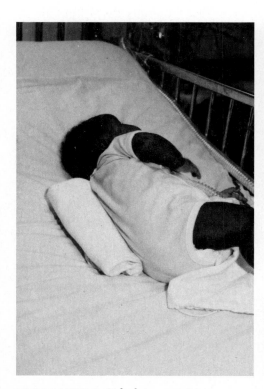

FIGURE 104.1 *Side lying position.*

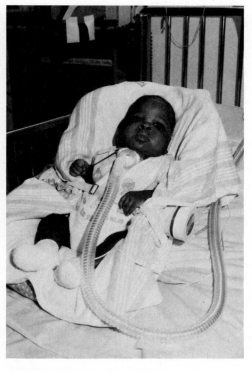

FIGURE 104.2 *Infant positioned in an infant seat.*

105

Respiratory Syncytial Virus: Nasal Washing for Culture

PSYCHOSOCIAL CONSIDERATIONS: Explain the procedure in developmentally appropriate terms. Reassure the child that the discomfort will last only for a moment and that you will help him or her hold still. Fully awaken the child prior to performing the procedure. Perform the procedure quickly. Explain to the child and family that they should insert nothing into the nose.

TIME: 2 to 3 minutes

PURPOSE

To obtain nasal secretions for the purpose of respiratory syncytial virus (RSV) screening.

OBJECTIVES

• To obtain a specimen of nasal mucous.
• To prevent injury.

EQUIPMENT

Gloves, nonsterile
Mask
Blanket for mummy restraint, if appropriate
For nasopharyngeal using a bulb syringe—RSV prep kit, which includes the following:

Phosphate-buffered saline (3 ml in a 15 ml test tube)
Plastic medicine cup (20 ml)
Ear bulb syringe, sterile
Culture swab

For nasopharyngeal using butterfly tubing:

3 ml syringe
Butterfly IV needle
Scissors, sterile
Saline (0.9% sodium chloride), 3 ml, sterile

For tracheal:

Specimen collection trap
Suction equipment
Culture media, as required for additional tests (for example, viral cultures)

ESSENTIAL STEPS

1. Prepare the child and family.
   Restrain the child, as necessary.
   Do not suction nares prior to the procedure.
2. Assemble the equipment.
3. Wash hands and put on gloves and mask.
4. For nasopharyngeal using a bulb syringe:

   Pour 3 ml of phosphate-buffered saline into a plastic medicine cup. Transfer saline to an ear bulb syringe.

   Position the child in a parent's lap, sitting up and facing forward. Instruct the parent to restrain the child as needed.

   Insert the tip of the bulb syringe into the child's naris and gently squeeze the syringe to instill the saline. Squeeze the bulb several times to move the saline in and out of the bulb and then remove saline from the naris.

   Evacuate the contents of the bulb syringe into the 15 ml test tube.

Collect a throat swab and place the swab into the 15 ml test tube.

Label the test tube. Place it in a plastic bag and send it *immediately* to the lab.

5. For nasopharyngeal using butterfly tubing:

Attach the syringe to the butterfly hub.

Cut the needle and phalanges off the end of the tubing using the sterile scissors.

Insert the end of the tubing into either naris, until slightly past the curve of the nasal passage. If tubing is difficult to insert or will not advance, try the other naris. If difficulty persists, stop the procedure and notify a physician.

Aspirate at least .2 ml of nasal secretions. Remove the tubing from the naris.

Aspirate approximately 2.8 ml of sterile saline into the syringe to make a solution.

Place the solution in an appropriate lab tube or medium.

Label the specimen. Place it in a plastic bag and send it *immediately* to the lab.

6. For tracheal:

Connect the specimen trap to the suction setup as described on the package.

Proceed with routine suctioning. Refer to "Suctioning: Endotracheal/Tracheostomy."

Disconnect the specimen trap and tubing and place the end of the latex tubing over the rigid end to seal the trap using a sterile technique.

Label the specimen. Place it in a plastic bag and send it *immediately* to the lab.

Skills Checklist

- ☐ Prepare the child and family.
- ☐ Assemble the equipment.
- ☐ Wash hands and put on gloves and mask.
- ☐ Obtain a specimen.
- ☐ Label the specimen. Place it in a plastic bag and send it to the lab.
- ☐ Document.

DOCUMENTATION

- Date.
- Time.
- Method used.
- Naris used.

POTENTIAL RELATED NURSING DIAGNOSES

Airway clearance, ineffective

Breathing pattern, ineffective

Infection: *high risk*

POTENTIAL RELATED MEDICAL DIAGNOSES

Respiratory distress

Pneumonia

Bronchiolitis

106 Restraints: Limb

PURPOSE

To safely and adequately restrain the limb(s) of a child in order to protect surgery sites, IV infusions, or tube placement or to prevent the child from injuring him- or herself or others.

OBJECTIVES

- To prevent injury to the child or surgical site.
- To maintain an IV or tube placement.
- To maintain circulation of the extremity.

EQUIPMENT

Plastic elbow restraints, if appropriate (see Figs. 106.1 and 106.2)

Soft restraints, if appropriate (see Figs. 106.3–106.7)

Leather wrist and ankle restraints, if appropriate

Four-point restraint, such as mummy or papoose board, if appropriate (see Fig. 106.8)

S SAFETY ISSUES

- **Leather restraints will probably have additional safety requirements. Check institution policy.**
- **Check circulation and movement of joints every 1 to 2 hours.**

PSYCHOSOCIAL CONSIDERATIONS: Explain the procedure in developmentally appropriate terms. Explain to the child why the restraint is necessary. Reassure the child that it is not a punishment. Release the restraints every few hours and hold the child. Allow for as much normal motion as possible; do not keep the child tied tightly so as to inhibit all movement.

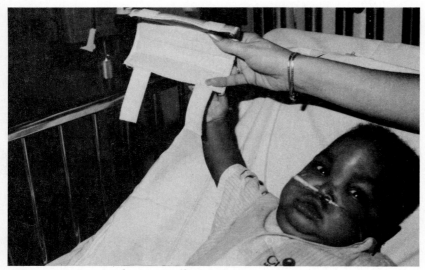

FIGURE 106.1 *Applying an elbow restraint.*

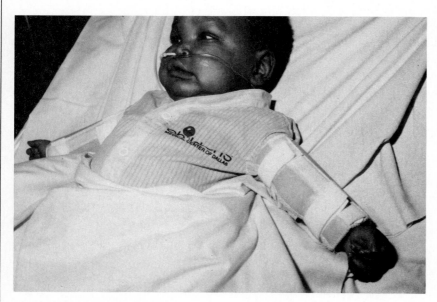

FIGURE 106.2 *Elbow restraint.*

ESSENTIAL STEPS

1. Prepare the child and family.

   Reassure the child that this is not a punishment.

   Explain to the family the necessity of limb restraints.

2. Assemble the equipment.

3. Wash hands.

4. Attach limb restraints to a secure object (*not* to the side rail); attach to the bed frame or springs or pin to the sheet. Evaluate if padding is needed. Use a nonslipping hitch knot to avoid impeding circulation. (Note: This does not apply to elbow restraints.)

5. Remove the restraint to assess skin and to perform range of motion (ROM) at least every 2 to 4 hours and PRN.

6. Check the area distal to the restraint for signs of circulatory impairment.

7. Reposition the child every 2 hours. Position the child on the side if there is a risk of vomiting or aspiration.

Skills Checklist

☐ Prepare the child and family.
☐ Assemble the equipment.
☐ Wash hands.
☐ Apply restraint(s).
☐ Remove restraint. Assess the skin and perform ROM.
☐ Check the area distal to the restraint for circulatory impairment.
☐ Reposition the child every 2 hours.
☐ Document.

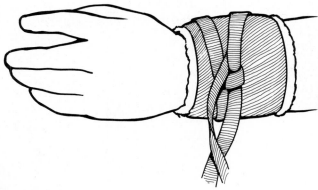

FIGURE 106.4 *Soft wrist restraint.*

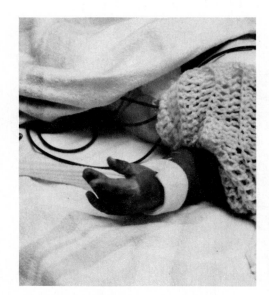

FIGURE 106.3 *Soft wrist restraint.*

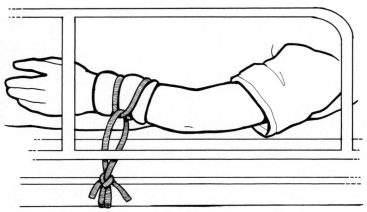

FIGURE 106.5 *Secured soft wrist restraint.*

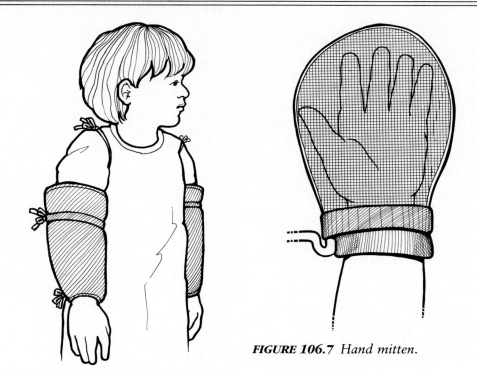

FIGURE 106.7 *Hand mitten.*

FIGURE 106.6 *Soft elbow restraints.*

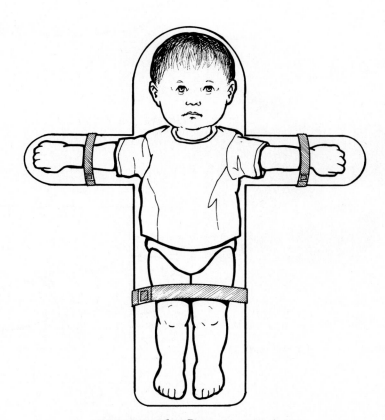

FIGURE 106.8 *Papoose restraint.*

DOCUMENTATION

- Reason for restraint.
- Type of restraint used.
- Skin condition and circulation status of the limb(s); any nursing interventions.
- Reason for removal of the restraints.
- Response to restraints.

POTENTIAL RELATED NURSING DIAGNOSES

Activity intolerance

Skin integrity, impaired: *high risk*

Mobility, impaired physical

Injury: *high risk*

POTENTIAL RELATED MEDICAL DIAGNOSES

Cleft lip and palate repair

IV medication infusion

Bryants' traction

Respiratory infections

Gastrointestinal diseases with nasogastric tube placement

REFERENCES

Mott, S., James, S., and Sperhac, A. 1990. *Nursing care of children and families.* Redwood City, Calif.: Addison-Wesley.

107 Safety: Electrical Guidelines

TIME: Varies

PURPOSE

To provide a safe environment.

To ensure that electrical hazards will be recognized and appropriate interventions instituted.

OBJECTIVES

- To maintain a safe environment.
- To prevent injury.

1. Check electrical equipment and power cords for signs of damage before use.
2. Use equipment that has a current safety inspection sticker. Check institution policy.
3. Disconnect electric cords by grasping the plug with dry hands and pulling straight out. Never pull on the cord.
4. Refer to "Pacemakers: External Cardiac" for safety guidelines for handling pacemaker wires.
5. When working with children who are electrically at risk (have monitor leads, fluid-filled catheters, pacing wires, and so on), never simultaneously touch the child and a metal surface of equipment that is plugged in.
6. If a child is temporarily disconnected from a cardiac/apnea monitor, remove all lead wires from the child.
7. Do not place containers with liquid in them on or near electrical equipment.
8. Do not block or cover equipment exhaust vents.
9. Avoid using extension cords. If necessary, use approved cords only.
10. Do not touch electrical equipment with wet hands or feet.

11. Unplug electrical equipment before immersing a child in water.

12. Avoid equipment and toys that could produce sparks.

13. If a piece of equipment may be unsafe:

    Remove it from the child's reach and disconnect it from its power source.

    Label it "defective." Note the date and describe the problem.

    Send the defective equipment to the appropriate area within the institution.

14. Be safety-conscious:

    Look for frayed cords.

    Look for long cords.

    Locate emergency outlets.

15. Ensure that equipment brought into the institution from home has been inspected by the appropriate department prior to use in the institution.

16. Prevent microshock:

    Turn equipment on before connecting it to the child.

    Disconnect equipment from the child before turning it off.

    Wear latex gloves when handling pacemaker wires, metal stopcocks, or conductive connections.

Skills Checklist

☐ Check equipment and cords for damage before use.
☐ Assess electrical outlets.
☐ Assess electrical equipment for safe functioning.
☐ Avoid having liquids around electrical equipment.
☐ Know and practice electrical safety steps.
☐ Remove any piece of equipment suspected of being unsafe from use.

POTENTIAL RELATED NURSING DIAGNOSES

Injury: *high risk*

POTENTIAL RELATED MEDICAL DIAGNOSES

Universal application

108 Safety: Patient

PSYCHOSOCIAL CONSIDERATIONS: Explain the procedure in developmentally appropriate terms. Discuss safety issues and rationale with the child and parents, as appropriate.

TIME: Varies

PURPOSE

To provide a safe environment in patient care areas.

OBJECTIVES

- To maintain a safe environment.
- To prevent injury.

 SAFETY ISSUES

- **All staff should be instructed in infant and child CPR and obstructed airway rescue.**

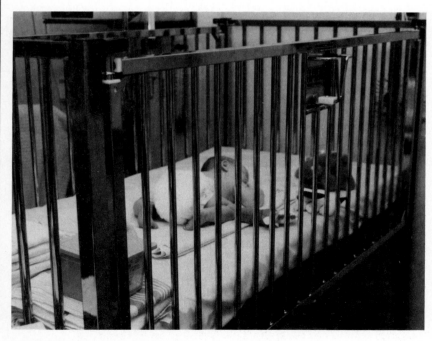

FIGURE 108.1 *Raised side rails.*

ESSENTIAL STEPS

1. Keep crib sides up when out of direct physical contact with the child. (See Fig. 108.1) Keep one hand on the child if turning away from the child.

2. Stay at the child's side when the child is on a stretcher, an exam table, scales, and so on. Use a safety strap when available.

3. Secure a plastic bubble top for the crib if the child can climb over the crib rails and if no adult is present. (See Fig. 108.2)

4. Ensure that each child has an identification band and, if applicable, an allergy band.

5. Use a plastic feeding bottle if the child holds his or her own bottle. Do not prop bottles.

6. Do not place an infant on the back after feeding. Place an infant on the side or abdomen unless contra-indicated, or sitting upright in an infant seat.

7. Place all used disposable needles, syringes, knife blades, lancets, and razor blades in a sharps disposal container.

8. Keep linen chutes and trayveyors locked.

9. Clarify any order in question before implementing it.

10. Do not warm compresses, formula, or baby food jars in microwave ovens.

11. Use *only* commercially manufactured pacifiers. Homemade pacifiers are not safe; they may separate.

12. Place only large bandages on infants, if necessary (especially for fingers and toes). Remove bandages as soon as possible.

13. Place any nondrinkable solutions in a screw-top specimen cup and label the contents.

14. Evaluate and use caution when giving children certain foods, especially hard candies, hot dogs, grapes, popcorn, or peanuts. Children may choke on these items.

15. Evaluate children's toys as to safety-related age appropriateness. Balloons are potential aspiration hazards because children like to bite them. Mylar balloons are potential electrical hazards because they conduct electricity.

16. Ensure that the child is supervised when in a highchair, playpen, wagon, and so on.

17. Ensure that all electrical outlets are plugged with outlet covers.

18. Position a child's crib away from outlets, switches, and so on.

19. Keep the patient areas clean and free of any potentially hazardous articles, such as cleaning materials, dangerous instruments, breakable items, and so on.

NOTE: Refer to the following nursing procedures for additional specific information: "Bathing the Child: Tub or Basin," "Medication Administration: General Procedure," "Medication Administration: IV," "Safety: Electrical Guidelines," and "Seizure Precautions."

DOCUMENTATION

• Any safety measure(s) implemented.

POTENTIAL RELATED NURSING DIAGNOSES

Injury: *high risk*

POTENTIAL RELATED MEDICAL DIAGNOSES

Any diagnosis requiring hospitalization

Skills Checklist

☐ Prepare the child and family.
☐ Assess the room for safety hazards.
☐ Implement appropriate interventions.
☐ Document.

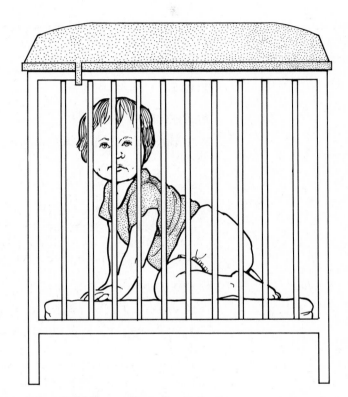

FIGURE 108.2 *Bubble top for crib.*

109 Seizure Precautions

- Inserting an airway may not be possible. The main concern is to prevent injury. Do not force an airway between clenched teeth or try to use fingers to separate the teeth.
- Turn the head to the side to facilitate drainage of secretions.
- Passively extend the neck or use the jaw thrust maneuver to open and maintain an airway, if appropriate.
- Do not move a child who is having a seizure, unless the child is in danger of falling or injuring him- or herself.

PSYCHOSOCIAL CONSIDERATIONS: Explain the procedure in developmentally appropriate terms. Explain that precautions are for safety reasons. Provide reassurance to the child to decrease anxiety.

TIME: 10 to 15 minutes

PURPOSE

To protect the child in the event of a seizure.

OBJECTIVES

- To maintain a patent airway.
- To provide safety measures to protect from injury.
- To provide privacy during a seizure.

EQUIPMENT

Oral airway, of appropriate size

Oxygen flowmeter with appropriate-size bag and mask

Padded side rails (for severe seizures)

Suction setup and appropriate-size suction catheter

Tonsil (yaunker) suction (large-diameter suction catheter for oral suction of the mouth)

ESSENTIAL STEPS

1. Prepare the child and family.
2. Assemble the equipment at the bedside.

  Tape the oral airway at the head of the bed.

  Assemble the bag and mask. Attach to the oxygen flowmeter.

  Pad side rails, if appropriate.

  Assemble the suction setup.

3. In the event of a seizure:

Provide privacy.

Note the time that the seizure begins. Observe all events of the seizure and note the time that the seizure ends.

Evaluate the need for oxygen or suctioning during the seizure. Initiate resuscitative action, if necessary.

Stay with the child until vital signs are stable and he or she is past the postictal state. Reorient the child as necessary.

DOCUMENTATION

• Time that seizure precautions were instituted.
• That seizure precautions were observed. Bag, mask, oxygen, suction checks.
• If a seizure occurs, all information about the seizure: time, duration, movements, injuries, aura, incontinence, vomiting, postictal state.

POTENTIAL RELATED NURSING DIAGNOSES

Airway clearance, ineffective

Anxiety

Body image disturbance

Fear

Growth and development, altered

Injury: *high risk*

Self-esteem disturbance

Social isolation

Skills Checklist

☐ Prepare the child and family.
☐ Assemble the equipment.
☐ Place the oral airway at bedside.
☐ Assemble the bag and mask. Check flowmeter.
☐ Pad side rails, if appropriate.
☐ Assemble the suction setup. Check function.
☐ Document.

POTENTIAL RELATED MEDICAL DIAGNOSES

Birth injury

Meningitis

Encephalitis

Epilepsy

Fever

Tumor

Trauma

Hemorrhage

Metabolic disorders

REFERENCES

Mott, S., James, S., and Sperhac, A. 1990. *Nursing care of children and families*. Redwood City, Calif.: Addison-Wesley.

EQUIPMENT

Tepid water (body temperature; should feel neither cold nor warm to the touch)

Washbasin or bathtub

Two washcloths or small towels

Dry towel or blanket

PSYCHOSOCIAL CONSIDERATIONS: Explain the procedure in developmentally appropriate terms. The child may be uncomfortable or irritable related to high fever. Older children may be fearful of a stranger seeing or touching genitalia. Talk in soothing tones.

TIME: 15 minutes

PURPOSE

To safely reduce a child's elevated temperature, usually for temperatures above 40°C (104°F).

OBJECTIVES

- To reduce body temperature slowly.
- To prevent injury or seizures.

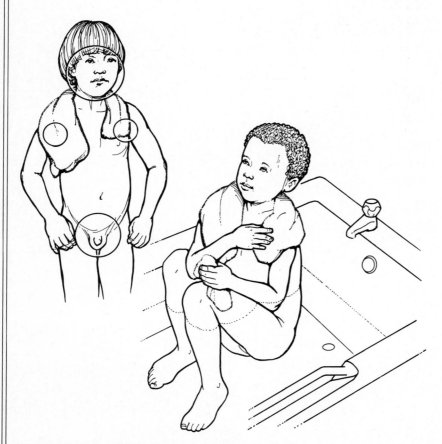

FIGURE 110.1 *Child taking a tepid sponge bath.*

ⓢ SAFETY ISSUES

- Do not use alcohol or cool water. Alcohol can lower the temperature too rapidly and may precipitate febrile seizures.
- This procedure is controversial and may not be used in all institutions.

ESSENTIAL STEPS

1. Prepare the child and family.
2. Assemble the equipment.
3. Wash hands.
4. Take vital signs.
5. Undress the child.
6. Bathe in a bathtub or on a bed using a basin of water. If using a bathtub, put only a small amount (1″ to 2″) of tepid water in the tub. Moisten a towel with water and place it around the child's upper body and shoulders. Dribble water over the towel and the child's legs. If the water cools to less than normal body temperature, add slightly warmer water.

7. Place tepid, moist cloths over areas where there are large superficial blood vessels, such as axillary and inguinal regions. Periodically change washcloths. (See Figs. 110.1 and 110.2)

8. Continue sponging for 15 minutes. If the child begins to shiver, stop the procedure. Following the bath, dry the child and dress in lightweight clothing.

9. Take the child's temperature immediately after discontinuing the procedure, again in 30 minutes, and then every 2 hours.

10. Repeat the sponging every 2 hours as necessary.

11. Notify the physician if the child's temperature does not respond within 1 hour.

DOCUMENTATION

- Time and duration of sponging.
- Name of physician and time contacted, as appropriate.
- Vital signs.
- Child's tolerance and response.

POTENTIAL RELATED NURSING DIAGNOSES

Hyperthermia

Infection: *high risk*

Body temperature, altered: *high risk*

POTENTIAL RELATED MEDICAL DIAGNOSES

Meningitis

Infection

Sepsis

REFERENCES

Mott, S., James, S., and Sperhac, A. 1990. *Nursing care of children and families.* Redwood City, Calif.: Addison-Wesley.

Skills Checklist

- ☐ Prepare the child and family.
- ☐ Assemble the equipment.
- ☐ Wash hands.
- ☐ Take vital signs.
- ☐ Undress the child.
- ☐ Place in a tub or apply tepid washcloths.
- ☐ Periodically change washcloths.
- ☐ Dry and dress the child to prevent chilling or shivering.
- ☐ Take the child's temperature.
- ☐ Document.

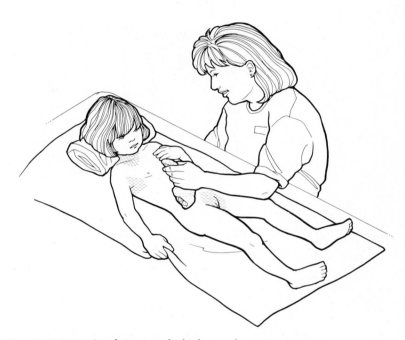

FIGURE 110.2 *Applying cool cloths to decrease temperature.*

111 Stool Specimen

PSYCHOSOCIAL CONSIDERATIONS: Explain the procedure in developmentally appropriate terms. Determine and use the individual child's word(s) for bowel movement. The physician may order a laxative or stool softener. The child may feel uncomfortable having a bowel movement in a bedpan. Place the bedpan over a toilet to increase comfort, or use a specipan, if appropriate.

TIME: 5 minutes upon defecation

PURPOSE

To collect a stool specimen for diagnostic purposes.

OBJECTIVES

• To collect a stool specimen (may be from a diaper, bedpan, specipan, or rectal swab).

EQUIPMENT

Gloves, nonsterile

Bedpan or specipan, as needed

Stool specimen cup

Tongue blade, if appropriate

Culture swab (not sufficient for ova and parasites), sterile

ESSENTIAL STEPS

1. Prepare the child and family.
2. Assemble the equipment.
3. Wash hands and put on gloves.
4. For a stool specimen other than a rectal swab:

   Obtain the stool specimen and place in a container. Send 1 to 2 gm for ova and parasites. Scrape stool from a diaper using a tongue blade, if appropriate.

   Label the specimen container.

   Send the specimen to the lab.
5. For a rectal swab (see Fig. 111.1):

   Insert the swab ½″ to ¾″ into the rectum.

   Place the swab in a culture tube.

   Label the top and bottom of the container (in case of separation). Place in a plastic bag and send the specimen to the lab.

DOCUMENTATION

- Time.
- Type of specimen obtained.

POTENTIAL RELATED NURSING DIAGNOSES

Skin integrity, impaired: *high risk*

Fluid volume deficit (diarrhea)

Infection: *high risk*

POTENTIAL RELATED MEDICAL DIAGNOSES

Diarrhea

Constipation

Tarry stools

Weight loss

Parasitic infection

REFERENCES

Mott, S., James, S., and Sperhac, A. 1990. *Nursing care of children and families.* Redwood City, Calif.: Addison-Wesley.

Skills Checklist

☐ Prepare the child and family.

☐ Assemble the equipment.

☐ Wash hands and put on gloves.

☐ Obtain a specimen.

☐ Label the specimen. Place in a plastic bag and send to the lab.

☐ Document.

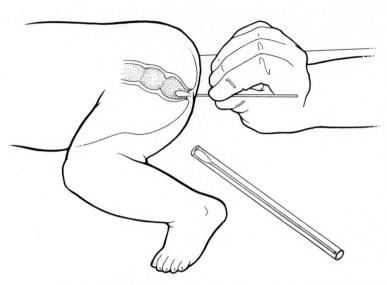

FIGURE 111.1 *Obtaining a stool specimen using a rectal swab.*

112 String Test

1. Prepare the child and family.
2. Assemble the equipment.
3. Wash hands.
4. Ensure that the child has been NPO since midnight the night before the test. Infants must be NPO 4 hours before the test.
5. Offer water to moisten the mouth and throat.
6. Pull approximately 15 cm (6" to 7") of thread from the capsule.
7. For a child old enough to swallow the capsule:

   Have the child swallow the capsule with water while holding the end loop of the thread.

   Secure the thread to the face with a piece of tape.
8. For infants and toddlers who cannot swallow capsules:

   Place the capsule between the index and middle fingers, holding the end of the thread in the other hand.

   Using a tongue blade to open the mouth, using the same hand holding the thread, quickly push the capsule down the child's oropharynx as deeply as possible.

PSYCHOSOCIAL CONSIDERATIONS: Explain the procedure in developmentally appropriate terms. Reinforce the importance of swallowing. Do not offer the idea that the child might gag (especially to toddlers and preschoolers). Talk in soothing tones to decrease fear. Avoid using terms like *snake* and *worm*. Comfort the child after the procedure.

TIME: 5 minutes

PURPOSE

To obtain a small sample of upper gastrointestinal (GI) contents for the diagnosis of *Giardia lamblia* or GI bleeding.

OBJECTIVES

- To obtain a sample of gastrointestinal contents.
- To prevent aspiration or trauma upon insertion.

EQUIPMENT

Water

Enterotest Pediatric Capsule, *or,* for older children, Enterotest Capsule (see Fig. 112.1)

Tape

Tongue blade (for infants and toddlers)

pH stick and color chart

Specimen cup, sterile

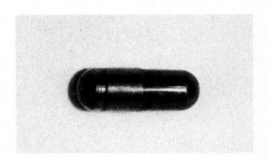

FIGURE 112.1 *Enterotest Capsule.*

After sitting the child upright to help prevent aspiration, offer water to drink immediately to help the capsule descend.

If the child gags and spits the capsule out, repeat the steps for 8.

Once the child has swallowed the capsule, tape the end loop to the face.

9. While the capsule is in place, keep the child NPO except for water as desired.

10. After 3 to 4 hours, remove the string. Instruct the child to open the mouth and raise the chin. Withdraw the string with a rapid but gentle pull.

11. To test for *Giardia:*

Verify duodenal placement by placing the string on a flat surface and, using the pH stick, touching the wet string at 3″ to 4″ intervals. Compare the color changes on the string to the color chart. (The esophagus is neutral; stomach, acid; duodenum, alkaline.)

If the distal end was in the duodenum, send the entire string to the lab in a sterile cup.

12. To test for GI bleeding: Determine the location of GI bleeding by measuring from the proximal end of the string or by noting relation to pH color changes.

13. Explain to the parents that they may see the small BB-like weights passed in the stool.

14. Label the specimen. Place in a plastic bag and send to the lab.

DOCUMENTATION

- Date and time the procedure was started.
- Position documented per pH.
- That the string was sent to the lab.
- Date and time the procedure ended.

Skills Checklist

☐ Prepare the child and family.
☐ Assemble the equipment.
☐ Wash hands.
☐ Ensure that the child was NPO for the proper amount of time.
☐ Offer water to moisten the mouth and throat.
☐ Pull 15 cm of thread from the capsule.
☐ For a child:
  • Have the child swallow the capsule.
  • Secure the thread to the face.
☐ For an infant:
  • Place the capsule in the oropharynx.
  • Give the infant water to sip.
  • Once swallowed, secure the thread to the face.
☐ Maintain NPO while the string is in place.
☐ Remove the string and test.
☐ Send the labeled specimen to the lab.
☐ Document.

POTENTIAL RELATED NURSING DIAGNOSES

Nutrition, altered, less than body requirements

Infection: *high risk*

Skin integrity, impaired: *high risk*

Tissue perfusion, altered, gastrointestinal

POTENTIAL RELATED MEDICAL DIAGNOSES

Diarrhea

Vomiting

Weight loss

Gastrointestinal bleeding

Giardia lamblia

Suctioning: Endotracheal/ Tracheostomy

PSYCHOSOCIAL CONSIDERATIONS: Explain the procedure in developmentally appropriate terms. A child may fear loss of breath or suffocation. Tell the child that you will give oxygen before and after the procedure. Do not prolong suctioning beyond 10 seconds. Speak soothingly while performing the procedure.

TIME: 5 minutes

PURPOSE

To remove excessive or thick secretions; to ensure that the airway is patent for the child with an endotracheal (ET) or tracheostomy (trach) tube.

OBJECTIVES

• To maintain a clear airway.
• To prevent injury or trauma.

EQUIPMENT

Oxygen flowmeter with appropriate-size bag and mask

Wall suction apparatus with suction canister and tubing

Suction catheter kit of appropriate size (refer to Table 113.1 for the catheter size); if only one glove is included in the kit, obtain a clean glove for the nonsterile hand

Water for irrigation of suction catheter when the child's secretions are thick, sterile

Goggles

Mask

Manometer for hand-ventilating with appropriate pressure (optional); pressure should usually be 20 to 30 cm of water in the nonventilated patient and equal to or slightly more than peak pressure in the ventilated patient

• Preoxygenate all children with inspired oxygen (FiO$_2$ 100%) before and following each pass of the suction catheter unless contraindicated by the physician's plan of care (for example, in cases of prematurity and chronic lung disease).

• Hand-ventilate all ventilated children before and following each pass of the suction catheter unless contraindicated by the physician's plan of care. Hand-ventilation is optional in most non-ventilated patients.

• Hyperventilate children with persistent pulmonary hypertension or with signs and symptoms of increased intracranial pressure (ICP) for 1 full minute prior to and following each passage of the suction catheter. If ICP monitors are being used, hyperventilate according to the readings.

• If the child becomes cyanotic and/or bradycardic during suctioning, hyperventilate and hyperoxygenate until condition returns to baseline.

• Suctioning is a sterile procedure: Use suction catheters one time only, unless the catheter is of the type that is covered with a sterile sleeve and can be reused.

• A sterile water bottle (for optional catheter irrigation) should be dated and timed when opened and changed every 24 hours.

TABLE 113.1 *Suction Catheter Sizes*

Tracheostomy Tube Sizes	Suction Catheter French Sizes
Shiley Pedi	French
00	6½
0	6½ to 8
1	8
2	8 to 10
3	10
4	10 to 12
Shiley Regular	French
4	10 to 12
6	14
8	14
Metal Trach	French
0	6½ to 8
2	10
3	10 to 12
4	12 to 14
5	14
6	14
7	14
8	14

Endotracheal Tube Sizes	Suction Catheter French Sizes
Oral/Nasal Uncuffed	French
2.5	6½
3.0	6½
3.5	6½ to 8
4.0	8
4.5	8 to 10
5.0	10 to 12
5.5	10 to 12
6.0	10 to 14
Oral/Nasal Cuffed	French
6.0	10 to 14
7.0	12 to 14
Cole Tube	French
2.5	6½
3.0	6½
3.5	6½ to 8
4.0	8

Skills Checklist

☐ Prepare the child and family.
☐ Assemble the equipment.
☐ Wash hands. Put on goggles and mask.
☐ Assess breath sounds.
☐ Test the equipment.
☐ Position the child.
☐ Open the suction catheter aseptically.
☐ Put on gloves.
☐ Pour sterile water into a container.
☐ Connect the catheter to a suction source.
☐ Preoxygenate the child.
☐ Suction.
☐ Give oxygen.
☐ Assess breath sounds.
☐ Document.

ESSENTIAL STEPS

1. Check the following equipment at the beginning of each shift:

   Oxygen flowmeter, ventilation bag, and mask; check function.

   Suction source; check function.

   Suction catheter kit of appropriate size.

   One sterile ET or trach tube of the same size as and another of one size smaller than the child's, taped to the head of the bed in an evident place. (Note: The soft Dow Corning Aberdeen tracheostomy tube does not have an obturator. The soft tip of this tube allows insertion without an obturator.)

   Sterile water for children with thick secretions.

2. Assess the need for suctioning.

   If the child is on bolus feedings, suction before feeding or 30 minutes to 1 hour after feeding, if possible.

If the child requires suctioning within the first hour after feeding or is on continuous drip feedings, a single shallow pass of the suction catheter into the airway may be sufficient to temporarily clear the airway. Manual aspiration of stomach contents may be necessary to prevent vomiting and the risk of aspirating if deep suctioning is required.

3. Prepare the child and family. Ensure that the ET or trach tube is secure.

4. Assemble the equipment.

5. Wash hands and put on goggles and mask.

6. Auscultate the child's breath sounds bilaterally and observe the respiratory effort.

7. Turn on the oxygen flowmeter at 7 to 10 L per minute.

8. Turn on the wall suction and test it with a thumb or finger to the mm/Hg setting indicated by the age and size of the child. (Refer to Table 113.2)

9. Place the child in a supine position. Elevate the head of the bed, if desired.

10. Open the suction catheter kit, leaving the catheter inside the sterile envelope.

11. Put on gloves.

12. Open the sterile basin and partially fill it with sterile water for catheter irrigation (optional).

13. Pull the sterile catheter out of the envelope, grasping the catheter with the sterile gloved hand.

14. Connect the wall suction tubing to the connector on the suction catheter. Touch the catheter connector with the nonsterile hand.

15. Place the child's head in the midline position.

16. Disconnect the child from the ventilator or other oxygen equipment.

17. Preoxygenate and ventilate the child as indicated by clinical condition.

18. To suction:

Hold the suction catheter with the sterile gloved hand. Maintain sterile technique.

Hold the child's head in midline position.

Tell the child that preparations are being made for insertion of the catheter.

Gently insert the catheter 3 to 5 cm. Do not apply suction during insertion of the catheter. (See Fig. 113.1)

Remove the catheter while applying continuous suction and twirling the catheter. (See Fig. 113.2) Remove within 5 to 10 seconds of insertion. If using an angled tipped caude catheter, do not twirl.

After each catheter insertion, oxygenate and ventilate the child as indicated by clinical condition.

Irrigate the catheter as needed, using sterile water.

Repeat the fourth through the seventh step of number 18 two times or until the quantity of aspirate is minimal.

Reconnect the child to the ventilator or return the child to an oxygen source.

If nasal and/or oral secretions are present, suction the mouth and nose. Do not reinsert the catheter into the trachea once it has been used to suction the mouth or nose.

Discard the catheter by enfolding it in a glove. Place both gloves in the trash.

Flush the suction tubing with water for irrigation.

Ensure that the child's ET or trach tube is appropriately secured.

TABLE 113.2 *Maximum Negative Pressure for Airway Suctioning*

Age	Negative Pressure (mm/Hg)
Infant (<1 year)	45–65
Child (1–6 years)	65–80
Older Child (>6 years)	80–110

Listen to breath sounds to assess the child's response to suctioning.

Notify a physician of any unusual events during suctioning, such as cyanosis, bradycardia, unexpected quality of aspirate, or difficulty passing the catheter.

DOCUMENTATION

- FiO$_2$ used for ventilation during suctioning procedure.
- Type (color and thickness) and amount of secretions; any changes.
- Quality of breath sounds after suctioning.
- Any adverse effects and name of the physician notified, as appropriate.

POTENTIAL RELATED NURSING DIAGNOSES

Airway clearance, ineffective

Breathing pattern, ineffective

Gas exchange, impaired

Anxiety

Fear

Communication, impaired

POTENTIAL RELATED MEDICAL DIAGNOSES

Bronchopulmonary dysplasia

Cardiothoracic surgery

Muscular dystrophy

Reye's syndrome

Near drowning

Trauma

Unconsciousness

REFERENCES

Carroll, P. 1988. Lowering the risks of endotracheal suctioning. *Nursing 88* 18 (May): 46–50.

Carroll, P. 1989. Safe suctioning. *Nursing 89* 19 (Sept.): 48–51.

Corvana, S. 1990. About tracheal tubes. *Nursing 90* 20(6) (June): 30.

Kaufman, J. 1988. What parents need to know about trach care. *RN* 51 (Oct.): 99–104.

Mapp, C. 1988. Trach care. *Nursing 88* 18 (July): 34–41.

Mott, S., James, S., and Sperhac, A. 1990. *Nursing care of children and families.* Redwood City, Calif.: Addison-Wesley.

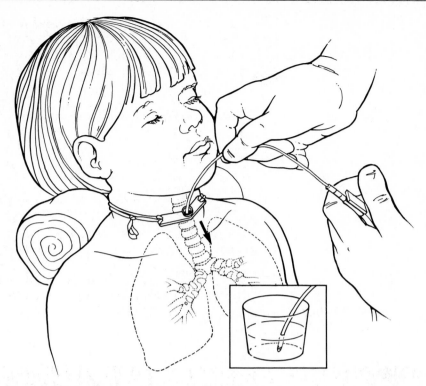

FIGURE 113.1 *Inserting the suction catheter.*

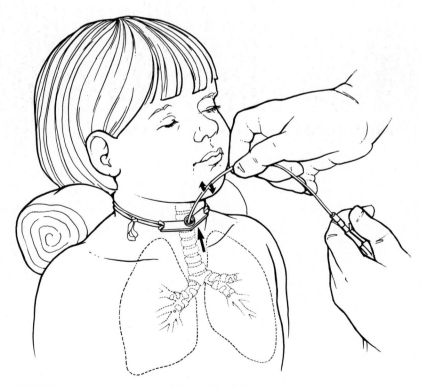

FIGURE 113.2 *Suctioning while withdrawing the catheter.*

114 Suctioning: Nasotracheal

PSYCHOSOCIAL CONSIDERATIONS: Explain the procedure in developmentally appropriate terms. The child may fear loss of breath or suffocation. Talk in soothing tones during suctioning.

TIME: 5 minutes

PURPOSE

To remove excessive or thick secretions from the child's airway.

OBJECTIVES

- To clear the child's airway.
- To prevent trauma.

EQUIPMENT

Oxygen flowmeter with appropriate-size bag and mask

Wall suction apparatus with suction canister and tubing

Suction catheter kit of appropriate size (refer to Table 114.1); if the kit includes only one glove, obtain a clean glove for the nonsterile hand

Water for irrigation of suction catheter when the child's secretions are thick, sterile

Goggles

Mask

Water-soluble lubricant

- Preoxygenate all children with inspired oxygen (FiO_2 100%) before and following each pass of the suction catheter unless contraindicated by the physician's plan of care (for example, in cases of prematurity or chronic lung disease).
- Children with persistent pulmonary hypertension should receive oxygen for 1 full minute before and following each passage of the suction catheter.
- Hyperventilate children with signs and symptoms of increased intracranial pressure (ICP) for 1 full minute prior to and following each passage of the suction catheter. If the child is on an ICP monitor, hyperoxygenate according to the readings.
- If the child becomes cyanotic and/or bradycardic during suctioning, hyperventilate and hyperoxygenate until condition returns to baseline.
- Suctioning is a sterile procedure: Use suction catheters one time only.
- A sterile water bottle (for optional catheter irrigation) should be dated and timed when opened and changed every 24 hours.

TABLE 114.1 *Catheter Sizes for Suctioning the Nonintubated Patient*

Age	Catheter Size
Newborn up to 6 months	5–6½
6 months up to 1 year	8
1 year up to 2 years	8–10
2 years up to 5 years	10
5 years up to 10 years	12
≥10 years	12–14

ESSENTIAL STEPS

1. Check the following equipment at the beginning of each shift:

   Oxygen flowmeter, ventilation bag, and mask; check function.

   Suction source; check function.

   Suction catheter kits of appropriate size.

   Sterile water for children with thick secretions.

2. Assess the need for suctioning.

   If the child is on bolus feedings, suction before feeding or 30 minutes to 1 hour after feeding when possible.

   If the child requires suctioning within the first hour after feeding or is on continuous drip feedings, a single shallow pass of the suction catheter into the airway may be sufficient to temporarily clear the airway. Aspiration of stomach contents may be necessary if deep suctioning is required.

3. Prepare the child and family.

4. Assemble the equipment.

5. Wash hands and put on goggles and mask.

6. Auscultate the child's breath sounds bilaterally and observe the respiratory effort.

7. Turn on the oxygen flowmeter at 7 to 10 L per minute. Blow-by is often sufficient to maintain oxygen levels.

8. Turn on the wall suction and test it with a thumb or finger to the mm/Hg setting indicated by the age and size of the child. (Refer to Table 114.2)

Skills Checklist

☐ Prepare the child and family.
☐ Assemble the equipment.
☐ Wash hands. Put on goggles and mask.
☐ Auscultate breath sounds.
☐ Test the equipment.
☐ Position the child.
☐ Open the equipment.
☐ Put on sterile gloves.
☐ Lubricate the catheter.
☐ Connect the suction catheter to the suction source.
☐ Preoxygenate the child.
☐ Insert the catheter.
☐ Suction while withdrawing the catheter. Give oxygen.
☐ Assess breath sounds.
☐ Document.

TABLE 114.2 *Maximum Negative Pressure for Airway Suctioning*

Age	Negative Pressure (mm/Hg)
Infant (<1 year)	45–65
Child (1–6 years)	65–80
Older child (>6 years)	80–100

9. Place the child in a supine position. Elevate the head of the bed, if desired.

10. Open the suction catheter kit, leaving the catheter inside the sterile envelope.

11. Put on gloves.

12. Open the sterile basin and partially fill it with sterile water for catheter irrigation (optional).

13. Pull the sterile catheter out of the envelope, grasping the catheter with the sterile gloved hand.

14. Place the catheter tip in the sterile water-soluble lubricant.

15. Connect the wall suction tubing to the connector on the suction catheter. Touch the catheter connector with the nonsterile hand.

16. Preoxygenate the child as indicated by clinical condition.

17. Suction:

Hold the suction catheter with the sterile gloved hand. Maintain sterile technique.

Estimate the length of the catheter to be inserted by holding the catheter parallel to the child's airway from the tip of the nose to the tracheal carina.

Hold the child's head in a midline position.

Tell the child preparations are being made for insertion of the catheter.

Gently insert the catheter. (See Fig. 114.1)

Do not apply suction during insertion of the catheter.

Remove the catheter while applying continuous suction and twirling the catheter. Remove the catheter within 5 to 10 seconds of insertion. If using an angled tipped caude catheter, do not twirl it.

After each catheter insertion, oxygenate the child as indicated by the clinical condition.

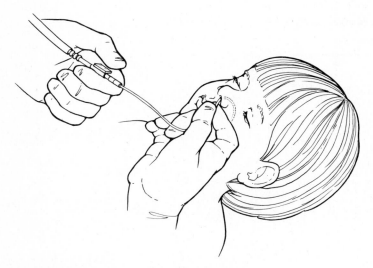

FIGURE 114.1 *Nasotracheal suctioning.*

If repeat suctioning is needed, allow the child to rest before repeating the fourth through the eighth step of number 17.

Irrigate the catheter as needed, using sterile water.

After the final tracheal suctioning and oxygenation, suction the mouth and the nose. Do not reinsert the catheter into the trachea once it has been used to suction the nose or mouth. (See Fig. 114.2)

Discard the catheter by enfolding it in a glove. Place both gloves in the trash.

Flush the suction tubing with water for irrigation.

18. Listen to breath sounds to assess the child's response to suctioning.

19. Notify a physician of any unusual events during suctioning, such as cyanosis, bradycardia, prolonged dyspnea, unexpected quality of aspirate, or difficulty passing the catheter.

DOCUMENTATION

- FiO_2 used for ventilation during suctioning procedure.
- Type (color and thickness) and amount of secretions; any changes.
- Quality of breath sounds after suctioning.
- Any adverse effects and name of the physician contacted, as appropriate.

POTENTIAL RELATED NURSING DIAGNOSES

Airway clearance, ineffective

Breathing pattern, ineffective

Anxiety

Fear

Injury: *high risk*

POTENTIAL RELATED MEDICAL DIAGNOSES

Cystic fibrosis

Rhinorrhea

Muscular dystrophy

Seizures

Bronchopulmonary dysplasia

Trauma

Unconsciousness

REFERENCES

Mott, S., James, S., and Sperhac, A. 1990. *Nursing care of children and families.* Redwood City, Calif.: Addison-Wesley.

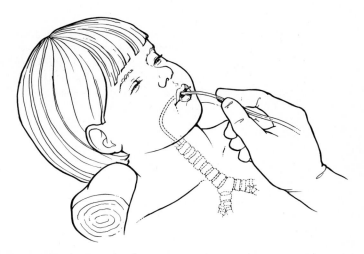

FIGURE 114.2 *Orotracheal suctioning.*

115 Suicide Precautions

PSYCHOSOCIAL CONSIDERATIONS: A suicidal child may be anxious and frightened. Loss of control and anger can heighten these fears. The child needs to feel safe and protected. Be aware of verbal and nonverbal cues that may indicate suicidal thoughts, such as giving belongings away, writing or talking about death, withdrawing, being depressed, and so on.

PURPOSE

To provide a safe environment and protection for the suicidal child admitted to a general unit.

OBJECTIVES

• To prevent the child from injuring self.

 SAFETY ISSUES

• Place any child who has attempted or is suspected of attempting suicide, or who has expressed suicidal ideation, under continuous observation immediately until seen by the physician.

• A physician's order is usually required for suicide precautions.

• Suicide precautions usually include:

   Continuous observation by a parent, a guardian, or hospital personnel until a staff psychiatrist has evaluated the child and made further recommendations.

   Search of the child's personal belongings and room.

   A psychiatric evaluation to recommend the level of care required.

ESSENTIAL STEPS

1. Prepare the child and family. Explain how and why searches will be done, hospital routine, visiting policy, what and how continuous observation will be done, and the need for restraints, if appropriate.

2. Assess the child's mental status, that is, orientation to person, place, and time. Assess short- and long-term memory.

3. Arrange for continuous observation by a parent, a guardian, or hospital personnel as long as the threat of self-harm exists.

4. Obtain an order for suicide precautions and psychiatric consultation. Psychiatric evaluation should include the level of care necessary:

1 on 1, for high risk of injury to self.

15-minute visual checks.

Routine care; no special precautions necessary.

5. Search the child and the child's room, including all personal belongings, with a family member present. Remove all items from the child's room that might be dangerous to the child, such as medications, glass objects, razors, belts, hard plastics, liquids (such as toiletry items), clothes hangers, and phone cords.

DOCUMENTATION

- That the room and body searches were done. Outcome of the room and body searches.
- Other pertinent observations and information.

POTENTIAL RELATED NURSING DIAGNOSES

Coping, ineffective individual

Fear

Anxiety

Hopelessness

Injury: *high risk*

Powerlessness

Social isolation

Violence, self-directed: *high risk*

Knowledge deficit (if associated with overdose)

Skills Checklist

☐ Prepare the child and family.

☐ Assess the child's mental status.

☐ Arrange for continuous observation.

☐ Obtain an order for suicide precautions and psychiatric consultation.

☐ Search the child and the room.

☐ Document.

POTENTIAL RELATED MEDICAL DIAGNOSES

Chronic illness

Incest

Abuse

Depression

REFERENCES

Mott, S., James, S., and Sperhac, A. 1990. *Nursing care of children and families*. Redwood City, Calif.: Addison-Wesley.

116 Suprapubic Percutaneous Bladder Puncture

PSYCHOSOCIAL CONSIDERATIONS: Explain the procedure in developmentally appropriate terms. Avoid using terms with mixed meanings, such as *stick into bladder*. Comfort and nurture the child after the procedure.

TIME: 10 to 15 minutes

PURPOSE

To obtain a urine sample in an aseptic manner.

OBJECTIVES

- To obtain a sterile urine sample when other methods are not acceptable.
- To reduce the risk of infection.
- To prevent injury and trauma.

EQUIPMENT

Gloves, nonsterile

Povidone-iodine solution *or,* if allergic to iodine, alcohol

22g or 23g needle and syringe, sterile

4″ × 3″ gauze, sterile

Adhesive bandage, as appropriate

Urine container *or* capped syringe

- Assess fullness of the bladder; may need to hydrate prior to the procedure.
- Assess for blood in the urine after the procedure.
- Assess the puncture site for bleeding.

ESSENTIAL STEPS

1. Prepare the child and family.
2. Assemble the equipment.
3. Wash hands and put on gloves.
4. Check the time of the last voiding.
5. Position the child on the back and restrain as necessary (See Figs. 116.1 and 116.2). Offer a pacifier to an infant, if appropriate. Apply pressure to the urethra to prevent voiding, if appropriate.

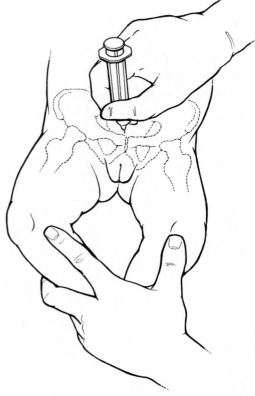

FIGURE 116.1 *Suprapubic bladder puncture.*

6. When the procedure is completed, apply pressure to the puncture site with a sterile gauze pad until oozing ceases.

7. Apply a bandage, as needed.

8. Label the specimen. Place the urine in a sterile urine container or a sterile capped syringe. Place it in a plastic bag and send it to the lab within 30 minutes.

DOCUMENTATION

- Time.
- Physician performing the tap.
- Appearance of the puncture site. Bandage applied, if any.
- Child's tolerance of the procedure.
- Amount and appearance of urine.

POTENTIAL RELATED NURSING DIAGNOSES

Hyperthermia

Anxiety

Fear

Infection: *high risk*

Injury: *high risk*

Skin integrity, impaired

Urinary elimination, altered

POTENTIAL RELATED MEDICAL DIAGNOSES

Fever

Seizure

Frequency of urination

Sepsis

Urinary tract infection

REFERENCES

Kulberg, A. 1983. Urinalysis and urine culture. *Topics in Emergency Medicine 5*, no. 1: 47–59.

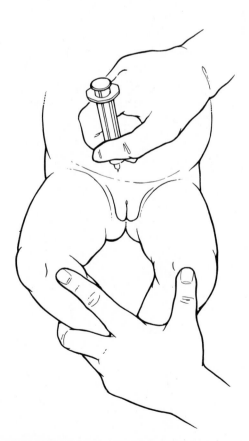

FIGURE 116.2 *Suprapubic bladder puncture.*

117 Surgical Preparation for the Inpatient

PSYCHOSOCIAL CONSIDERATIONS: Children fear the unknown. Explain what will happen in developmentally appropriate terms. Avoid using terms with mixed meanings, such as *cut into, cut off, stick,* and *shot.* Describe to the child what he or she will see, feel, and hear. To decrease fear of the unknown, let the child play with masks, gowns, induction masks, incentive spirometers, and so on.

TIME: Varies with the individual child and family; preparation may start prior to admission

PURPOSE

To prepare the hospitalized child and the child's family for impending surgery.

To administer and document optimal preoperative care.

OBJECTIVES

- To explain preoperative and postoperative care.
- To decrease anxiety.
- To increase compliance through education.

EQUIPMENT

Preoperative teaching materials
Preoperative checklist

SAFETY ISSUES

- Ensure that a surgical consent form has been signed and witnessed. This may be listed on the preoperative checklist.

ESSENTIAL STEPS

1. Prepare the child and family psychologically through appropriate preop teaching. Discuss such things as the surgery, postoperative pain management, medications and side effects, NPO status, and activity.
2. Prepare the child physically.
3. The day before the procedure, place a preop checklist in the front of the child's chart. This checklist provides guidance in actual tasks to be performed.
4. Initiate and complete as many checklist tasks as possible.
5. Request that the pharmacy and central supply send medications or supplies needed for surgery.
6. Contact the anesthesiologist regarding questions about preop medication orders. (Refer to Table 117.1)

7. Notify the surgeon and/or anesthesiologist and surgery charge nurse if the child:

> Has an elevated temperature (above 37.8°C, 100°F) or other abnormal vital signs.
>
> Has abnormal lab values, such as a decreased number of platelets, decreased hemoglobin or hematocrit levels, or an increased white blood cell count.
>
> Has a complete blood count more than 72 hours old, if applicable.

8. Remove all of the following: earrings, hair devices, nail polish, contact lenses, jewelry, and any prosthesis. Check for loose teeth and note on the checklist and on the front of the chart if any exist.

9. Have the child void. Take vital signs.

10. Administer preop medication.

11. After administering preop medication, instruct the child to stay in bed.

12. Raise the side rails on the crib or bed.

13. Reassess the child's vital signs and level of consciousness approximately 10 minutes after giving preop medication to check for possible reaction. Continue to assess every 10 to 15 minutes until the child goes to surgery.

Skills Checklist

☐ Prepare the child and family.
☐ Complete the checklist.
☐ Document.

TABLE 117.1 *Preoperative Medications: Examples*

ANTICHOLINERGICS:	
Atropine sulfate	0.005 to 0.03 mg/kg IM or IV (maximum 1.5 mg)
Scopolamine	0.005 to 0.01 mg/kg IM
Glycopyrrolate (Robinul)	0.0025 to 0.01 mg/kg IM
SEDATIVES–HYPNOTICS:	
Diazepam (Valium)	0.4–0.6 mg/kg PO (maximum 15 mg)
Droperidol (Inapsine)	0.15 mg/kg IM
Hydroxyzine (Vistaril)	0.5–1.0 mg/kg PO, IM, or IV
Medazolam (Versed)	0.05–0.1 mg/kg IV, IM, or PO
Pentobarbital (Nembutal)	2–6 mg/kg IM, PO, or PR
Promethazine (Phenergan)	0.2–1.0 mg/kg IM or IV
Secobarbital (Seconal)	1–4 mg/kg IM, PO, or PR
Triazolam (Halcion)	0.06 mg, 0.125 mg, 0.25 mg, or 0.5 mg PO
NARCOTICS:	
Morphine sulfate	0.1–0.2 mg/kg IM
Meperidine (Demerol)	0.5–1.5 mg/kg IM
MISCELLANEOUS DRUGS:	
Metoclopramide (Reglan)	0.1 mg/kg IV or 0.1–0.15 mg/kg PO
Sodium citrate and citric acid solution (Bicitra)	15–30 cc PO

KEY: IM = intramuscular; IV = intravenous; PO = by mouth; PR = per rectum.

Client Teaching

What Children Need to Know about Surgery

A. About preoperative scrubs and cleaning procedures: how many to expect and how they will feel.

B. That the child will have nothing to eat or drink after a certain time.

C. About preoperative medications: how they will make the child feel—sleepy, dizzy, dry-mouthed, and so on.

D. About the ride to surgery: method of transportation, how long it will take, whether it will include an elevator ride.

E. About the preanesthesia room: What the staff and equipment will look like.

F. When the parent(s) will leave the child.

G. Where the parent(s) will wait for the child.

H. That operating room personnel will be wearing gowns and masks.

I. That the child will be asleep and will not feel anything during surgery.

J. That the child will wake up as soon as surgery is over.

K. That the child will wake up in the recovery room. Some children may go directly to the critical care area from surgery.

L. The specifics of dressings, treatment devices, and tubes; how the child will look; what the child will feel.

M. What will happen upon return to the hospital room or other planned location: what the child will be expected to do, such as cough or breathe deeply.

N. Approximately how long the child will remain in the hospital.

O. What to do if there is pain.

P. About preoperative injection—but don't prepare too far in advance or early in the preoperative instruction; the idea may cause anxiety.

Q. That the child will be checked frequently after surgery, but that that does not mean something is wrong.

R. If tours of an operating suite, recovery room, or the critical care area are appropriate.

DOCUMENTATION

- Date each item on the preop checklist was completed. (For nonapplicable items, initial and write NA in the item space.)
- Time, amount, and route of medication given.
- Document informing the child and parents of side effects of the medication.
- Vital signs.
- That teaching was performed.
- Notification of physician regarding:

  Abnormal labs.

  Abnormal temperature or other abnormal vital signs.

POTENTIAL RELATED NURSING DIAGNOSES

Fear

Anxiety

Injury: *high risk*

Coping, ineffective individual

POTENTIAL RELATED MEDICAL DIAGNOSES

Universal application

REFERENCES

Mott, S., James, S., and Sperhac, A. 1990. *Nursing care of children and families.* Redwood City, Calif.: Addison-Wesley.

118 Suture and Staple Removal

SAFETY ISSUES

- **Ensure that the wound is approximated before removing staples or sutures.**

PSYCHOSOCIAL CONSIDERATIONS: Explain the procedure in developmentally appropriate terms. Removal of sutures or staples can be psychologically traumatic. Tell the child that crying or yelling is okay, but not moving. Explain to the child that the procedure may sting or that the child may feel a pulling sensation.

TIME: 5 to 10 minutes

PURPOSE

To safely remove sutures or staples from an incision or incisions.

OBJECTIVES

- To remove staples or sutures.
- To maintain approximation of incision.
- To provide a clean environment.

EQUIPMENT

Gloves, sterile

Povidone-iodine or alcohol solution or swabs

Suture removal kit, including sterile scissors, 2″ × 2″ gauze, povidone-iodine ointment, and forceps—if appropriate

Staple removal kit, including a staple remover, povidone-iodine ointment, and 2″ × 2″ gauze pads—if appropriate

Normal saline (0.9% sodium chloride), sterile

Cotton balls, if applicable

ESSENTIAL STEPS

1. Prepare the child and family.
2. Assemble the equipment.
3. Wash hands and put on gloves.
4. Clean the incision with povidone-iodine or alcohol solution or swabs.
5. To remove a plain interrupted (single) suture (see Fig. 118.1):

   Pull the knot of the suture away from the skin with forceps.

   Cut the suture between the knot and the skin.

   Pull the suture out by the knot with forceps.

   Remove every other suture. (Note: This method allows the nurse to ascertain whether or not the incision will remain approximated. Do not pull a contaminated visible part of a suture back through the skin.)

   If the incision remains approximated, remove the remaining sutures.

Clean the incision line with normal saline, if appropriate.

Apply povidone-iodine ointment and a dressing, if applicable.

6. To remove a plain continuous suture (see Fig. 118.1):

Cut the suture opposite the knot; then cut the next suture at the same side and place.

Pull the knot with forceps to remove the suture.

Use this same method down the incision line. Note that there will be no knot to grasp for the later sutures; grasp the suture where the knot had been on the first suture.

Clean the incision line with normal saline, if appropriate.

Apply povidone-iodine ointment and a dressing, if applicable.

7. To remove a mattress interrupted suture (see Fig. 118.1):

Cut the suture visible at the opposite side of the knot.

Grasp the knot with forceps and pull gently.

Continue the process.

Clean the incision line with normal saline, if appropriate.

Apply povidone-iodine ointment and a dressing, if applicable.

Plain Interrupted Suture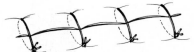

Plain Continuous or Continuous Running Suture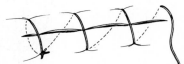

Mattress Interrupted Suture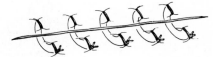

Mattress Continuous Suture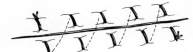

Blanket Continuous Suture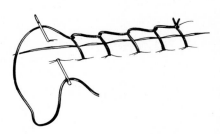

FIGURE 118.1 *Types of sutures.*

8. To remove a staple (see Figs. 118.2 and 118.3):

Fit the lower part of the staple remover under the staple.

Squeeze the handles of the remover.

Slowly lift the staple out.

Continue removing staples following the first through third step of number 8. If the incision begins to separate, remove every other staple, if appropriate. Remove remaining staples 1 to 2 days later.

Clean the incision with normal saline, if appropriate.

Apply povidone-iodine ointment and a dressing, if applicable.

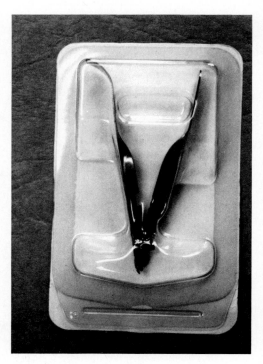

FIGURE 118.2 Staple remover.

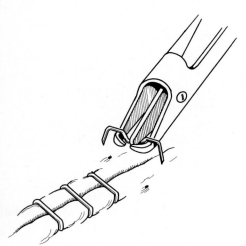

FIGURE 118.3 Removing a staple.

DOCUMENTATION

- Time and date.
- Appearance of the incision.
- Incision care given.
- Dressing and/or ointment applied.
- Ease or difficulty of removal.
- Child's response.

POTENTIAL RELATED NURSING DIAGNOSES

Infection: *high risk*

Skin integrity, impaired: *high risk*

Anxiety

POTENTIAL RELATED MEDICAL DIAGNOSES

Trauma

Surgery

119 Throat Culture

EQUIPMENT

Blanket (for use as a mummy restraint), if necessary

Tongue blade, if necessary

Gauze (optional)

Culture swab (culterette), sterile

PSYCHOSOCIAL CONSIDERATIONS: Explain the procedure in developmentally appropriate terms. Avoid using terms with mixed meanings, such as *stick into the throat*. Do not pretend to see things in the child's throat that do not exist. Let the child handle the equipment and see the soft cotton swab used as a culturette. Encourage parents to stay during the procedure as possible.

SAFETY ISSUES

• **Do not perform immediately after the child has eaten as doing so may induce vomiting.**

TIME: 2 to 3 minutes

PURPOSE

To obtain a throat culture to check for the presence of pathogens.

OBJECTIVES

• To obtain a throat culture.
• To prevent trauma.

ESSENTIAL STEPS

1. Prepare the child and family.
2. Assemble the equipment.
3. Wash hands.
4. Restrain the child as necessary. Use a mummy restraint or ask another person to hold and distract the child.

5. Ask the child to open the mouth, stick the tongue out, and say "ahh." Use a tongue blade and/or gauze to hold the tongue down, if necessary.

6. Swab only the back of the throat with a sterile swab. Try to touch across the left and right tonsils. Do not touch the tongue or oral mucous membranes. (See Fig. 119.1)

7. Return the swab to a sterile container.

8. Label and send the specimen to the lab immediately.

DOCUMENTATION

- Time.
- Type of culture.

POTENTIAL RELATED NURSING DIAGNOSES

Infection: *high risk*

Anxiety

Fear

POTENTIAL RELATED MEDICAL DIAGNOSES

Infection

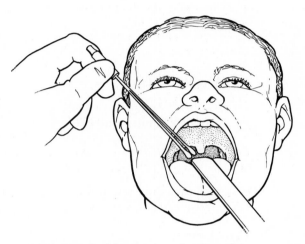

FIGURE 119.1 *Obtaining a throat culture.*

120 Total Parenteral Nutrition: Discontinuation

PSYCHOSOCIAL CONSIDERATIONS: Explain the procedure in developmentally appropriate terms. Answer questions honestly. Encourage the child and parents to voice concerns.

TIME: Varies

PURPOSE

To assure safe cessation or cycling of total parenteral nutrition (TPN) therapy.

OBJECTIVES

• To wean the child from TPN.
• To prevent injury and trauma.
• To prevent hypoglycemia.

EQUIPMENT

Gloves, sterile

Smooth-edge clamps

Povidone-iodine swabs *or* alcohol swabs

2″×2″ gauze

3 ml syringe with 25g ⅝″ needle

Heparin (units/ml vary from 10 to 100, per institution policy)

Injection cap

Lancet

Tape

Chemstrips

• The rate of the TPN infusion may be decreased gradually over several days as the rate and concentration of enteral feedings are progressively increased. To do this, begin by turning off TPN for 1 hour; progressively increase the length of time the TPN is turned off, such as for 1½ hours, then 2 hours, and so on. Monitor glucose levels during off times.

• The TPN can be discontinued rapidly over 1 hour. During rapid discontinuation, decrease the rate by 25% of the original rate every 15 minutes. At the conclusion of the hour, either heparin-lock the catheter or infuse another prescribed fluid (such as a blood product).

• Monitor blood glucose the first two or three times the TPN is rapidly decreased. If glucose levels are stable, further glucose monitoring is not necessary unless indicated per the physician's plan of care.

• To restart the infusion during cycled TPN, gradually increase the infusion over 1 hour by increasing the rate by 25% of the ordered rate every 15 minutes.

ESSENTIAL STEPS

1. Prepare the child and family.
2. Assemble the equipment.
3. Wash hands.
4. Begin decreasing the rate of TPN infusion 1 hour before infusion is to be discontinued.
5. At the conclusion of the hour, heparin-lock the catheter. Refer to "Central Venous Catheter: Heparin Lock/Cap Change."
6. Tape the extension tube and catheter securely to the dressing.
7. To determine blood glucose levels, check a Chemstrip 30 minutes after the TPN is discontinued.
8. If the Chemstrip is between 80 and 100 mg/dL, continue to monitor the Chemstrip at least each hour.
9. Notify the physician if the Chemstrip is less than 80 mg/dL.

DOCUMENTATION

- The process of discontinuation of the TPN.
- Blood glucose results.
- Child's tolerance of discontinuation.
- Supportive enteral feedings given.

Skills Checklist

☐ Prepare the child and family.
☐ Assemble the equipment.
☐ Wash hands.
☐ Decrease TPN infusion rate.
☐ Monitor glucose.
☐ Heparin-lock the catheter.
☐ Check glucose level 30 minutes after the TPN is discontinued.
☐ Document.

POTENTIAL RELATED NURSING DIAGNOSES

Infection: *high risk*

Injury: *high risk*

Trauma: *high risk*

POTENTIAL RELATED MEDICAL DIAGNOSES

Malabsorption syndrome

Anorexia

Nutritional deficiencies

Total Parenteral Nutrition and Lipid Therapy: Monitoring

PSYCHOSOCIAL CONSIDERATIONS: Explain the procedure in developmentally appropriate terms. Allow the child to express concerns and feelings. Explain why you must take blood samples and check the catheter site. Younger children may benefit from therapeutic play with a doll or puppet.

TIME: Continuous

PURPOSE

To assure safe administration of total parenteral nutrition (TPN) and lipid therapy and the early recognition of complications.

OBJECTIVES

• To monitor TPN and lipid infusion(s).
• To prevent injury and trauma.

EQUIPMENT

Testape
Routine supplies for blood sampling and CVC care
Chemstrips
Pump

 SAFETY ISSUES

• Unless otherwise specified in a physician's plan of care, routine monitoring of children receiving TPN therapy should include:

   Daily weights.

   Strict intake and output.

   Vital signs at least every 8 hours.

   Testape of all urine specimens.

   Inspection of the central venous catheter (CVC) exit site during routine dressing changes.

Routine TPN laboratory blood studies, which should include sodium, potassium, calcium, phosphorus, total and direct bilirubin, prealbumin, ammonia, blood urea nitrogen (BUN), alanine aminotransferase (ALT), and albumin.

   Daily measurements of triglyceride levels during the infusion of lipids.

• Inspect the IV infusion and CVC dressing or peripheral catheter site hourly.

• Measure blood glucose levels (via Chemstrip and/or serum glucose levels) when the TPN is abruptly discontinued.

• Use an infusion pump for all TPN and lipid infusions. Monitor the volume of solution administered hourly.

ESSENTIAL STEPS

1. Prepare the child and family.
2. Assemble the equipment.
3. Wash hands.
4. Monitor the child. Report significant results to the physician. If the *urine* is positive for glucose, follow-up may include:

Results	Follow-up
+1	Notify a physician
+2	Perform Chemstrip, notify a physician
≥+3	Perform Chemstrip, notify a physician, obtain STAT blood glucose

5. Inspect the peripheral TPN site for evidence of infiltration:

   Inspect the site each hour for the presence of pain, swelling, blanching, induration, or infection.

   Assess for the presence or absence of gravity flow at least each shift and any time the patency of the IV is in doubt or any evidence of infiltration exists.

If infiltration occurs:

Discontinue the IV.

Elevate the area until swelling recedes.

Do not apply hot or cold compresses.

Notify the physician.

Observe the site closely for evidence of skin breakdown.

Contact the physician to evaluate the site if skin breakdown occurs.

6. During routine dressing changes, assess the CVC exit site for erythema, induration, skin breakdown, and/or drainage. If evidence of infection is present, culture the site and notify the physician.

7. Monitor the child's temperature at least every 8 hours. Notify the physician if the temperature is greater than 38.5°C (101.3°F). As per the physician's plan of care, assist with standard workup for suspected CVC/TPN-related sepsis, which may include:

Peripheral and central blood cultures.

CVC exit site cultures.

Complete blood count with differential.

Urine culture and sensitivity.

8. If the child is receiving lipid therapy, obtain the triglyceride level at least every other day during lipid infusion.

9. Obtain routine TPN labs by venipuncture every week.

DOCUMENTATION

- Infusion of TPN and/or lipids.
- Appearance of CVC dressing.
- Appearance of CVC exit site or peripheral venipuncture site.
- Evidence of complications, such as fever or glucosuria.
- Nursing interventions.
- Child's weight.

Skills Checklist

- ☐ Prepare the child and family.
- ☐ Assemble the equipment.
- ☐ Wash hands.
- ☐ Monitor lab values.
- ☐ Monitor for signs of infiltration.
- ☐ Monitor urine.
- ☐ Monitor weight.
- ☐ Monitor vital signs.
- ☐ Monitor peripheral IV site or CVC exit site for signs of infection.
- ☐ Document.

- Rate of TPN and lipid infusions.
- Glucose concentration of TPN and fat concentration of lipid emulsion.
- Volume and type of all enteral intake.
- Urine Testape results.
- Stool volume and stool record, if ordered.

POTENTIAL RELATED NURSING DIAGNOSES

Injury: *high risk*

Fluid volume excess

Infection: *high risk*

Trauma: *high risk*

Skin integrity, impaired

POTENTIAL RELATED MEDICAL DIAGNOSES

Short bowel syndrome

Anorexia

Malabsorption syndrome

Nutritional deficiencies

Ruptured appendix

REFERENCES

Mize, and Allen, S. 1990. Total parental nutrition in *Essentials of Pediatric Intensive Care*, edited by D. Levin and F. Morriss, St. Louis, Mo.: Quality Medical Publishing, Inc.

Mott, S., James, S., and Sperhac, A. 1990. *Nursing care of children and families.* Redwood City, Calif.: Addison-Wesley.

Testerman, E. 1989. Current trends in total parenteral nutrition. *Journal of Intravenous Nursing* 12, no. 3: 152–62.

122 Tracheostomy Care: General

PSYCHOSOCIAL CONSIDERATIONS: Explain procedures in developmentally appropriate terms. Avoid using terms with mixed meanings, such as *suction out* and *suck out*. These terms can increase anxiety. The child may fear not being able to breathe during suctioning. Speak to the child in reassuring terms. Count during suctioning to provide a time frame for when the suctioning will be complete.

PURPOSE

To maintain a patent airway.

To promote healing of a new tracheostomy site.

To maintain skin integrity.

To decrease the risk of wound infection.

OBJECTIVES

- To provide guidelines of care for a tracheostomy.
- To implement safe care of a tracheostomy.

SAFETY ISSUES

- Keep a trach tube of the same size and type as the child's, a trach tube one size smaller, an oxygen bag, a mask, and a suction setup at bedside. Keep bag-to-trach adapters at bedside to use with metal trach tubes.

- Change trach ties as needed, at least every other day.

- Follow trach site care procedures every 8 hours.

- Change disposable inner cannulas every 8 hours.

- The physician usually orders the extent of tracheostomy care to be performed within the first 72 hours postoperatively.

- Do not perform trach care procedures for at least 30 minutes prior to or following a feeding, except for children receiving continuous drip feeds.

- Some institutions prefer normal saline instead of hydrogen peroxide (H_2O_2) to clean wounds, because H_2O_2 may damage tissue.

NOTE: Refer to the following procedures for Time, Equipment, Essential Steps, and Documentation:
- Emergency Procedures
- Changing Trach Ties
- Trach Site Care
- Inner Cannula Care (Nondisposable)
- Inner Cannula Care (Disposable)

Emergency Procedures

TIME: Varies

EQUIPMENT

Oxygen flowmeter with appropriate-size bag and mask

Trach tube of appropriate size and type

Suction catheter of appropriate size

Shoulder roll, if appropriate

Gloves, nonsterile

Gauze, if appropriate

ESSENTIAL STEPS

1. Prepare the child and family.
2. Assemble the equipment.
3. For an obstructed tracheostomy:

    In the case of an acute tracheostomy (7 days or less following a tracheostomy):

    > Suction the child. Refer to "Suctioning: Endotracheal/ Tracheostomy."

    > Attempt bag-to-trach ventilation with 100% oxygen (O_2).

    > If the tube remains plugged, attempt to ventilate through a face mask.

    > Activate an emergency page for a physician or call code team, if appropriate.

    > If no physician is available to help and the child's condition is deteriorating, replace the tube.

    >> Cut the old ties and remove the old trach tube, if present.

    >> Gently pull up on stay sutures to establish an airway.

    >> Gently replace or reinsert the trach tube.

    > Hand-ventilate the child with 100% O_2 after changing.

    > Suction as indicated.

    In the case of chronic tracheostomy (more than 7 days following a tracheostomy):

Skills Checklist

Changing Trach Ties

☐ Prepare the child and family.
☐ Assemble the equipment.
☐ Wash hands and put on gloves.
☐ Apply new ties.
☐ Remove old ties.
☐ Document.

Trach Site Care

☐ Prepare the child and family.
☐ Assemble the equipment.
☐ Wash hands and put on gloves.
☐ Remove the soiled dressing, if applicable.
☐ Clean the area, including the tube perimeter and the flanges.
☐ Dry.
☐ Apply a new dressing, if applicable.
☐ Document.

Inner Cannula Care (Nondisposable)

☐ Prepare the child and family.
☐ Assemble the equipment.
☐ Wash hands.
☐ Remove the soiled dressing, if applicable.
☐ Remove the inner cannula.
☐ Put on gloves and clean the inner cannula.
☐ Rinse.
☐ Suction.
☐ Reinsert the inner cannula.
☐ Apply a new dressing, if applicable.
☐ Document.

Inner Cannula Care (Disposable)

☐ Prepare the child and family.
☐ Assemble the equipment.
☐ Wash hands and put on gloves.
☐ Remove the soiled dressing, if applicable.
☐ Remove the inner cannula and dispose of it.
☐ Suction.
☐ Insert the new cannula.
☐ Apply a new dressing, if applicable.
☐ Document.

Suction the child. Refer to "Suctioning: Endotracheal/Tracheostomy."

Attempt bag-to-trach ventilation with 100% O_2.

If the tube remains plugged, refer to "Tracheostomy Tube Change."

4. If the trach tube has been removed:

In the case of an acute tracheostomy (7 days or less following a tracheostomy):

Position the child on a shoulder roll.

Cover the stoma with a gauze and hold in place with a finger.

Hand-ventilate the child with 100% O_2 through a face mask.

Activate an emergency page for a physician.

In the case of a chronic tracheostomy (more than 7 days following a tracheostomy):

Refer to the procedure for "Tracheostomy Tube Change."

Notify a physician, if appropriate.

DOCUMENTATION

- Sequence of events.
- Name of the physician notified.
- Interventions.
- Child's response.

Changing Trach Ties

TIME: 5 to 10 minutes

EQUIPMENT

Gloves, nonsterile

Twill tape

Scissors

ESSENTIAL STEPS

1. Prepare the child and family.
2. Assemble the equipment.
3. Wash hands and put on gloves.
4. If using the two-tie method:

Take two pieces of twill tape and fold an end of each one lengthwise about 1″ to 1½″. (See sixth step in number 4 to determine length of tape.)

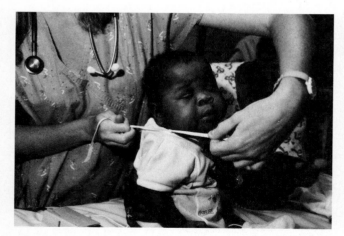

FIGURE 122.1 *Tying the tracheostomy tie using the one-tie method.*

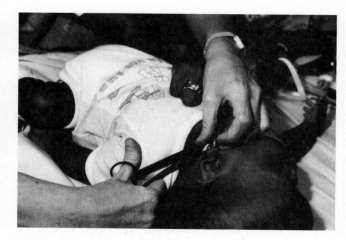

FIGURE 122.2 *Cutting the old ties.*

Cut a small slit (¼″) lengthwise at the fold.

Take the slit end of the new tie and slip it under and through the hole on the flange of the long end of the trach tube.

Pull the tie through the slit portion of the tie while immobilizing the trach tube.

Repeat first through fourth step in number 4 for the other new tie.

Tie the new ties at the side of the neck securely in a double knot; ties should be snug enough to minimize trach tube movement, but loose enough for a little finger to be slipped between the tie and the child's neck.

Cut the soiled ties and discard.

5. If using the one-tie method:

Cut a single piece of twill tape that is long enough to go around the child's neck twice.

Slip one end through the front side of the flange opening.

Pass the string behind the child's neck and through the back side of the opposite flange opening.

Pass the string again behind the child's neck and tie the new ties at the side of the neck securely in a double or square knot; ties should be snug enough to minimize trach tube movement but loose enough for a little finger to be slipped between the tie and the child's neck. (See Fig. 122.1)

Cut the soiled ties and discard. (See Fig. 122.2)

Check the tightness of the ties. (See Fig. 122.3)

6. Assess the skin.

DOCUMENTATION

- That trach ties have been changed.
- Assessment of the skin.

Trach Site Care

TIME: 5 to 10 minutes

EQUIPMENT

Gloves, nonsterile

Cotton-tip applicators, sterile

Half-strength hydrogen peroxide (H_2O_2) *or* normal saline (0.9% sodium chloride), sterile, *or* water, sterile

Trach dressing, if indicated

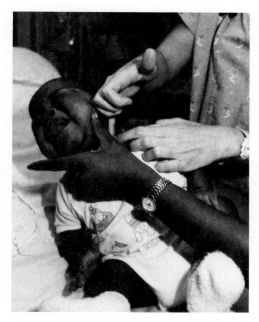

FIGURE 122.3 *Checking the tightness of the new ties.*

ESSENTIAL STEPS

1. Prepare the child and family.
2. Assemble the equipment.
3. Wash hands and put on gloves.
4. Remove the soiled trach dressing, if applicable.
5. Using cotton-tip applicators and half-strength H_2O_2 or normal saline, clean around the stoma site. Then clean the skin surfaces around and under the tube flanges.
6. Clean the tube perimeter and flanges with half-strength H_2O_2 or normal saline.
7. With dry applicators, normal saline, or sterile water, remove any excess H_2O_2 and debris.
8. Apply a new tracheostomy dressing, if ordered. If trach dressing is needed, use only the precut dressings; cutting 2″×2″ or 4″×4″ pads can leave loose threads that could get into the stoma site or be aspirated.

DOCUMENTATION

- That trach site care has been completed.
- Observations.

Inner Cannula Care (Nondisposable)

TIME: 1 to 10 minutes

EQUIPMENT

Trach care kit which may include a brush for cleaning, containers for solutions, and sterile gloves

Half-strength hydrogen peroxide (H_2O_2)

Normal saline (0.9% sodium chloride), sterile

Suction catheter of appropriate size

ESSENTIAL STEPS

1. Prepare the child and family.
2. Assemble the equipment.
3. Wash hands.
4. After opening the trach care tray, pour half-strength H_2O_2 into one basin and normal saline into another.
5. Remove the soiled trach dressing and discard, if applicable.
6. Remove the inner cannula and place it in the half-strength H_2O_2 or normal saline. (For ventilator-dependent patients, disconnect the ventilator, quickly insert a clean inner cannula, and lock the cannula in place. Immediately reconnect the ventilator.)
7. Put on sterile gloves.
8. Using the brush for cleaning, clean the inside and outside of the inner cannula with half-strength H_2O_2 or normal saline.
9. Rinse the inner cannula with normal saline.
10. Lay the inner cannula on the sterile surface to dry.

11. Remove the gloves and suction through the outer cannula using sterile technique. Refer to "Suctioning: Endotracheal/ Tracheostomy."

12. Reinsert the inner cannula and lock in place.

13. Apply a new dressing, if ordered. If trach dressing is needed, use only the precut dressings; cutting 2″×2″ or 4″×4″ pads can leave loose threads that could get into the stoma site or be aspirated.

DOCUMENTATION

- That cannula care has been completed.
- Observations.

Inner Cannula Care (Disposable)

TIME: 5 to 10 minutes

EQUIPMENT

Gloves, nonsterile
Suction catheter of appropriate size
Replacement disposable inner cannula
Trach dressing, if indicated

ESSENTIAL STEPS

1. Prepare the child and family.
2. Assemble the equipment.
3. Wash hands and put on gloves.
4. Remove the soiled trach dressing and discard, if applicable.
5. Remove and discard the inner cannula. Open the package of the new inner cannula maintaining sterility.
6. Suction through the outer cannula using sterile technique. Refer to "Suctioning: Endotracheal/ Tracheostomy."

7. Insert the replacement inner cannula and lock into place.

8. Apply a new dressing, if ordered. If trach dressing is needed, use only precut dressings; cutting 2″×2″ or 4″×4″ pads can leave loose threads that could get into the stoma site or be aspirated.

DOCUMENTATION

- That cannula care has been completed.
- Observations.

POTENTIAL RELATED NURSING DIAGNOSES

Anxiety
Skin integrity, impaired: *high risk*
Infection: *high risk*
Gas exchange, impaired
Airway clearance, ineffective

POTENTIAL RELATED MEDICAL DIAGNOSES

Bronchopulmonary dysplasia
Near drowning
Muscular dystrophy
Trauma

REFERENCES

Lineweaver, W., McMorris, S., Soucy, D., and Howard, R. 1985. Cellular and bacterial toxicities of topical antimicrobials. *Plastic and Reconstructive Surgery* 75, no. 3: 394–96.

Mott, S., James, S., and Sperhac, A. 1990. *Nursing care of children and families.* Redwood City, Calif.: Addison-Wesley.

123 Tracheostomy Tube Change

PSYCHOSOCIAL CONSIDERATIONS: Explain the procedure in developmentally appropriate terms. Explain that the child can hold his or her breath during removal and insertion of the tube; this will decrease the sensation of not being able to breathe. Provide constant reassurance.

TIME: 10 to 15 minutes for set up; 2 to 3 minutes for change

PURPOSE

To prevent respiratory compromise due to potential or partial plugging from secretions.

OBJECTIVES

- To maintain a patent airway.
- To prevent injury.

EQUIPMENT

Gloves, nonsterile (sterile if using sterile technique)

Blanket(s) for roll(s) or mummy restraint

Suction catheter

Suction equipment

Tracheostomy tube of identical size and type to the child's

Twill tape

Ambu bag with tracheostomy adapter and appropriate-size face mask

Oxygen (O_2)

Scissors

SAFETY ISSUES

- The surgeon does the initial trach tube change (usually on the seventh day posttracheostomy).
- Keep a trach tube identical in size and type to the child's, another of one size smaller, a bag, and a mask at bedside.
- Use a new trach tube each time the trach tube is changed unless otherwise indicated.
- Do not change a trach tube within 1 hour of a feeding, except in emergency situations. The changing could cause vomiting and risk possible aspiration. Preferably, the change should be done early in the morning before any feedings or 2 to 3 hours after feeding.

ESSENTIAL STEPS

1. Prepare the child and family.
2. Assemble the equipment.
3. Have two people present if possible to assist with an active child.
4. Wash hands and put on gloves.
5. Place the child in a supine position with a roll under the shoulders, or, if an older child, in a semisitting position. The head should be in a midline position. Put rolls on either side of the head to maintain the position in a very small child. Mummy wrap an infant.
6. Suction, if indicated.
7. Prepare the new trach tube:

   Secure the trach ties to the clean trach tube.

   Insert the obturator inside the new trach tube. If the trach tube has an inner cannula, the obturator cannot be inserted into the outer cannula until the inner cannula has been removed. The inner cannula will need to be reinserted once the new tube has been placed. (Note: Infants under 1 year of age may become hypoxic with the use of an obturator. The tip of the tracheostomy tube can be inserted into the stoma, maintaining a patent airway without use of an obturator.)

If the trach tube has a cuff, inflate the cuff to check for leaks; then deflate before insertion.

8. Bag the child with 100% O_2 (or 40% over the child's ordered concentration, if appropriate).

9. Deflate the cuff if present, cut the ties around the child's neck, and remove the old trach with one hand, using an outward, downward motion. If the child can tolerate it, observe the trach stoma at this time for skin integrity and use a wet washcloth to clean the stoma and surrounding area. If secretions are bubbling from the stoma, suction the stoma.

10. With the other hand, take the new trach tube, holding it with a thumb over the obturator and a forefinger underneath one wing tip and

keeping the tube sterile prior to insertion. Insert gently into the tracheostomy using an inward, downward motion. Once the tube is in place, hold onto it and pull out the obturator. Inflate the cuff if present. (See Figs. 123.1 and 123.2)

Skills Checklist

☐ Prepare the child and family.
☐ Assemble the equipment.
☐ Wash hands and put on gloves.
☐ Position the child.
☐ Secure trach ties to the new tube. Insert obturator.
☐ Check the cuff.
☐ Bag the child.
☐ Remove the old tube.
☐ Observe the trach stoma.
☐ Insert the new tube.
☐ Reoxygenate the child.
☐ Assess the child and secure the tube.
☐ Document.

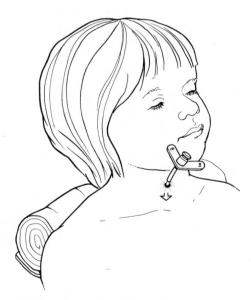

FIGURE 123.1 *Insertion of a new tracheostomy tube.*

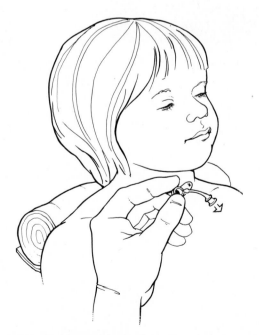

FIGURE 123.2 *Removing the obturator.*

11. Allow the child to reoxygenate, or bag the child if appropriate and suction if necessary.

12. For ventilator-dependent children:

Disconnect the ventilator.

Bag the child with 100% O_2.

Deflate the cuff, if present.

Change the trach tube as in Steps 9 and 10 and inflate the cuff if present.

Reoxygenate with 100% O_2 and then reconnect the ventilator.

13. Assess the child for respiratory distress, such as cyanosis, difficulty in breathing, or significant bleeding. Auscultate for breath sounds bilaterally anterior and posterior.

While the second person stabilizes the trach, tie the trach ties securely using a square knot and another half knot. (See Figs. 123.3 and 123.4)

14. If the trach tube will not go back in:

Call a physician STAT.

Remain calm. There is more time than might be expected.

If the tube won't go back in because secretions or collapse of skin folds prevent visualization of the stoma, retract the skin down on the neck just below where the stoma should be (second or third tracheal ring). The stoma should appear.

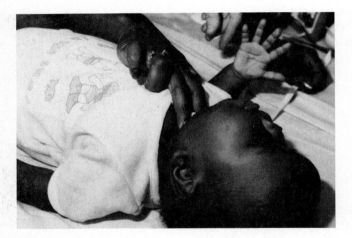

FIGURE 123.3 *Securing the tracheostomy tube.*

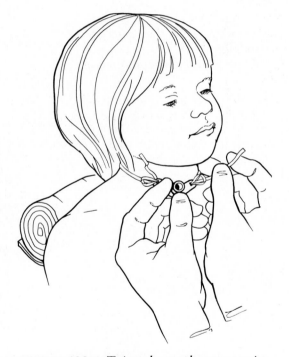

FIGURE 123.4 *Tying the tracheostomy ties.*

If the tube won't advance because the child is crying, blow in the child's face. The child will take a breath. Or give an infant a pacifier. Ask older children to take a breath, or try to insert on the inspiration of a cry.

If the appropriate-size trach tube does not fit, insert the next smaller size.

If the smaller size trach tube does not advance, insert a suction catheter into the stoma to establish an airway. Blow-by O_2 helps to increase oxygenation.

If all else fails, cover the stoma with a finger and hand-ventilate the child with 100% oxygen through a face mask.

DOCUMENTATION

- Date and time of tube change.
- Size of trach tube.
- Any problems with removal and reinsertion of tube.
- Assessment of trach stoma site.
- Child's response.
- That trach tube (size and type), bag, and mask are at bedside.

POTENTIAL RELATED NURSING DIAGNOSES

Airway clearance, ineffective

Breathing pattern, ineffective

Gas exchange, impaired

Anxiety

POTENTIAL RELATED MEDICAL DIAGNOSES

Lye ingestion

Bronchopulmonary dysplasia

Strictures—subglottic stenosis

Laryngotracheal malasia

REFERENCES

Mott, S., James, S., and Sperhac, A. 1990. *Nursing care of children and families.* Redwood City, Calif.: Addison-Wesley.

124 Traction

OBJECTIVES

- To immobilize and maintain alignment of particular bones.
- To prevent further injury or trauma.

EQUIPMENT

For skin traction:

    Traction, as specified by the physician; refer to traction manual

    Benzoin, if appropriate

    Tape

For skeletal traction:

    Traction, as specified by the physician; refer to traction manual

    Hydrogen peroxide *or* normal saline (0.9% sodium chloride), sterile, *or* povidone-iodine

    Applicators, sterile

    2″×2″ gauze, sterile

    Antimicrobial ointment

PSYCHOSOCIAL CONSIDERATIONS: Explain the procedure in developmentally appropriate terms. Avoid using terms with mixed meanings, such as *hang*. Provide diversional activity for the immobilized child. Provide things to play with to release aggression and energy, such as clay, punch-a-ball, play-doh, or a cobbler's bench and wooden hammer. Utilize the trapeze to maximize self-mobility when appropriate.

TIME: Varies

PURPOSE

To immobilize the body and maintain alignment to relieve pressure, muscle spasms, and/or pain, and/or to reduce a fracture.

S   SAFETY ISSUES

- **Perform a neurovascular assessment at least every 2 hours. The assessment should include peripheral pulses, color and temperature of the extremity, capillary refill, and sensations.**
- **Be aware of problems caused by immobility, such as pressure sores and thrombophlebitis.**
- **Never remove weights from skeletal traction.**
- **Note that halo vests can impair lung expansion and cause respiratory distress.**

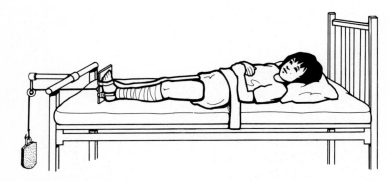

FIGURE 124.1 *Bucks extension.*

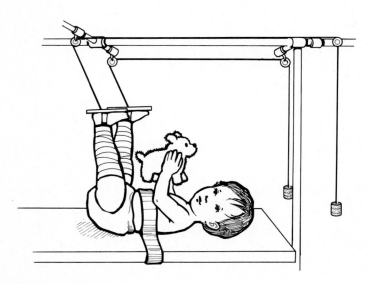

FIGURE 124.2 *Bryant traction.*

ESSENTIAL STEPS

Skin Traction

1. Prepare the child and family.

2. Assemble the equipment.

3. Review the traction manual for setup.

4. Wash hands.

5. Apply one of the following types of skin traction:

   Bucks—to immobilize the leg. (See Fig. 124.1)

   Bryant—to reduce a fracture or dislocated hip. The child must be less than 2 years of age and weigh less than 30 lb. (See Fig. 124.2)

   Russell—to immobilize a hip or knee or reduce fractures of the femur. (See Fig. 124.3)

   Cervical—to immobilize the cervical spine. (See Fig. 124.4)

6. Assess circulation in the extremities. Check capillary refill, color, motion, temperature, pulse, and sensation for each extremity in traction.

7. Weights should swing freely and knots should be taped.

8. If the traction pulls the child down in the bed, apply a vest or a sheet to keep the child in place.

9. Rewrap skin traction every 8 hours or according to the physician's plan of care. Avoid wrapping too tightly over pulse points or the Achilles tendon.

Skills Checklist

Skin Traction

☐ Prepare the child and family.

☐ Assemble the equipment. Review the traction manual.

☐ Wash hands.

☐ Apply traction.

☐ Assess skin integrity and circulation.

☐ Check weights.

☐ Rewrap skin traction every 8 hours.

☐ Document.

Skeletal Traction

☐ Prepare the child and family.

☐ Assemble the equipment. Review the traction manual.

☐ Wash hands.

☐ Note alignment.

☐ Assess circulation.

☐ Assess and clean the pin site.

☐ Check weights.

☐ Document.

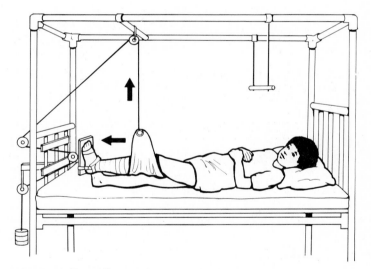

FIGURE 124.3 *Russell traction.*

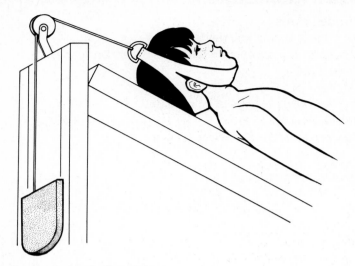

FIGURE 124.4 *Cervical traction.*

Skeletal Traction

1. Prepare the child and family.
2. Assemble the equipment.
3. Review the traction manual.
4. Wash hands.
5. Use one of the following types of skeletal traction:

   Crutchfield tongs. (See Fig. 124.5)

   Ninety-ninety.

   Balance suspension. (See Fig. 124.6)

   Halo vest.
6. Note alignment to determine if the traction is correct.
7. Observe extremities for circulation. Check capillary refill, color, motion, temperature, sensation, and pulse for each extremity in traction.
8. Assess the pin insertion site. Note especially redness, swelling, discharge, or pin movement.
9. Clean the pin sites with hydrogen peroxide, sterile saline, or povidone-iodine, using sterile applicators.
10. Dry with sterile gauze.
11. Apply antimicrobial ointment. Repeat pin care every 8 hours or according to the physician's plan of care.
12. Weights should swing freely and knots should be taped.

DOCUMENTATION

- Skin integrity.
- Neurovascular assessments.
- Pin site appearance and care, if applicable.
- Weight(s), in pounds.
- Type of traction.

POTENTIAL RELATED NURSING DIAGNOSES

Activity intolerance

Constipation

Infection: *high risk*

Injury: *high risk*

Skin integrity, impaired: *high risk*

POTENTIAL RELATED MEDICAL DIAGNOSES

Fracture

Surgery

Congenital defect

Trauma

REFERENCES

Mott, S., James, S., and Sperhac, A. 1990. *Nursing care of children and families.* Redwood City, Calif.: Addison-Wesley.

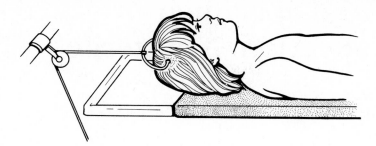

FIGURE 124.5 *Crutchfield tongs.*

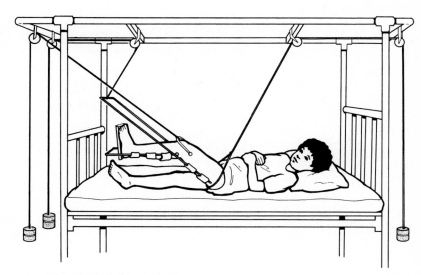

FIGURE 124.6 *Balance suspension.*

125 Urine Specimen Collection: Nonsterile

PSYCHOSOCIAL CONSIDERATIONS: Determine and use the individual child's terms for voiding and urine. Explain the procedure in developmentally appropriate terms. The child may fear having genitalia exposed to a stranger. Have parents or a significant other remain with the child to provide reassurance.

TIME: 3 to 5 minutes for collection (longer if a urine bag is used)

PURPOSE

To collect a nonsterile, voided urine specimen.

OBJECTIVES

- To obtain a sample of urine.

EQUIPMENT

For a routine collection (for most lab tests except culture):

    Gloves, nonsterile

    Water and cotton balls

    Urine bag and/or specimen cup

For a clean catch (for noncatherized culture or according to the physician's plan of care):

    Gloves, nonsterile

    Povidone-iodine solution *or,* if the child is iodine-sensitive, another approved antiseptic

    Cotton balls

    Water, sterile

    Syringe and needle, sterile

    Urine bag *or* specimen cup, sterile

    4″×4″ gauze, sterile

ESSENTIAL STEPS

1. Prepare the child and family. If possible, give the child 60 to 90 ml of liquid to drink. Infants and young children generally void within 30 minutes of ingesting liquids.
2. Assemble the equipment.
3. For a routine specimen collection:

    Wash hands and put on gloves.

    Clean genitalia with water. For an uncircumcised male, retract the foreskin just enough to visualize

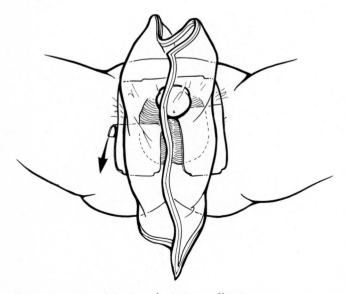

FIGURE 125.1 *Nonsterile urine collection.*

the meatus for cleaning; then allow the foreskin to return to cover the meatus.

If the child is toilet trained, have him or her void in a nonsterile cup.

For male infants, apply the urine bag around the base of the penis; it is not necessary to contain the scrotum in the bag. (See Fig. 125.1) For female infants, apply the urine bag around the vulva. Be sure the lower edge of the bag opening is above the anal orifice. Make sure the adhesive is securely applied, to prevent leakage. (If desired, place sterile cotton balls in the bag. When the urine enters the bag, the cotton will absorb it. This prevents all the urine from draining out of a loose bag. The cotton can be squeezed using aseptic technique and the urine removed.) Apply a diaper loosely. Check the urine bag every 30 minutes for urine. If the adhesive becomes moist, the bag will not remain in place. Place the collected specimen in a nonsterile cup.

4. For a clean-catch specimen:

Wash hands and put on gloves.

If the child is toilet trained, collect the specimen in the following manner:

For the uncircumcised male child, retract the foreskin to visualize the meatus. Clean with the antiseptic in a circular motion from the glans to the base. Wipe the same area with

Skills Checklist

Routine Specimen Collection
☐ Prepare the child and family.
☐ Assemble the equipment.
☐ Wash hands and put on gloves.
☐ Clean genitalia with water.
☐ Use a nonsterile cup or apply a urine bag.
☐ If using a urine bag, place the collected specimen in a nonsterile cup.
☐ Label the specimen. Place it in a plastic bag and send to the lab.
☐ Document.

Clean-Catch Specimen Collection
☐ Prepare the child and family.
☐ Assemble the equipment.
☐ Wash hands and put on gloves.
☐ Clean genitalia with povidone-iodine solution or another antiseptic.
☐ For a toilet-trained child:
  • Have the child begin to void.
  • Catch midstream urine.
☐ For an infant:
  • Clean and assess the skin.
  • Apply a urine bag.
  • Clean the port with povidone-iodine and withdraw urine with a sterile syringe and needle.
  • Place urine in a sterile cup.
☐ Label the specimen. Place in a plastic bag and send it to the lab.
☐ Document.

Normal Urine Lab Values:

White Blood Cells: few
Bacteria: none
Red Blood Cells: none
Casts: 0–1
Epithelial Cells: few
pH
   Newborn: 5–7
   >1 month: 4.5–8
Glucose: <2.8 mmol/d
Color: straw

sterile water to prevent contamination of urine with antiseptic, which might alter the lab results. After initiation of urination, insert the sterile specimen cup into the stream, collecting a minimum of 5 ml. Withdraw the cup before urination ceases. Do not touch the cup to any part of the skin. Keep the lid and the inside of the cup clean. Pull the foreskin back down in the uncircumcised male.

For the female, clean with the antiseptic from front to back, once down each labia and once down the middle. Do not go back over the area with the same cotton ball. Wipe with sterile water. Have the child spread the labia during urination and collect as in second step of number 4.

If the child is not toilet trained, clean as in second step of number 4 and dry with sterile gauze or allow to air dry. Apply a sterile urine bag as for a routine collection. Because it is questionable whether the urine bag is still sterile after 30 to 45 minutes, remove the bag if the child has not voided in that time, repeat the cleaning, and apply a sterile bag.

After collection, clean the perineal area to remove any remaining antiseptic. Assess the skin; antiseptic and adhesives are harsh and can cause skin irritation.

To obtain a specimen from an external pediatric urine bag, clean the port with a povidone-iodine or alcohol swab and withdraw urine with a sterile syringe and needle. Transfer urine to a sterile cup.

5. Label the specimen. Place it in a plastic bag and send it to the lab.

DOCUMENTATION

- Method of collection (routine or clean catch).
- Time and date of collection.
- Amount and characteristics of specimen.
- That specimen has been sent to lab.

POTENTIAL RELATED NURSING DIAGNOSES

Hypothermia

Urinary elimination, altered

POTENTIAL RELATED MEDICAL DIAGNOSES

Urinary tract infection

Kidney infection

Preoperative surgical analysis

Fever of unknown origin

Universal application

REFERENCES

Mott, S., James, S., and Sperhac, A. 1990. *Nursing care of children and families.* Redwood City, Calif.: Addison-Wesley.

Urine Specimen Collection: Sterile Catheterization

PSYCHOSOCIAL CONSIDERATIONS: Determine and use the individual child's words for urine and voiding. Explain the procedure in developmentally appropriate terms. The child may fear having genitalia exposed to a stranger. Have another person hold the legs and provide reassurance. A family member may be allowed to remain with the child.

TIME: 5 minutes for setup
10 minutes for performance

PURPOSE

To obtain a sterile urine specimen.

OBJECTIVES

- To maintain sterility during urine collection.
- To collect a sample of urine for culture and/or sensitivity.
- To prevent external contaminants from entering the bladder.
- To prevent physiological and/or psychological trauma.

EQUIPMENT

Catheterization tray, including sterile drapes, sterile gloves, antiseptic solution, cotton balls, sterile lubricant, forceps, and a receptacle (see Fig. 126.1)

Urinary catheter of appropriate size— for collecting a straight catheterization specimen

Povidone-iodine swab *or* alcohol swab, sterile syringe, and a 25g needle—for a child with an indwelling catheter

ESSENTIAL STEPS

1. Prepare the child and family.
2. Assemble the equipment.
3. Wash hands.
4. For a straight catheterization specimen:

   Open the package using sterile technique.

   Place the drapes on the child under the hips and around the penis or perineal area.

   Open the catheter and place on a sterile field.

   Put on sterile gloves.

   Open the antiseptic solution. Pour over cotton balls.

   Open the lubricant and coat the end of the catheter.

   Pick up the cotton ball with forceps and clean the penis or vulva.

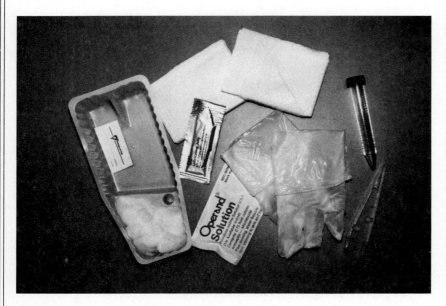

FIGURE 126.1 *Catheter kit contents.*

For a male: Clean in a circular motion from the tip of the penis toward the abdomen. Pick up the penis with the nondominant hand. Do not touch any part of the skin with the hand holding the forceps; keep this hand sterile.

For a female: Separate the labia with the nondominant hand, exposing the urinary meatus. (See Fig. 126.2) Clean from the clitoris toward the rectum, using one cotton ball for each labia and one down the middle. Use forceps to pick up the cotton balls to avoid contamination of the fingers. Do not go back up from the rectum to the urinary meatus.

Once the area is clean, pick up the lubricated catheter with the sterile hand and insert the catheter until urine returns. To insert the catheter into a penis, hold the penis at a 90° angle to the body. The urinary meatus in females may be hidden or deviated to one side, or close to the vaginal opening. If the catheter is inserted into the vagina, leave it in place. Insert a second sterile catheter into the meatus using the first catheter as a guide. Maintain sterile technique. (See Fig. 126.3) Place the open end of the catheter in a sterile receptacle.

Skills Checklist

Straight Catheterization Specimen
- [ ] Prepare the child and family.
- [ ] Assemble the equipment.
- [ ] Wash hands.
- [ ] Place drapes.
- [ ] Open the catheter and place on a sterile field.
- [ ] Put on gloves.
- [ ] Soak cotton balls in antiseptic.
- [ ] Apply lubricant to the catheter.
- [ ] Clean external genitalia.
- [ ] Insert the catheter with sterile-gloved hand.
- [ ] Collect urine in a container.
- [ ] Remove the catheter.
- [ ] Dispose of the equipment.
- [ ] Label the specimen. Place in a plastic bag and send to the lab.
- [ ] Document.

Indwelling Catheter
- [ ] Prepare the child and family.
- [ ] Assemble the equipment.
- [ ] Wash hands.
- [ ] Clean the port closest to the child.
- [ ] Withdraw the specimen.
- [ ] Transfer the specimen to a sterile container.
- [ ] Label the specimen. Place in a plastic bag and send to the lab.
- [ ] Document.

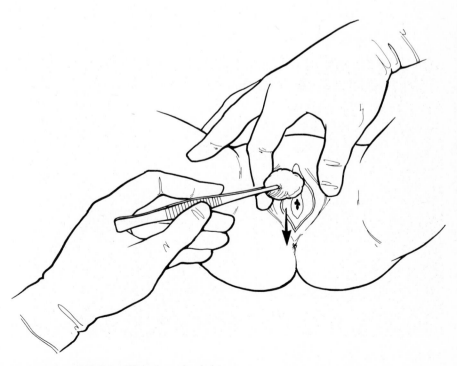

FIGURE 126.2 *Cleaning the labia.*

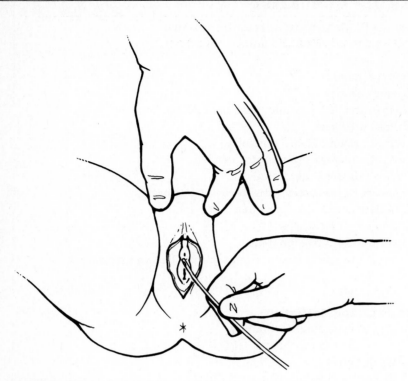

FIGURE 126.3 Inserting the catheter.

Depending on the laboratory requirements and the tests ordered, collect 5 to 30 ml of urine.

Once the required amount is obtained, withdraw the catheter gently but firmly. Squeeze the catheter while withdrawing to prevent urine from flowing back. Continue emptying the bladder if desired before removing the catheter. Dispose of the equipment.

5. For the child with an indwelling catheter:

Clean the port on the urinary drainage bag system closest to the child with a povidone-iodine or alcohol swab.

Insert a sterile syringe with a 25g needle into the port and withdraw the specimen (1 to 5 ml).

Transfer the specimen to a sterile container.

6. Label the specimen. Place it in a plastic bag and send to the lab.

DOCUMENTATION

- Time and date of specimen collection.
- Amount and characteristics of specimen.
- Size and type of catheter used.
- Child's tolerance of the procedure.
- That the specimen has been sent to lab.

POTENTIAL RELATED NURSING DIAGNOSES

Infection: *high risk*

Hyperthermia

Urinary elimination, altered

POTENTIAL RELATED MEDICAL DIAGNOSES

Urinary tract infection

Kidney infection

Preoperative surgical analysis

Fever of unknown origin

REFERENCES

Mott, S., James, S., and Sperhac, A. 1990. *Nursing care of children and families.* Redwood City, Calif.: Addison-Wesley.

Normal Urine Lab Values:

White Blood Cells: few
Bacteria: none
Red Blood Cells: none
Casts: 0−1
Epithelial Cells: few
pH
    Newborn: 5−7
    >1 month: 4.5−8
Glucose: <2.8 mmol/d
Color: straw

127 Ventriculostomy Catheter Care

PSYCHOSOCIAL CONSIDERATIONS: Explain the procedure in developmentally appropriate terms. Avoid using terms with mixed meanings. The child may be confused related to increased intracranial pressure. Make explanations simple and clear. Do not tell the child that *fluid will be drained off the brain.* The child may envision a drain such as in a bathtub and believe that his or her brain may be pulled out.

TIME: 15 minutes

PURPOSE

To maintain a closed system during drainage and/or removal of cerebrospinal fluid (CSF).

OBJECTIVES

- To maintain a closed system.
- To reduce the risks of infection.
- To prevent injury or trauma.

EQUIPMENT

To remove CSF:

    Gloves, sterile

    30 ml syringe

    One of the following:

        23g or 25g needle and stopcock

        23g or 25g butterfly and smooth-edge clamps

    Two povidone-iodine swabs *or* two alcohol swabs

To change the ventriculostomy bag and tubing:

    Gloves, sterile

    Bile bag

    Two povidone-iodine swabs *or* two alcohol swabs

    Two 2″×2″ gauze pads, sterile

    Smooth-edge clamp

    Adhesive tape

SAFETY ISSUES

- Monitor neurological status frequently.
- The neurosurgeon will usually specify postinsertion:

    Drainage of CSF (continuous, intermittent, or none).

    Level of the ventriculostomy drainage bag.

    Position of the child (head of bed elevated or child supine, for example).

- The ventriculostomy bag is usually emptied when it is approximately half full. Maintain a *closed system* and use sterile technique.

ESSENTIAL STEPS

1. Prepare the child and family.
2. Assemble the equipment.
3. Wash hands.
4. To remove CSF during continuous or intermittent drainage:

    Open the equipment onto a sterile field.

    Put on gloves.

    Attach the syringe to the stopcock and then attach the needle to the stopcock *or* attach the butterfly to the syringe.

    Clean the needle port of the bile bag with povidone-iodine or alcohol swabs.

    Insert the needle into the port to withdraw CSF.

Use the stopcock when additional CSF needs to be withdrawn, or use the smooth-edge clamp to clamp the butterfly tubing before disconnecting the syringe to empty it. Maintain a closed system and *do not* repuncture the port.

5. To change the ventriculostomy bag and tubing:

Open the equipment onto a sterile field.

Put on gloves.

Connect the bag and tubing.

Clean the tubing connector site with two povidone-iodine or alcohol swabs for 30 seconds. Dry the connection with two sterile gauze pads.

Clamp the tubing adjacent to the child. Disconnect the old tubing and reconnect the new tubing.

Remove the clamp.

Secure all connections by applying adhesive tape.

Secure the ventriculostomy bag to the level ordered by the neurosurgeon.

DOCUMENTATION

- Date and time.
- Type of procedure performed.
- Amount, color, and consistency of CSF removed from the bag.
- Position of the child and the ventriculostomy drainage bag.

POTENTIAL RELATED NURSING DIAGNOSES

Injury: *high risk*

Fluid volume deficit

Infection: *high risk*

Skin integrity, impaired: *high risk*

Tissue perfusion, altered, cerebral

Skills Checklist

Removing CSF
☐ Prepare the child and family.
☐ Assemble the equipment.
☐ Wash hands.
☐ Open the equipment onto a sterile field.
☐ Put on gloves.
☐ Clean the port of the bile bag.
☐ Insert the needle into the port of the bile bag.
☐ Withdraw CSF.
☐ Remove the needle.
☐ Document.

Changing the Bag and Tubing
☐ Prepare the child and family.
☐ Assemble the equipment.
☐ Wash hands.
☐ Open the equipment onto a sterile field.
☐ Put on gloves.
☐ Connect the bag and tubing.
☐ Clean the connector site.
☐ Clamp the tubing.
☐ Disconnect the old tubing and connect the new tubing.
☐ Remove the clamp.
☐ Secure the connections with tape.
☐ Secure the ventriculostomy bag.
☐ Document.

POTENTIAL RELATED MEDICAL DIAGNOSES

Increased intracranial pressure

Intracranial monitoring

Head trauma

Postsurgical procedure

REFERENCES
Tilem, D., and Greenberg, C. S. 1988. Nursing care of the child with a ventriculostomy. *Journal of pediatric nursing* 3, no. 3: 188–93.

TIME: 10 to 15 minutes

PURPOSE

To establish baseline clinical parameters as a basis for detecting alterations in the child's condition.

To serially monitor temperature, pulse, respiration, and blood pressure.

To evaluate the degree of abnormality in the child's cardiopulmonary state.

OBJECTIVES

* To obtain accurate vital signs.
* To prevent injury or trauma.

EQUIPMENT

Thermometer (glass or electronic; can be an ear thermometer)

Water-soluble lubricant (for taking a rectal temperature)

Watch with a second hand or a digital watch

Stethoscope

Blood pressure cuff, appropriate size

    The cuff width should cover half to two-thirds of the length of the child's upper arm or thigh

    The inner *bladder length* should be approximately the same circumference as the extremity, without overlapping

Sphygmomanometer or an electronic blood pressure machine

PSYCHOSOCIAL CONSIDERATIONS: Explain the procedures in developmentally appropriate terms. Avoid using terms with mixed meanings. Allow the child time to handle the equipment prior to a procedure. Do not take the blood pressure (B/P) or temperature of a sleeping child.

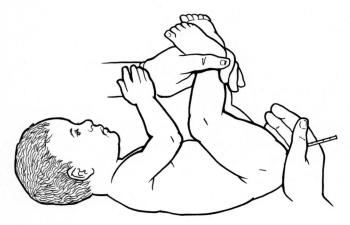

FIGURE 128.1 Taking a temperature rectally.

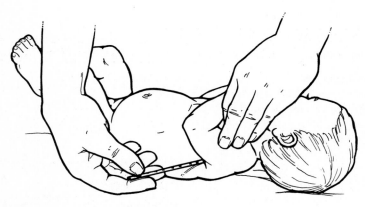

FIGURE 128.2 Taking an axillary temperature.

SAFETY ISSUES

- Vital sign measurements include temperature, apical heart rate, respiratory rate, and blood pressure.
- Do not leave a thermometer in an unattended child.
- When possible, take the child's temperature through the oral, axillary, or ear route as these are less invasive and traumatic than the rectal route.
- Generally, antipyretics are ordered for temperatures ≥38.5°C (101.3°F).

ESSENTIAL STEPS

1. Prepare the child and family.
2. Assemble the equipment.
3. Wash hands.
4. Take the child's temperature (see Figs. 128.1 and 128.2):

   Refer to Table 128.1 to determine the appropriate technique (oral, rectal, axillary, or ear) and type of thermometer.

   If using an electronic thermometer, refer to the manufacturer's instructions.

   Use a new probe cover for each use of the thermometer.

   For oral method:

   Hold in place until the thermometer beeps.

   If the measurement is questionable, check the child's temperature with a glass thermometer.

Skills Checklist

- ☐ Prepare the child and family.
- ☐ Assemble the equipment.
- ☐ Wash hands.
- ☐ Obtain vital signs:
  - Temperature.
  - Heart rate.
  - Respiration.
  - Blood pressure.
- ☐ Document.

For rectal method:

Lubricate the tip of the probe cover.

Insert the probe. Distance is age-dependent.

Hold in place until the thermometer beeps.

For axillary method:

Refer to the manufacturer's instructions.

For ear method:

Refer to the manufacturer's instructions.

TABLE 128.1 *Thermometer Applications*

ELECTRONIC THERMOMETERS		GLASS THERMOMETERS	
PATIENT POPULATION		**PATIENT POPULATION**	
Oral:	>2 years	Oral:	>6 years
Rectal:	>1 month	Rectal:	>1 month
Axillary:	Not accurate unless a special 5-minute technique is used. See manufacturer's recommendations.	Axillary:	No age limitations.
CONTRAINDICATIONS		**CONTRAINDICATIONS**	
Oral:	Postop oral surgery	Oral:	Postop oral surgery
Rectal:	Prolapsed rectum	Rectal:	Prolapsed rectum
	Imperforate anus		Imperforate anus
	Newborn <1 month		Newborn <1 month
	Premature baby		Premature baby
	Severe diarrhea		Severe diarrhea
	Bleeding tendency, i.e., leukemia, thrombocytopenia		Bleeding tendency, i.e., leukemia, thrombocytopenia

If using a glass thermometer:

Shake the mercury below 34°C (94°F) before using.

For oral method:

Place under the child's tongue.

Instruct the child to close his or her lips around the thermometer.

Leave the thermometer in place for *5 minutes.*

For rectal method:

Lubricate the tip of the thermometer.

Insert into the rectum.

Hold the thermometer in place for approximately *5 minutes.*

For axillary method:

Place the thermometer well into the axilla.

Leave in place for *5 minutes.*

Remove the thermometer. Read and record the temperature.

Clean and store the thermometer.

Notify the physician of any abnormal temperature.

5. Obtain apical pulse measurements (see Fig. 128.3):

Place the stethoscope over the point of maximum cardiac impulse (PMI). For a child more than 8 years of age, this point is usually located at the fifth left intercostal space at the midclavicular line. In younger children, the PMI may be located higher and more medially.

Count the pulse for 1 full minute, noting the rate and rhythm.

Auscultate for abnormal heart sounds (murmurs, rubs, clicks, or gallops).

When evaluating for a pulse deficit, palpate the artery pulse while auscultating the apical heart rate to determine any difference.

Pulses of other arteries (such as femoral, pedal, temporal, or carotid) may be palpated to evaluate peripheral perfusion.

Notify the physician of any pulse abnormalities.

6. Measure respiration:

Auscultate for normal, abnormal, and/or absent breath sounds. (See Fig. 128.4)

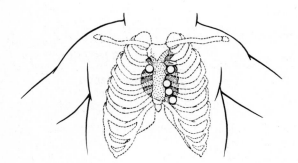

FIGURE 128.3 *Apical pulse points.*

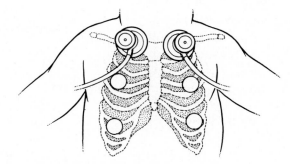

FIGURE 128.4 *Auscultation of the lungs.*

Count the number of respirations for 1 full minute. Note the rate, depth, and character of respirations.

Observe movements of the chest. Assess symmetry. In children under 7 years of age, the movement is abdominal. In older children, the movement is thoracic.

Observe for signs of respiratory distress, such as retractions, flaring, or grunting.

Observe abdominal movements in infants. Paradoxical abdominal movement (such as when the abdominal wall rises with inspiration while the chest wall retracts) is abnormal except in premature infants.

Notify the physician of any abnormal rates or characteristics and of any respiratory distress.

7. Measure the blood pressure:

If using the auscultation method (see Fig. 128.5):

Wrap the cuff around the upper arm.

Center the rubber bladder over the brachial artery without overlapping the edges.

Locate the brachial artery pulse in the antecubital fossa. The arm should be at heart level.

Place the diaphragm of the stethoscope over the brachial artery pulse.

Inflate the cuff.

Deflate the cuff, noting systolic and diastolic pressures.

If using the palpation method (may be used when unable to auscultate B/P; see Fig. 128.6):

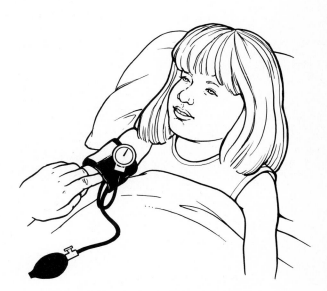

FIGURE 128.6 *Palpating a blood pressure; finger placement.*

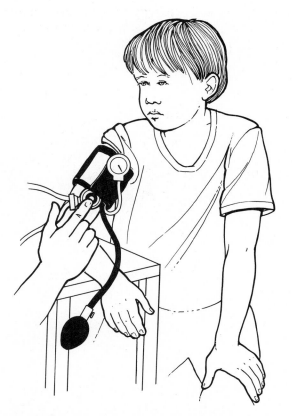

FIGURE 128.5 *Auscultating a blood pressure; stethoscope placement.*

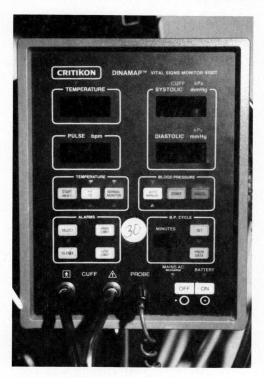

FIGURE 128.7 *Electronic blood pressure machine.*

Wrap the cuff.

Palpate the brachial or radial artery.

Inflate the cuff.

As air is let out, palpate for the onset of an arterial pulsation. Record this number over a p (for example, 90/p) to indicate that the pressure was obtained by palpation.

If using the Doppler method:

Obtain a Doppler.

Record Doppler systolic pressures over D (for example, 60/D).

If using an electronic blood pressure machine, refer to the manufacturer's instructions. (See Fig. 128.7)

For cuff measurement and positioning at the thigh:

The cuff size should be proportionately wider and longer than that for the arm.

While the child is lying face down, apply the cuff with the bladder over the posterior aspect of the midthigh.

If the child is unable to lie face down, obtain the pressure reading with the child supine, by flexing the knee just enough to permit application of the stethoscope over the popliteal space.

Place the stethoscope over the popliteal fossa to obtain the reading.

The larger bladder usually records systolic pressure in the thigh of 10 to 40 mm/Hg higher than that in the arm, but the diastolic pressure is essentially the same for both.

For cuff measurement and positioning at the calf:

The cuff size will be approximately the same size as for the arm.

Position the distal border of the cuff at the malleoli.

Auscultate over the posterior tibial on the dorsalis pedis artery.

DOCUMENTATION

- Vital signs.
- Route used for temperature.
- Abnormal vital signs, along with the name and time of the physician notified.

POTENTIAL RELATED NURSING DIAGNOSES

Hyperthermia

Anxiety

Fear

Pain, acute

Injury: *high risk*

POTENTIAL RELATED MEDICAL DIAGNOSES

Universal application

REFERENCES

Mott, S., James, S., and Sperhac, A. 1990. *Nursing care of children and families.* Redwood City, Calif.: Addison-Wesley.

EQUIPMENT

Scales (when possible, use the same scale each time for a given child)

Scale paper or baby blanket, if appropriate

Detergent or disinfectant cleaning agent

Warmer lights, if appropriate

PSYCHOSOCIAL CONSIDERATIONS: Explain the procedure in developmentally appropriate terms. Avoid using terms with mixed meanings. Make the child feel safe and secure. Cold scales may startle an infant.

TIME: 5 minutes

PURPOSE

To obtain an accurate weight.

To provide data for:

Determining the child's response to formula, hyperalimentation, fluid therapy, and diuretics.

Determining the correct medication dosage.

Determining the child's growth and developmental rates.

Baseline on admission.

OBJECTIVES

- To obtain a weight.
- To determine changes in weight.

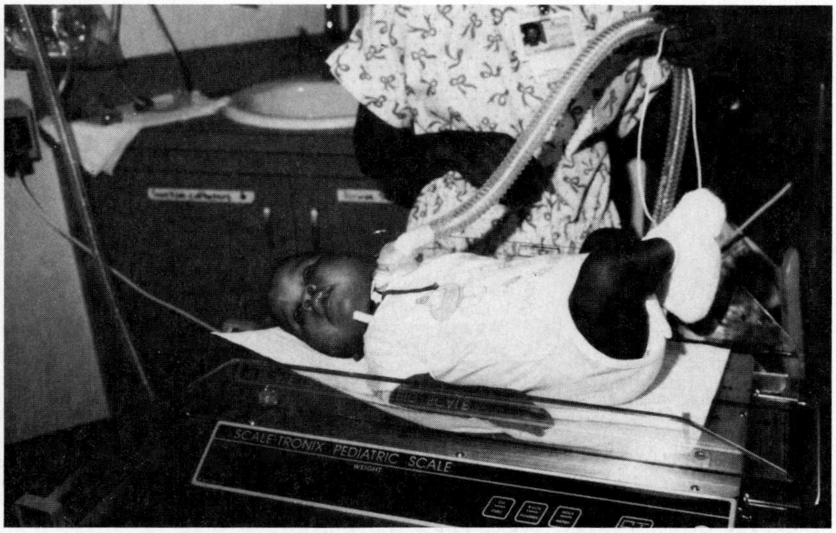

SAFETY ISSUES

- Daily weights are usually required for:

  An infant under 1 month of age.

  A premature infant. Stable premies may be weighed less often to decrease handling and stimulation.

  A failure-to-thrive child.

  A child with chronic renal failure.

  A child with a cardiac condition.

  A child receiving diuretics.

  A child with gastrointestinal problems.

  A child with cystic fibrosis.

  A diabetic child.

  A child with bulemia or anorexia nervosa.

  A child on total parenteral nutrition.

  An infant under 1 year of age and on IV therapy.

- Measure weights in metric units.
- Obtain weights prior to breakfast or at approximately the same time each day.
- Weigh infants nude.

FIGURE 129.1 *Weighing on an infant scale. (Note that infants generally are not weighed while wearing clothing.)*

ESSENTIAL STEPS

1. Prepare the child and family.
2. Assemble the equipment.

   Place paper or a baby blanket on the scale if appropriate.

   Balance or "zero" the scale prior to weighing each child. If not using an electronic scale, weigh the scale paper or baby blanket separately and subtract from the total body weight.

3. Wash hands.
4. Weigh the child on the appropriate scale. Weigh the child without clothes or with only underwear. It is important to use the same scale, time, and attire consistently. Ensure privacy. Protect the infant from falling while on the scale. The room should be warm to avoid chilling. (See Figs. 129.1, 129.2, 129.3, 129.4, and 129.5)
5. Clean the scale with detergent or a disinfectant cleaner, if appropriate.

DOCUMENTATION

- Weight.
- If weight was taken with an IV board, endotracheal tube, and so on, so that discontinuation of these things can be taken into account as a legitimate weight loss.
- Time.
- Type of scale used, if appropriate.

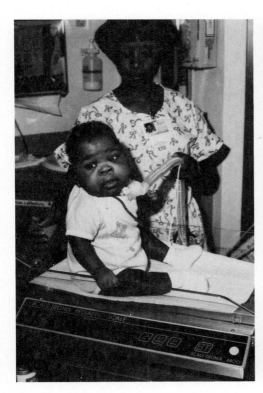

FIGURE 129.2 Weighing on an infant scale.

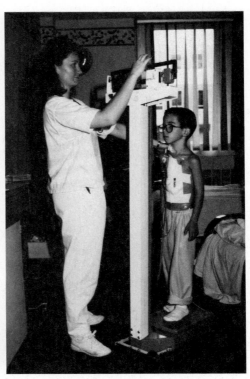

FIGURE 129.3 Weighing on a bedside scale. (Weigh older children in minimal attire.)

369

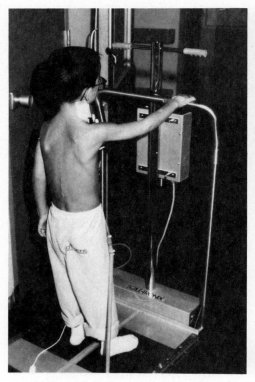

FIGURE 129.4 *Weighing on a bedside scale. (Weigh older children in minimal attire.)*

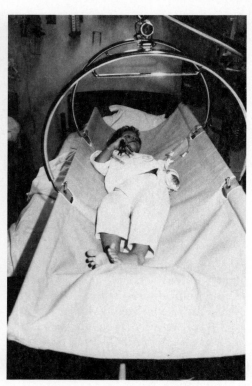

FIGURE 129.5 *Weighing on an overbed scale. (Note that infants are generally not weighed while wearing clothing.)*

POTENTIAL RELATED NURSING DIAGNOSES

Fluid volume deficit

Fluid volume excess

Nutrition, altered, less than body requirements

Nutrition, altered, more than body requirements

Tissue perfusion, altered

Cardiac output, decreased

Urinary elimination, altered

Hypothermia

POTENTIAL RELATED MEDICAL DIAGNOSES

Anorexia

Weight loss

Cardiovascular disease

Renal disease

Bulemia

Prematurity

Failure to thrive

Malabsorption

Index